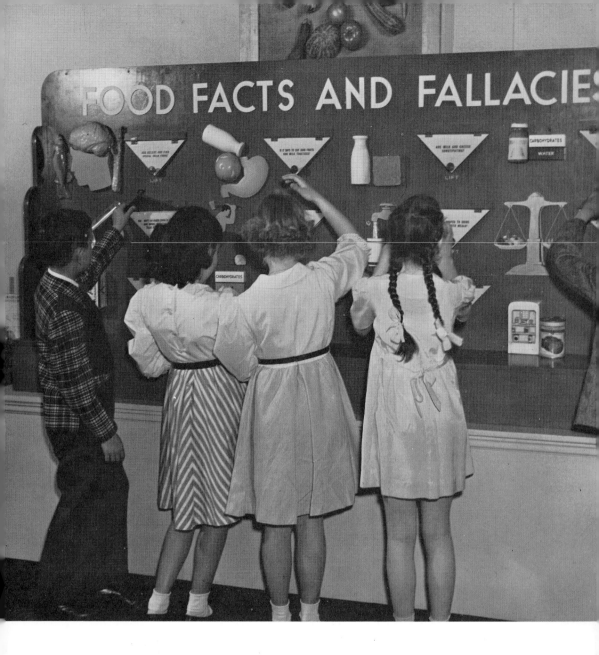

third edition

W. B. SAUNDERS COMPANY
Philadelphia-London-Toronto

health education in the elementary school

68664

CARL E. WILLGOOSE, Ed.D.
Boston University

W. B. Saunders Company: West Washington Square
Philadelphia, Pa. 19105

12 Dyott Street
London W.C. 1

1835 Yonge Street
Toronto 7, Ontario

Health Education in the Elementary School

Print No.:   4   5   6   7   8   9

PREFACE TO THE THIRD EDITION

When Alfred North Whitehead wrote that ". . . there is only one subject matter for education, and that is life in all of its manifestations," he was admonishing educators to look beyond the obvious topical facts, units, and lesson plans of the moment and take a broader view of education. Essentially, this means that teachers of all subjects, including health education, must inquire into the nature of the concomitant learnings and the numerous behaviors that are linked in some way with the subject matter material. The multidisciplinary nature of health instruction makes this even more important.

Health education is becoming stronger nationally. Perhaps the most significant of recent changes are the number of inquiries coming from school superintendents and school boards relative to what constitutes an adequate program of health teaching. Today, an increased emphasis is being given to significant and explicit health education experiences—experiences which relate to the immediate activities of day-to-day living at each grade level. Thus, such vital areas as mental health, smoking, alcohol, drugs, and sex and family living education are taught as a part of a unified health instruction program in order that youngsters may gain an early sensitivity for the fragility and preciousness of human life. The long range objective is to develop a personal awareness of the potentialities of a fully awakened human being. It is expected that, in the next decade, many more people will place optimal health on a higher level in their individual value systems and demonstrate their moral vitality by acting according to what they know. Currently, there are too many people who know what to do but fail to do it. Their health practices do not reflect their health knowledge.

Informed and energetic classroom teachers of health education have a clear contribution to make to the attitude-behavior dimension. Hopefully, this may be accomplished through normal curriculum-development activity in which teachers evaluate content by age-grade level, experiment with various methods and materials for teaching specific health topics, and periodically evaluate the results of teaching. In this way health instruction will continue to move at an accelerated speed from a "do-gooder" activity to a carefully organized and programmed part of the total school curriculum.

CARL E. WILLGOOSE

Boston, Mass.

PREFACE TO THE FIRST EDITION

There is no person in the American public school system better fitted to make a significant contribution to the health of school-children than the classroom teacher in the elementary school. This teacher alone holds the key position for improving child health. With her interest, enthusiasm, and professional understanding the school health program moves ahead. Without her support, however, the health education program never really gets started.

The potential ability of the classroom teacher in the field of health is related to a knowledge and understanding of the topic. The teacher of today knows the characteristics of healthy children, and what this means in terms of ability to learn. She knows the interrelationship of physical, mental and emotional health, as well as the health needs of the child in the community. She knows how to detect health abnormalities and refer them to proper medical service personnel for effective follow-up. And she knows *how* to teach health at the various grade levels.

In short, the classroom teacher needs some preparation in the field of school health. The primary purpose of this book is to help in the preparation. Here, successful teaching methods in education have been applied specifically to health instruction. The more successful procedures have been coupled with usable instructional materials and teaching aids to provide the elementary teacher with the where-withal to carry on a stimulating and fruitful program. The goal is to improve both health status and health behavior.

The early chapters of the book are concerned with the general topic of school health and the health status of the child. They stress the detection and referral role of the classroom teacher and her unique opportunity to function efficiently with the school health service personnel. Then follows a reference to the school environment and its effect on general behavior and learning. No attempt has been made in these early chapters to be complete in dealing with school health service and healthful school environment. These are major areas of study in themselves. They are briefly presented here so that the elementary schoolteacher can see the bearing they have on total school health and their relationship to health instruction in the classroom.

The major part of the book is specifically concerned with health instruction. It is designed to furnish the elementary teacher with a quantity of orderly and practical information to be of help in planning, carrying out and evaluating health teaching. In fact, any person concerned with health teaching will find this book useful. This includes the health supervisor, the dental hygienist, the nurse-teacher and the full-time teacher of health. But the classroom teacher will be helped most, for this is her book.

The author is indebted to a number of colleagues, students, and authors for their help in providing suggestions and materials. Suggestions by Dr. R. Lee Martin and Professor Helen Buckley relative to the elementary curriculum are gratefully acknowledged. Special thanks go to my family for being so patient and to Mrs. Virginia Smeltzer for typing the manuscript.

CARL E. WILLGOOSE

Oswego, N.Y.

CONTENTS

The Nature
and Scope of
Health Education

*He that has health has hope, and
he that has hope has everything.*

—ARABIAN PROVERB

Any worthwhile endeavor has an underlying philosophy—a point of view which substantiates whatever is planned for in the scheme of things to come. In all ages men have philosophized about the world they hope to make. Each succeeding generation has talked about the great deeds left to be done, the new frontiers to conquer, and the utopias yet to be fashioned. And each age has had its great statesmen, teachers and architects, who were remembered as great because they did more than dream, hope, and struggle. They got things done; they possessed a "vitality for doing."

Man's health has always represented that certain something—that specific capacity or wherewithal *to do* that exists somewhere between his loftiest thoughts and his real deeds. This is the *sine qua non*, the indispensable quality in man. With this wherewithal or capacity to perform, man is able to strive and struggle through life seeking to achieve a certain happiness.

This is accomplished "not by acquiescing with what is but by struggling for something else, not by accepting but by doing, not by receiving but by giving, not by rest but by activity."[1] Life, by its very nature, is activity. Any stable happiness, therefore, is related to the ability of the organism to be active. Weak muscles, poor hearing or vision, diseased tissues, or an emotional disturbance weaken the organism and curtail its ability to be active.

Health Defined in the Good Life

Health has been defined in many ways. From what has already been said, however, it might well be defined as "the capacity for activity"—any and all activity. In fact it is so firmly related to all activity that the World Health Organization of the United Nations defines it as "a state of complete physi-

[1] Lawton, Shailer U., and Rogers, Frederick R. *Educational Paths to Virtue*—I. Newton, Mass.: Pleiades Co., 1937, p. 47.

1

cal, mental and social well-being, and not merely the absence of disease and infirmity."[2]

One of the most revealing definitions of health was written several decades ago by Jesse Feiring Williams of Columbia University. He defined health as "the quality of life that enables the individual to live most and to serve best."[3] Health, therefore, is a condition that permits happy, successful living. Even man's ability to be charitable depends upon it, for charity consists of giving of oneself without thought of return — something in which the most virtuous person is limited when he is ill or below par.

As important as it is to life, health can hardly be labeled as one of life's goals. It is, however, a necessary factor that influences the degree to which life goals or objectives are reached. It is the kind of thing that caused Duncan Spaeth to write:

> While health itself is not the finest flower in life, it is the soil from which the finest flowers grow.

Good health is so obvious to a thinking person that it is often dismissed as elemental. It is typical therefore that when man experiences illness, disease, and defects which interfere with his immediate ambitions, he awakes to the primary importance of personal well-being. After getting out of a sickbed, Schopenhauer wrote:

> The greatest of follies is to neglect one's health for other virtues in life.

Perhaps it is time to ask the question: what is modern man's health potential? Theoretically, it ranges from complete lack of health (death) at one end of a continuum to optimal health at the other end. It is frequently a fluctuating state. Hoyman classifies man's health status into five levels[4] (See p. 3).

The observation that a state of health has far-reaching consequences was clearly illustrated by Julian Huxley, when he said that ". . . the highest and most sacred duty of man is seen as the proper utilization of the untapped resources of human beings."[5] Involved here is the whole of man's capacity for expression. It is multidimensional — anthropological, biological, psychological, economic, and even political. This gives support to the concept of an "ecology of health" where all human relationships between a community and its environment are health related. Moreover, there is a personal responsibility of the individual for his own health and the health of the community. As far back as the seventeenth century John Donne expressed this viewpoint beautifully when he stated in part: "No man is an Island, entire of itself; every man is a piece of the Continent, a part of the main . . . any man's death diminishes me, because I am involved in mankind."[6]

Just as early philosophers and teachers were concerned with man's well-being, contemporary writers and statesmen have pointed to the need for more attention to man's health. In 1956 President Dwight D. Eisenhower called a Physical Fitness Conference to ascertain ways and means of improving the total fitness of American youth. Fitness was discussed in its broad meaning of total fitness. During the decade that followed, the President's Council on Physical Fitness was established and widely accepted na-

---

[2] Constitution of the World Health Organization, *Chronicle of the World Health Organization, 1:*29-43; Geneva: World Health Organization, 1947, p. 3.

[3] Williams, Jesse F. *Personal Hygiene Applied*, 8th ed. Philadelphia: W. B. Saunders Company, 1946.

[4] Hoyman, Howard S. "Our Modern Concept of Health," *Journal of School Health, 32:* 253-264, September 1962.

[5] Quoted by Theodosius Dobzhansky in *Biological Basis of Human Freedom.* New York: Columbia University Press, 1956.

[6] For an expanded treatment of this topic see Leo Kartman, "Human Ecology and Public Health," *American Journal of Public Health,* 57:737-750, May 1967.

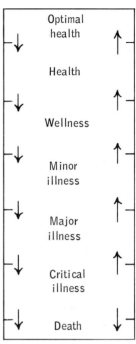

Health — from suboptimal level to optimal health*

Wellness — subhealth levels ranging from low-level to high-
level wellness

Minor illness — incipient or subclinical; milder illnesses and
disabilities

Major illness — incipient or subclinical; diseases and disabilities of a more serious nature

Critical illness — grave illness to approaching death

* The level at which an individual's living approaches his full desirable potentialities (e.g., Dr. Albert Schweitzer, Grandma Moses, Konrad Adenauer).

tionally. It was instrumental in making operational a number of health and physical education programs. One of its strongest supporters was President John F. Kennedy, who in 1962 spoke forcefully on this point: "We do not want a nation of spectators. We want a nation of participants in the vigorous life."

Through the years of the early sixties there was overwhelming support for government and school-community programs designed to raise the health of the citizenry. Strong recommendations came from such groups as the American Medical Association, the American Public Health Association, the Educational Policies Commission of the National Education Association, and the White House Conference on Health. It was at this conference that both private and public health physicians reported that "educated patients" are much better patients; they understand something about their own health and follow the recommenda-

tions of their physicians, and recover sooner from illness. On more than one occasion it was effectively brought out that the health-educated layman is a necessary ingredient in present-day society.

Health from Past to Present

Man's apparent concern for his health, welfare, and survival has not always been so noticeable and scientific as it appears to be today.

The gradual decrease over the centuries of magic guesswork, incantation, and superstition, together with the corresponding rise in applied scientific knowledge represents a magnificent process of slow evolution. Sound ideas were practiced side by side with unsound treatments and rituals. As in all ages of man, only a minority knew the truth, and they had to work uphill in the face of customs, habits, and ignorance. In prehistoric times, and even today in some parts of the world, evil spirits were "scared away" because of the general belief that they caused sickness. Yet these same prehistoric people discovered that certain herbs and other plants were quite good for numerous disorders. As far back as 4500 B.C. along the Nile in Egypt, Imhotep was practicing medicine in Luxor and Karnak. By 2500 B.C., surgical operations were being performed with the "help" of Thoth, the god of medicine. Today, thousands of Egyptians in the same region wear the scarab beetle charm about the neck to ward off disease and encourage fertility.

The constant struggle for light over darkness has been, and always will be, a continuing one. This is well demonstrated by early Hebrew law relating to communicable disease, isolation, quarantine and cleanliness. The books of the Bible—Leviticus and Deuteronomy—are rich in illustrations of early health recommendations and practices. This is further illustrated by a 500 year period of ancient Greek and Roman history (300 B.C. to 200 A.D.). It was Hippocrates who taught that each disease arises from a natural cause. It was the Athenian youth who took good care of their bodies and worshiped the goddess Hygeia under the guidance of priest-physicians. It was Galen, the Greek physician and writer, who experimented widely in physiology but was looked down upon by the Roman citizens of the period. Yet the Romans were really interested in health and developed many practical surgical instruments to be used on wounded gladiators and soldiers. They made more progress in sanitation, plumbing and sewer construction than almost any other civilization over the years. The Roman aqueduct is still considered a masterpiece of engineering.

During the disease-ridden Middle Ages, advancement in hygiene and medicine was somewhat retarded. Hospitals were organized for the care of the sick, but it was not until the tail end of the fifteenth and beginning of the sixteenth centuries that scientific advancements began to be noticeable. By the seventeenth century Leeuwenhoek and his microscope opened a previously invisible world to man. Witchcraft reached a new high but alchemy slowly gave way to chemistry. By the middle 1700's all physical and biological sciences were making great strides. Scientists were no longer hidden for protection but were looked upon with some degree of respect. Uncleanliness was everywhere, in the streets, in the hospitals and in the homes.

In the nineteenth century all kinds of medical discoveries and changes in hygienic practices took place. In the face of high death rates from infectious diseases, a number of significant discoveries occurred. Some of these were the clinical thermometer, the stethoscope, the x-ray, radium, the antiseptic method and anesthesia. It was proved once and for all that communicable diseases are caused by microorganisms which enter the body from without, that insects carry malaria and yellow fever, and that the universal practice of healthful living not only improves one's resistance to tuberculosis and other diseases but it also improves total health.

The twentieth century, building upon the past, has produced much of what is known and practiced today. Health promotion activities may go down in history as the greatest single contribution of the twentieth century. Federal, state, school, and community health programs have flourished. The man in the street—the common man—has not only felt the impact of this, but has actually taken part in the promotion program. He has had a hand in hospital organization, maternal education, the mental hygiene movements, and school health education. He knows something about heart disease, allergies, psychological stress, cancer, brain surgery, obesity, disease-carrying insects, blood transfusions, the

science of nutrition, longevity, streptococcus and staphylococcus bacilli,
antibiotics, tranquilizers, sodium fluoride and fluoridation, and countless
other items related to disease. His dollars have supported the fight to bring
poliomyelitis under control, to pursue
the cause of multiple sclerosis, muscular dystrophy, and coronary occlu-
sions. His personal sacrifices on the
local level to raise money for the Community Chest or United Fund, or to
give blood, have given him an insight
and appreciation for the place of health
in modern society.

Thus the average citizen is gradually
moving from superstitions and ignorance to a somewhat scientific viewpoint regarding health. A democratic
education calling for an enlightened
citizenry has done much to promote
this awakening and movement away
from darkness and indifference toward
light and understanding. But all the
health battles are not won yet. In fact,
the battle has just gotten under way.
The health needs of the people are extensive, and the implications for educators are great indeed.

The Need for Education for Health

The more complex civilization becomes, the less valid is instinctive behavior, and the more man must depend
upon the processes of education to
guide him. To survive he must use
modern knowledge and techniques
from the health sciences. By so doing
he can protect himself from many diseases, compensate for others and bol-
ster deficiencies of structure and function that he might attain and preserve
a relative fitness unheard of centuries
ago. Modern man has to make a critical
choice. Either he includes valid health
information and healthful activity in
his life or he suffers the inevitable
consequence.

It is not difficult to make a long list of
the reasons *why there is a need for
health education.* Some of the more
significant reasons are as follows:

The Changing Times. Nothing
stands still. Change, like night and
day, is an absolute. And Western civilization, in addition to reaping the sweet
fruits of progress, is suffering from the
spoils. In a society where speed, status,
comfort, and economic success are
high marks of achievement, it is not
uncommon to find men and women
who cannot adjust to the increasing
pressures. They keep plugging along,
lacking an apparent sense of values.
Some become overfed and underactive. And, while others become com-
placent and simply vegetate from year
to year with few goals in life to stimulate the best in them, there are others
who literally "burn" themselves out in
a life packed with situations generat-
ing insecurity, fear, anxiety, worry,
jealousy, anger, and hatred. Resulting
tensions refuse to stay bottled. They
make their presence known in headaches, indigestion, gastrointestinal
upsets, restlessness, sleeplessness, irritability, and fatigue.

Society today is anything but peace-
ful and serene. Even with a careful
education for health, it is most difficult
to achieve balance in living and to obtain an attitude of mind conducive to
total well-being. Western civilization
is characterized by the spectacle of
man fighting for perfection while
knowing little about where he is
headed. His efforts all too often do not
produce the peace of mind he seeks.
Instead they result in more cholesterol
to cause coronary disease, increased
secretions to cause gastric ulcers,
blood pressure to cause cerebral hem-
orrhage, and frustrations leading to the
doors of the mental institution. Reduced to its simplest terms, survival
depends on the physical-mental-spiri-
tual balance. Moreover, it depends on
how one *travels* toward the goals of
life, perhaps more than whether or not
he ever arrives.

Value Illness. The concern for
health by official bodies and profes-
sionals in health-related fields is at an

all-time high. This does not mean that the average citizen is well informed or has permitted his value system to be disturbed to any substantial degree. Although individual health status has improved, there are still thousands of people suffering from what Maslow refers to as "value illness."[7] This is the negative element behind drug addiction, alcoholism, illegitimacy, corruption, graft, and numerous irregularities in all walks of private and public life. The adult citizen *knows* what to do but is not *moved* to the state of doing it. This is illustrated continually in the field of health behavior where the knowledgeable individual is simply indifferent to the consequences of his own acts. He is not actively immoral, antisocial, or destructive in intent; he is simply amoral. His own moral principles and standards of right and wrong actions somehow do not compel him to act in keeping with what he knows is best.

Norman Cousins, editor of the *Saturday Review*, cites an alarming example of this value illness when he discusses his conversation with a doctor friend who is a heavy smoker.[8] The doctor reports that he did not need all the government publications to convince him that smoking can cause cancer or bronchitis or various forms of heart disease. The evidence was admittedly plain to him in his daily visits to the hospital wards. Moreover, he was able to reinforce his feelings by noting that he had seen enough lung surgery to recognize the difference between the pink healthy tissue of the non-smoker and the discolored tissues of smokers.

This caused Cousins to ask a question.

"You know all this and yet you yourself will continue to smoke?"

"Yes."

"Why?"

At this point the doctor replied that he supposed he was like many of his own patients. After being advised to give up smoking because of its detriment to good health and longevity, the patients did not really care whether they lived a fewer number of years. Neither did the doctor.

Here, says Cousins, is a problem far more serious than the problem leading up to it. Involved here are the ultimate questions a society has to ask about itself. Cousins asks: "What are the basic values of its people? How much sensitivity do they have to the fragility and preciousness of life? How shallow or profound is their awareness of the potentialities of a fully awakened human being? What connections do they see between a respect for life and healthy development of the society itself?"

The significance of such questions strikes at the very roots of an educational program, for few items can be more dangerous to the nation than the attitude by any sizable portion of its people that they really do not care whether they live well or poorly, or whether they live long or die early. Perhaps man is indeed his own greatest enemy. (Said Pogo: "We have met the enemy and they are us.")

World-Wide Conditions. Ultimately the thoughts of all men must be geared to conditions the world over. More people live in mud huts than in any other type of dwelling; more travel by foot (or by burro) than any other way; most have a life expectancy less than half that of the people in the United States; most mothers see half their children die before reaching maturity; more people get sick without a physician's help available than those who have even rudimentary medical care. In short, most of the world's peoples are in the "have not" stage. It is encouraging, however, to know that evidence is available to indicate that in the long run improved health

---

[7] Maslow, Abraham H. *Toward a Psychology of Being*. Princeton, New Jersey: D. Van Nostrand Co., Inc., 1962.

[8] Cousins, Norman. "The Danger Beyond Smoking," *Saturday Review*, January 25, 1964.

practices in one area of the globe have a favorable effect on other areas. This is also true in terms of health education ideas, for these ideas spread sometimes as quickly as new vaccines, sanitary practices, and wonder drugs.

The effectiveness of the World Health Organization is demonstrated by the large number of countries embarking upon health protection and education programs. Some of the world goals and accomplishments in a single year's time are impressive.

Improved communication and transportation have brought the people of the world closer together. Consequently, the health and welfare of the other fellow is more the worry of the ordinary citizen than ever before. Man may glory in his individuality, but it does not separate him from the universal self — the oneness of man. In fact the healthiest person alive today owes his enviable status to the practices of his friends and neighbors. In a complex society the welfare of the majority is directly affected by the welfare, knowledge, and understanding of the minority.[9] In short, education for health is the concern of the individual on both a local and a world-wide basis.

American Health Statistics. The health of the American people is well on the rise and has been for some time. Much of this is due to vast achievements in medical research, spectacular progress in the field of antibiotics, discoveries in the area of hormones, and other similar advances. Also, Americans spend over 30 billion dollars a year on health care.

In addition to these medical factors, a large share of credit should be given to public health and school health practices. The reduction in the tuberculosis death rate, for instance, represents one of man's finest accomplishments. At the start of the century the annual death rate in the United States

from tuberculosis was 194 for each 100,000 persons. Today it is less than five. Such a favorable picture has been brought about by a number of factors and not solely by medical care and research. It is related to such items as better housing, improvement in nutrition, public health education, and a generally higher standard of living. The significance of education is further illustrated by the death rate from appendicitis; it has been reduced approximately 60 per cent over a 20 year period, due primarily to an enlightened public — a public that does not run for a cathartic every time there is a stomach or abdominal pain.

It is true that health in America is becoming a "social accomplishment". Deaths from pneumonia have declined over 90 per cent in 20 years. Deaths from rheumatic fever are down, as is the sickness rate for practically all infectious diseases. Life expectancy is the highest ever. Under the mortality rate prevailing around the year 1900, the expectation of life at birth was not quite 50 years. By 1930 the figure had risen to 60 years; in 1955 it was 69.5 years. In 1961 it was 70.8.[10] As in earlier years white females have the best record of longevity. In 1955 it was 73.6 years. In 1966 it was almost 75. Thus since the turn of the century almost 25 years have been added to the expected lifetime. Coincident with the reduction in over-all mortality during the present century is the rapid reduction in newborn deaths. In 1900 to 1902, 24 per cent of newborn white males and 21 per cent of white females failed to survive to their twentieth birthday. Now, less than 2.5 per cent are likely to die before that age.[11] (See Figure 1-1.)

---

[9] Willgoose, Carl E. "Health, Welfare and Religious Freedom," *School and Society,* 73 (1893):198, March 31, 1951.

[10] Metropolitan Life Insurance Company. "Gains in Longevity Since 1900," *Statistical Bulletin,* 38:4, July 1957. See also Vol. 43 (January 1962) and Vol. 48 (August 1967).

[11] Metropolitan Life Insurance Company. "Infant Mortality in the United States and Abroad," *Statistical Bulletin,* 48:3-6, May 1967.

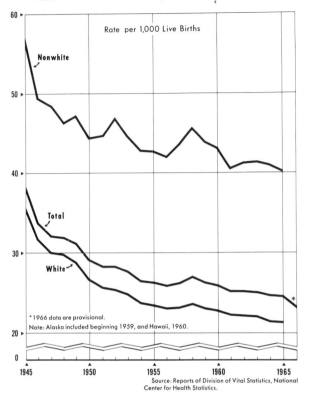

TREND IN INFANT MORTALITY, UNITED STATES, 1945-1966

Figure 1-1 Reduction in infant mortality (Metropolitan Life Insurance Co., *Statistical Bulletin* No. 48, May, 1967.)

Medical science has made spectacular progress in the last 20 years. The danger of infection through surgery has been greatly reduced. Low cost vaccines are very effective against serious illness. Regular medical examinations and early treatment prevent disease and disability in thousands of individuals. Vast numbers of people leave hospitals well who would have died two decades ago. And the average stay in the hospital for an appendectomy is five and a half days. It was 14 days 20 years ago.

Although much of this presents a pleasant health and welfare picture, there are problems ahead. They are growing problems, for the population of the United States will increase to 210 million by 1970 and 250 million by 1985. Moreover, with the skyrocketing suburbs, the growth of the cities, and the extensive shifts in population, new health adjustments will have to be made in many areas. Rapidly growing communities, for example, find that they have to develop or expand medical and public health facilities and services. These changes include hospitals and their associated services, the private practice of medicine, voluntary health associations, and the programs of local health departments. Health needs, therefore, are far from declining.

Significant Health Problems. In spite of health education and medical science efforts to make changes in the lives of the citizenry, the staggering statistics underscore the fact that the task ahead is great indeed. Moreover, the degenerative diseases of the adult population frequently have their roots in the day-to-day health practices of children and youth. Proper practices, established early in life, tend to reduce mortality and morbidity rates at all age

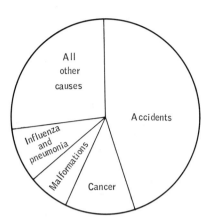

Figure 1–2 Pie graph illustrating causes of child deaths, 5 to 14 years of age.

levels. Childhood deaths, however, represent a significant statistic, particularly in the five to fourteen year age period. (See Figure 1–2.)

Some of the more prominent health problems are as follows:

Heart disease is the nation's number one killer with almost a million deaths a year (Figure 1–3). Coronary arterial disease is on the rise, but it can

be reduced when people know enough to watch their weight and limit their consumption of fats, seek diversion and tension-free recreation to attain a sound attitude of mind, and engage in a moderate amount of physical activity. Mortality and morbidity from heart disease is two to three times as high among people who do not realize the importance of physical activity and fail to get regular exercise. From the Framingham Heart Study, where there has been continuous evaluation of 5127 adults in one community since 1949, it has been shown that there is a clear association of coronary heart disease with age, blood pressure, serum cholesterol, weight, and cigarette smoking.[12] This is confirmed by the results of a study of 88 per cent of the entire community of Tecumseh, Michigan, where it was discovered that the maintenance of desirable body weight is an effective method to con-

[12] Friedman, Gary D., et al. "An Evaluation of Follow-Up Methods in the Framingham Heart Study," *American Journal of Public Health*, 57: 1015-1024, June 1967.

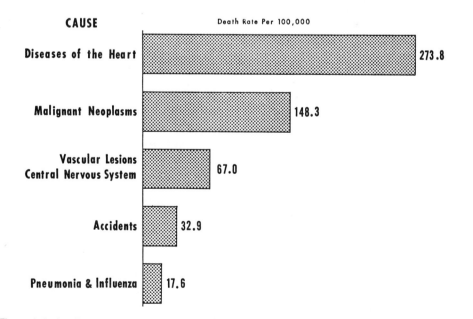

Figure 1–3 Leading causes of death per hundred thousand cases. (Metropolitan Life Insurance Company, *Statistical Bulletin*.)

trol blood cholesterol levels.[13] Of major importance, therefore, is the specific role of education. People must learn to recognize the symptoms of heart disease or cancer or any other disease and see their physicians early.

Mental disorders have increased so fast that present day figures indicate that one person in ten will enter a mental institution or receive some kind of psychiatric care before he dies. Also, approximately 50 per cent of all hospital beds in the United States are occupied by mental patients. Children are especially involved. About 400 out of 100,000 children under age 18 require psychiatric care as out-patients each year. Moreover, mental disorders are considered a significant factor in numerous physical illnesses, are strongly associated with suicide, and are often found to be implicated in accidents. In addition to causing considerable suffering and family disruption, mental illness exacts a financial toll of over two billion dollars a year for health care, and several billions of dollars more in annual loss to industry.

Because of better treatment and rehabilitation, there has been some decline in the number of patients. This advance has been offset by the number of people seeking treatment sooner. Also, the alcoholic, the retarded, and the brain damaged are being served.

Poor health in a society has many manifestations. Suicide, for example, was the cause of over 20,000 deaths in the United States in 1967, compared with over 10,000 homicides. This fact in itself should prompt more attention to be focused on the type of behavior that leads to an individual's self-destruction. But the 20,000 figure does not tell the whole story of suicide. Because of the moral and religious stigma attached to suicide, many such cases are

undoubtedly not recorded. Also, it is difficult to determine what percentage of other violent deaths, including the 52,000 annual automobile deaths, are caused by a conscious or subconscious desire to end life. Medical and safety authorities are almost unanimous in the belief that some percentage of all categories of violent death are in reality suicides. Moreover, almost half the suicides occur within three months of an emotional crisis, and about 40 per cent of the men and 20 per cent of the women kill themselves because of ill health. The rising rate has led to the recognition of a major medical and public health problem. Existing suicide prevention centers have been effective in saving lives each year and have demonstrated the importance of public education in detecting the potential suicide. Many suicides can be averted if unusual depression or signs of mental illness are recognized and properly treated.

The need for a formal educational approach to prevent and reduce poor mental health is evident. Experience has taught that preventive mental health services can reduce mental illness, alcoholism, divorce, suicide, emotional disturbances, juvenile crime, and employment problems. In view of the huge population increases expected in the years ahead, it is obvious that the man of today is faced with a herculean task in building and staffing the hospitals, clinics, or jails which people with these mental health problems would require.

The real solution is to *prevent* the disorders through combined efforts of lay and professional people. This is not easy, for our way of life with its emphasis on personal status, speed, and materialism tends to produce individuals with a disturbed sense of values. Balance in living is frequently difficult to attain. Large numbers of people are basically unhappy. They are looking for relief—"a way out". In 1967 the pharmaceutical industry

---

[13] Montoye, H. J., Epstein, F. H., and Kjelsberg, M. D. "Relationship Between Serum Cholesterol and Body Fitness," *American Journal of Clinical Nutrition*, 18:397-406, 1966.

spent more money on developing new tranquilizers, stimulants, sedatives, and analgesics than on any other kind of drug. Even earning a living fails to satisfy large segments of the population, for man is further removed from the goods produced as technology advances. His effort is only a partial contribution, and his identification with the product grows dimmer and dimmer. The frustrations and resentments that pile up at the workbench move along into the family circle, the neighborhood council, the polling place, and the social gathering. The worker cannot change his personality, his lack of self-esteem, his sense of impotence, his boredom — in short the patterns imprinted on him by his job — as easily as he sheds his overalls.

Cancer, a malignant neoplasm, is killing about 305,000 Americans a year. It is calculated that about six out of every 24 persons will develop cancer; of this number two will be saved, one will die who could have been saved, and three will die who cannot presently be saved. Significantly, the high death rate could be reduced by 33 per cent if proper treatment were started in time. Recent studies show that nearly 60 per cent of people treated early for cancer live at least five years.[14] Unfortunately, 40 per cent of the women with breast cancer do not seek help until it is too late. Thousands could be saved if men, women, and children would have an adequate medical examination each year. As it is, over 500,000 new cases of cancer are being discovered yearly.

Getting the public to accept the fact of cancer openly and do something about it in time is primarily a health education job. Today, pregnant women discuss it in mothers' classes, and children discuss it in the schoolroom. Posters like the one in Figure 1–4 help to get the message across. In lung cancer, the single biggest problem is a lack of knowledge of how to motivate smokers to stop smoking and to fore-

---

[14] National Advisory Cancer Council. *Progress Against Cancer 1966*. Washington, D.C.: U.S. Public Health Service, 1967.

Figure 1-4 Lung cancer and smoking. (Courtesy American Cancer Society.)

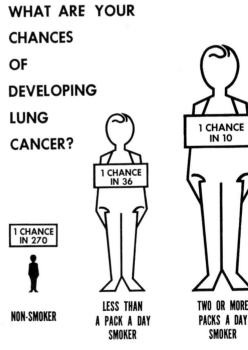

WHAT ARE YOUR CHANCES OF DEVELOPING LUNG CANCER?

1 CHANCE IN 270
NON-SMOKER

1 CHANCE IN 36
LESS THAN A PACK A DAY SMOKER

1 CHANCE IN 10
TWO OR MORE PACKS A DAY SMOKER

stall young people from acquiring the smoking habit. Simply telling them that 12 times as many smokers die of emphysema as non-smokers is not the answer. Educational programs in the schools, coupled with the efforts of the U.S. Public Health Service and the National Clearinghouse for Smoking and Health, may prove helpful during the next several years.

In addition to causing cancer, coronary heart disease, chronic bronchitis, and emphysema, cigarette smoking cuts several years off the life expectancy of millions of Americans. Smokers at every age pay a high risk price — 22 per cent of heavy smokers can expect to be hospitalized during any given 24-month period, as compared to only 14 per cent of non-smokers.

Hopefully, this situation will be helped by the Federal Communications Commission ruling that broadcasters who carry commercials which promote cigarette smoking as attractive and enjoyable must also provide "a significant amount of time" for messages on the harmful effects of cigarette smoking.

The over-all *physical fitness* of youth is another concern of parents and teachers. American youth are physically softer than those in many other countries. Youngsters in general lead a rather sedentary existence. Research indicates that civilization plays strange tricks. Many of the youth of the land are lacking the physical wherewithal to participate in vigorous, growth-stimulating activities. They simply have not been exposed to first rate health and physical education programs. Muscular weakness and lack of physical fitness are linked to a life lacking in muscle-building chores, with rich foods, bus and automobile transportation, more spectator rather than participation activities, more TV viewing, less walking, labor-saving devices, apartment living, and lack of adequate play space. Education to meet the loss of fitness is a constant need. It is almost an axiom that the more complex civilization becomes, the less valid is instinctive behavior and therefore the greater becomes the need of education to preserve health.

The need for proper programs of physical activity is of paramount concern to teachers of young children. Adults can hardly be expected to change their sedentary ways of living if in their early years of formal education they did not acquire an appreciation for physical skills and the need for regular exercise throughout a lifetime. Walking and bicycling, according to the eminent heart specialist, Dr. Paul

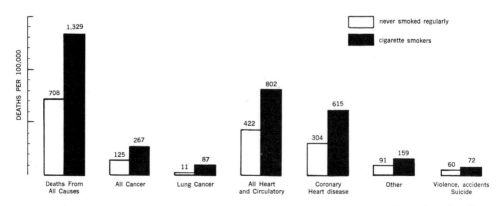

Figure 1–5 Findings of the Hammond Study (Courtesy U.S. Public Health Service, *The Facts about Smoking and Health*, 1968.)

Dudley White, are simple and practical exercises that should be a part of one's plan of normal living.

It has been demonstrated by the President's Council on Physical Fitness that physically underdeveloped children can be readily identified and given vigorous developmental activity to increase their level of physical fitness. A project involving over 200,000 schoolchildren in five states revealed that where a school had a physical education program prior to its selection in the project, the average physical fitness test failure was 25 per cent. In schools that had no program, however, the average rate of failure was 46 per cent. In all schools, swift improvement was achieved when below-average students were given individual attention.

Millions of people have *poor teeth*. In fact, about 95 per cent of the population suffers from this condition. The average number of unfilled cavities is five per head. Also, 26 million people have lost all of their teeth. Obviously, the American mouth is a disaster area that could be improved if gum stimulators and toothbrushes were properly used. The high rate of periodontal disease, caused by an accumulation of tartar which results in swelling and inflammation (68 million adult Americans have this disorder), is largely due to the fact that early symptoms are ignored and neglected.

Tens of thousands of children have serious difficulties with their teeth. Half the children in the country under 15 have never been to a dentist. It is true that poverty, ignorance and indifference have something to do with dental decay statistics, but there are numerous examples of well-educated parents with moderate to high incomes whose children's teeth are no better than the average.

By the time the average child reaches school, he has one to three carious teeth. At age 12 or 13 he has five permanent teeth attacked by caries. The decay rate rises sharply in the intermediate grades. (See Figure 1-6.) It is evident, too, that fluoridation of the water supply is highly significant. Yet, large numbers of people continue to resist a move in this direction because of entrenched beliefs and general misinformation. Although the effectiveness of water fluoridation has been amply demonstrated, this procedure is only now beginning to have

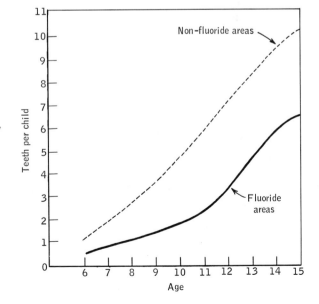

Figure 1-6 Relationship of tooth decay in children to age and fluoridation.

the impact that might be expected. From 1961 to 1966 the number of people drinking fluoridated water increased by 20 million. When large cities such as New York, Chicago, Philadelphia, Baltimore, Cleveland, Washington, St. Louis, and Detroit fluoridate their water, the impact is significant. Today, approximately 50 per cent of the U.S. community water supplies are fluoridated.

Fluoridation of the drinking water not only reduces tooth decay up to 70 per cent, but it is a tremendous money saver. In ten years Chicago's fluoridated water supply has saved parents more than two million dollars in dental costs for children under 14, and at the same time has reduced tooth decay by 67 per cent. This financial saving is dramatically illustrated by the findings of a two-city study in New York State where the mean cost for dental care per child in Kingston (non-fluoridated water) was more than double that in Newburgh (fluoridated water).[15]

The benefits from public water fluoridation programs greatly reduce the hazard of malocclusion, especially severe malocclusion which may be regarded as physically handicapping. Also, research is beginning to indicate that fluorides slow the course of periodontal disease by retarding bone destruction. Rheumatoid arthritis and osteoporosis – abnormal porousness of bone – are lower in areas where there is a high fluoride content in the water.

The staggering need for dental care, with an estimated backlog of 1,000,-000,000 untreated carious lesions in teeth in America would make one feel that the dentists are overworked. Yet surveys have indicated that only 40 per cent of the dentists are reported to have an overload. It has been conser-

vatively estimated that if all the dentists devoted their time exclusively to filling teeth, five years would be required to take care of the backlog alone. Education to get more people to see their dentists regularly must involve both the general public and the school personnel. Only a cooperative effort in the years ahead will improve the situation to any degree.

Accident statistics overwhelm the average reader. *Accidents* are the greatest threat to life and limb in childhood and call for an education of the public through school and community health agencies. This is recognized today as a necessity if man is to survive in a society demanding ever increasing human adaptability. Considerable adaptation takes place at an early age. Adaptation to physical strains, psychological stresses and hazardous situations is to be considered by parents and teachers alike. Here are some impressive findings:

Fifty-two million people a year are injured in some kind of an accident, and another 104,000 are killed.

Accidents are the chief cause of death in children ages five to 14 years. Over 7500 deaths occur yearly.

Over four million non-fatal injuries occur annually in and about the home.

Sports and recreation account for approximately 5200 fatalities and a great many more serious injuries annually.

More than 8000 people die by drowning each year. Over half the people in the U.S. cannot swim well enough to save themselves in an emergency (National Safety Council).

Motor vehicle accidents take about 52,000 lives a year and inflict disabling injuries on an additional 1,800,000 persons in the United States. Another 1,500,000 are injured but not disabled.

Socially maladjusted individuals are more likely to be involved in acci-

15 Ast, David B., et al. "Time and Cost Factors to Provide Regular, Periodic Dental Care for Children in a Fluoridated and Nonfluoridated Area," *American Journal of Public Health,* 57: 1635-1642, September 1967.

dents than are those without such difficulties.

The National Safety Council estimates that if seat belts were used consistently by all drivers and passengers, the incidence of serious injury could be reduced by one third and between 8000 and 10,000 lives could be saved annually.

55 million bicycles ridden in the United States today are connected with an annual loss of 700 lives. Four out of five such fatalities are believed to be associated with the disregard of safe practices. Safety authorities estimate that between 120,000 and 150,000 persons sustain disabling injuries in such mishaps in a single year.

Firearm accidents claim a toll of about 2400 lives a year.

Annually some 1500 pedestrians, five to 14 years of age, are killed in traffic. Injuries, which are a better indicator of the seriousness of the problem, show that 50,000 schoolchildren are injured in pedestrian accidents every year.

Medicines cause most accidental poisonings in children, and aspirin heads the list. (See Figure 1–7.) Children under five who swallowed aspirin were the victims in one-fourth of all cases of accidental poisoning reported

in 1966 to the National Clearinghouse for Poison Control Centers.

Tetanus (lockjaw) is almost entirely preventable by vaccination, but only one person in four bothers to get the preventive tetanus toxoid shots. Half of the 450 tetanus patients reported in the United States each year still die unnecessarily.

The need for education for safe living is great indeed. It must begin early with children. While adults have a high incidence of motor vehicle and firearms accidents, and often discuss ways of reducing them, it becomes most difficult to talk to the excitement-loving, venturesome youngsters who are repelled by the idea that being safe means avoiding unnecessary risks. So they have needless accidents while pursuing their day-to-day activities.

Childhood curiosity, like childhood enthusiasm, needs guiding. For example, every 24 hour period more than 750 children in the United States are poisoned by their own curiosity, which impels them to gulp aspirin and sleeping pills, sip floor polish and kerosene, swallow kitchen detergents, rubber cement and cosmetics, and gnaw peeling paint from furniture and walls. Children, it has been said, will eat just about anything—and there

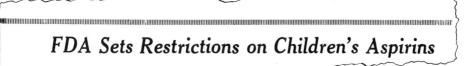

FDA Sets Restrictions on Children's Aspirins

United Press International

WASHINGTON — The Food and Drug Administration (FDA) said Monday that all children's aspirin bottles sold next July 1 will contain no more than 36 tablets each in an effort to reduce accidental overdoses.

The restriction was one of several steps announced jointly by the FDA and 32 drug firms

after a conference aimed at curbing childhood deaths and illnesses.

The F.D.A.'s action followed by exactly six weeks the death in Exeter, N.H., of a two-year-old boy from an overdose of candy-flavored aspirin.

At the time, Dr. Joel Alpert, head of the child health division at Children's U— about

die each

Figure 1–7 An historic action for child safety.

are some 15,000 substances which are, to some extent, poisonous.

The *problems of aging* are many. People are living longer; the population is growing older. It is not at all unrealistic to base training of children now in school on the probability that a high percentage will live past 90 and many beyond 100 years. It was uncommon for children in 1900 to know their grandparents. Today's average fifth-grader probably will live to see his great-grandchildren in the fifth grade. Many will see the birth of great-great-grandchildren. All of this will make for greater changes in family relationships. It will also place increased value on the continuous application of proper health knowledge all through the years.

The effects of *air and water pollution* are shocking. As man discovers new sources of energy, he seems to add new pollutants involving huge economic losses and lowered health for himself. Approximately 90 per cent of our urban population lives in localities which have heavily polluted waterways and air pollution hazards—

from radiation, smoke, smog, fumes, and chemicals. According to the U.S. Public Health Service, the ten cities with the dirtiest air in 1967 were, in order of pollution, New York, Chicago, Philadelphia, Los Angeles, Cleveland, Pittsburgh, Boston, Newark, Detroit, and St. Louis. There is abundant evidence to show that the bigger the city, the greater the air pollution and the number of deaths. (See Figure 1–8.)

That there is something obnoxious in the air becomes more evident as statistics from air sampling stations pile up. These make the automobile a top-ranking culprit, one which produces roughly one-half of the contaminants found in the air. In Los Angeles County in one year, automobiles released 965 tons of hydrocarbons, 250 tons of nitrogen oxides, 19 tons of sulfur dioxide, 6850 tons of carbon monoxide, and 27 tons of aerosols. Other methods of transporation rank second, followed by the petroleum industry, combustion of fuels, use of organic solvents, metals, chemicals, incineration of refuse, and minerals.

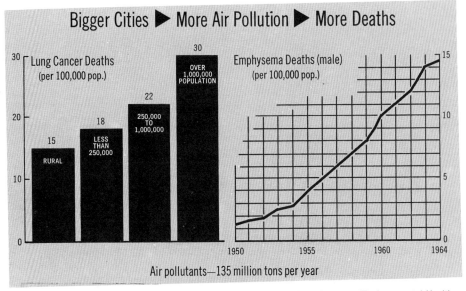

Figure 1–8 Air pollution and the population explosion (Report of Task Force on Environmental Health and Related Problems, *A Strategy for a Livable Environment*, U.S. Dept. Health, Education and Welfare, Washington, D.C., June, 1967.)

Severe air pollution triggers illness and may bring about premature death to thousands of people. Even "ordinary" levels of air pollution can cause coughing, sneezing, wheezing, and suffering. Short range discomfort may be followed by long range disease. Bronchitis, emphysema (a deteriorating lung condition sometimes marked by heart enlargement and impairment of heart action), and lung cancer are more prevalent in areas of high air contamination. A careful check of total deaths in New York City by day of occurrence indicates periodic peaks in mortality which are associated with periods of high air pollution.[16] Temperature inversion conditions and low wind speed permit air pollution to build up to high levels.

Although it is known that cigarette smoking and air pollution are separate causes of emphysema, it has now been shown that the combined effect is even more deadly. Smoking, however, has a greater chance of influencing emphysema than air pollution, for it has been found that the percentage of emphysema is higher among moderate smokers not exposed to pollution than among nonsmokers exposed to pollution.

Cleaning up America's polluted waters is a task for government at all levels and for industry in every community. But the education of the citizen is required if water pollution control programs are to continue to be implemented. Man has made numerous bodies of water so bacteria-ridden that he cannot drink it, so oily and irritant that he cannot swim in it, so unsupportive of life that he cannot fish in it, and so malodorous and filled with refuse and old junk that he cannot contemplate its once natural beauty.

Today, even noise pollution is a health hazard in industry and in the community. Exposure to severe noise causes hearing loss, and in many cities today noise levels exceed standards found injurious in industry.[17] Only an educated consumer will demand a reduction in noise levels in the home or on the street. Therefore, the problems of air, water, and noise pollution need to be discovered and worked on by children in the classroom if hopeful changes are to occur in the future.

Overweight has been a health problem in civilized countries for a number of years. An individual should know that it is to his advantage to reach his desirable or "ideal" weight and stay there the rest of his life. However, about three out of five men in their fifties are overweight. Half of the women beyond the age of 40 are more than 10 per cent above their desirable weight. Even half the men in their thirties are at least 10 per cent above their optimum weight. Studies at the University of Washington School of Medicine indicate that the teenage population is 20 to 30 per cent overweight and that girls are more frequently overweight than boys. Studies by Harvard University personnel show that young obese girls are significantly less active than non-obese children.[18] Not only are these children underactive and overfed, they do not exert energy to do *anything* often enough. They are passive and altogether too dependent on their parents.

Alcoholism is a serious illness affecting 6,500,000 people in America. Not only does it do incalculable damage to personal and family life (a leading cause of separation, divorce, desertion, and emotional problems), it shortens the life span by 12 years. Moreover,

---

[16] McCarroll, James, and Bradley, William. "Excess Mortality as an Indicator of Health Effects of Air Pollution," *American Journal of Public Health*, 56:1933-1942, November 1966.

[17] Dougherty, J. D., and Welsh, O. L. "Community Noise and Hearing Loss," *New England Journal of Medicine*, October 6, 1966.

[18] See report by B. A. Bullen, R. B. Reed, and J. Mayer in the *American Journal of Clinical Nutrition*, 14:211, 1964.

alcoholism is involved in 50 per cent or more of the automobile accident deaths that occur each year. One-third of all arrests in this country are for public drunkenness. There is a growing viewpoint that if people are going to drink (70 per cent do), then they should have some alcohol education. Drinking patterns and the responsibilities of those who drink need wide discussion.

Absenteeism everywhere has been slowly climbing. The annual rate for industrial absenteeism is now 6 per cent, an all-time high. The acute diseases such as colds and upper respiratory illnesses account for half of the current absenteeism; chronic debilitating disease accounts for the other half. Because of this, more than ten billion dollars a year is drained from the economy. Studies among high absentees show that they tend to be unhappy, discontented, egocentric, and generally unhealthy. Conversely, the worker with few absences tends to be happy and contented, outgoing, and reasonably well.

In New York City 65 per cent of school absences are caused by health problems. Preventable school absences in this one city cost upwards of five million dollars annually in state aid.

Sex-Related Problems. There is a massive accumulation of evidence to indicate that one of the foremost health-related problems of the century is the widespread lack of knowledge and understanding of human sex and sexuality.

Since 1958 the venereal disease rate has increased 500 per cent despite the fact that it should be common knowledge that syphilis and gonorrhea can be cured with penicillin. Much of the increase has been among children between the ages of 12 and 19 years. Society has been slow to act. In 1940 the U.S. Surgeon General could not even use the word syphilis in a radio broadcast. Almost 30 years later the word still causes adults to blush, and sixth graders to ask what it is. In New York City, where syphilis doubled among teenage boys in an eight-year period, a study showed that 32 per cent did not know that it could be cured, and 60 per cent did not know that venereal disease is transmitted through sexual intercourse. Keeping sex information "under wraps" has been exactly the wrong thing to do.

Since 1940 teenage marriages have risen 500 per cent, and studies indicate that 50 to 80 per cent of teenage wives are pregnant at the time of marriage. The divorce rate in such marriages is three times as high as that for individuals married after 21.[19]

Illegitimate births among girls in the 14 to 19 age group are more than double what they were 25 years ago. In Chicago alone there are approximately 115 pregnant girls under the age of 15 who appear each month at the Chicago Board of Health Clinic. Moreover, if present rates continue, in the state of Connecticut one 13-year-old girl in every six will become pregnant out of wedlock before her twentieth birthday.[20] The "every sixth teenage girl" figure is estimated to be about the same on a national basis. It is undoubtedly low, because it underestimates the number of pregnant girls who lose their babies through spontaneous and induced abortion. It also omits unmarried girls who have erroneous information entered on the birth certificate.

In Buffalo, the out-of-wedlock births

---

[19] Ferber, Ellen, and Sofokidis, Jeanette H. "Goodbye to the Birds and Bees: What's Happening," *American Education*, November 1966, p. 16.

[20] See article by Ruth and Edward Brecher, "Every Sixth Teenage Girl in Connecticut," (reprinted by *SIECUS*, 1790 Broadway, New York, New York 10019), based on material gathered from the Connecticut State Department of Health, 1966.

increased more than threefold between 1950 and 1965.[21] Most significant, however, was the twofold increase in births to girls under 17 years
of age. Studies show that very few of
these girls understand conception and
the sex function. In fact, one wonders
how enlightened the six and one-half
million American women are who take
birth-control pills 20 days of every
month.

The school systems in several of the
larger cities have been concerned
with the sex education of pregnant
and unwed girls. The growing number
of such students has caused problems.
By 1968 the special school for pregnant secondary school girls in Baltimore had 895 girls and had to turn
away 1200 more for lack of room.

Although unwed mothers and pregnant girls are being helped and children with venereal disease are being
treated, very few school systems are
providing a comprehensive sex education curriculum for students of both
sexes in grades one to 12. This is most
unfortunate, for this is a society in
which chaperones and supervision of
youth are unfashionable, the young
people are left on their own with easy
access to privacy, children of all ages
are totally vulnerable to the onslaughts
of commercial exploitation of sex,
news media report all kinds of sordid
sexual occurrences, and sex misinformation comes from many questionable
sources. Until this void is filled with
a quantity and quality of factual knowledge, the young person will continue
to remain very defenseless about
sex. Studies show that boys and girls
do not want sexual license; they crave
information and explanations. They
seek standards which will help them
understand the role of sex as a part of

their total personality. And they want
to talk about it—in the way that they
talk about any other topic in the school
curriculum. Kirkendall, in calling for
sex education, makes this need quite
clear when he says:

> The chief determinant of sexual con-
> duct is not factual information but the
> general feeling of satisfaction and
> worth which the individual has been
> able to develop about himself as a
> person. One's pattern of sexual be-
> havior is a reflection of one's total
> life pattern. An individual who feels
> he is accomplishing something with
> his life . . . will not be driven by guilt,
> anxiety or compulsion to engage in
> sex with little regard for what this
> means to other persons or to his total
> situation. In other words, he is in a
> position to direct and manage his
> sexuality.[22]

Considerably more attention will be
given to program planning in the area
of sex and family living education in
Chapter 7. (See page 156.)

Superstitions. There is a wide
variety of superstitions in existence
throughout the world. They are based
in some cases on old wives' tales, and
in other cases on pure magic. Rich and
poor alike believe them, and contrary to what might be expected, they
are a part of the daily existence of the
bright scholar as well as of the dull and
ignorant. Superstitions are difficult to
combat because they are concealed
beneath the veneer of education. It
has been succinctly stated that man
surveys the world about him, clutch-
ing science with one hand, hoping for
its benefits, yet holding firmly with
the other hand to the superstitions of
the ages. One sees the figure of Samuel
Pepys, famous diarist of the 1600's,
headed for home with a rabbit's foot

---

[21] Anderson, Ursula M., et al. "The Medical,
Social and Educational Implications of the
Increase in Out-of-Wedlock Births," *American
Journal of Public Health*, 56:1866-1873, Novem-
ber 1966.

[22] Kirkendall, Lester A. "Sex Education,"
Discussion Guide No. 1, published by Sex In-
formation and Education Council of the U.S.,
October 1965, p. 9.

in one pocket and a copy of Hooke's "Book of Microscopy" in the other.

Gullibility. This is a nation of healthy people. It is also a nation of tub thumpers, pill takers, television addicts, neurotics, and helpless individuals. Probably more people are "lost" in terms of what to do for themselves along health lines than most people realize. Newspaper advertising on the one hand and television ads on the other keep heads turning from this product to that product like a mass of humanity watching a tennis match. Americans have been accused of buying everything and anything if it is supposed to be "good for you." Nearly 20 billion pills are consumed each year. This averages out to about one hundred pills annually for every man, woman, and child in the country. Most pills, of course, are taken from necessity and render an important service in conquering or checking disease and improving personal efficiency. Millions of pills and gallons of patent medicines are devoured for imaginary illness brought on by gullibility. Parents are gullible and so are their children; they require a better understanding of health. When a knowledge of the human body and its requirements grows, gullibility begins to fade away.

Fads, Diets, and Quackery. Mature people are sometimes like the classmates of the little girl in the fourth grade who comes to school with a pretty red ribbon in her hair. Before the week is out, half of her girl friends in the class will be seen sporting attractive ribbons in their hair.

On almost any street in the community friendly neighbors spread the word that something helped them with their aches and pains. Some people subject themselves to such things as vitamin pills, steam baths, spinal manipulations, or blackstrap molasses and yogurt simply because their friends think it good for them. No thought of securing qualified medical attention has entered their minds. Dieting becomes popular for awhile, then it may give way to the use of a certain toothpaste or cigarette. People want to swallow a pill, suck a skim milk or lemon juice wafer or chew mint-flavored gum, eat what they please and still lose weight. They do not know that it may even be harmful. For example, diabetics and individuals with high blood pressure or heart disease should take tablets only upon the advice of a physician. People are always waiting for the "miracle drug," and, if tranquilizing drugs work for one person's illness, the attitude of the man on the street is often: "Why won't it work for my troubles, too?"

Cults and quackeries may be more serious than fads, for they tend to confuse the public as to their relationship with science. People practicing certain cults and quackery often believe they have a "cure," and they make what they have to offer sound powerfully scientific, especially to the person who is in need of help. The quack is hard to place behind bars because he often claims that he is not dispensing medicines. As long as he does not prescribe drugs or practice surgery, he seems to be safe in many states today. But his influence in spreading health misinformation is great indeed. Public and school health education can do much to curtail fads, cults, and quackeries.

Misconceptions. Honest people exist everywhere who are misled by their erroneous beliefs. Misinformed parents have stood by and watched their children play with a mad dog who was supposed to be perfectly safe because he was not foaming at the mouth. People are under all kinds of common misconceptions. Some border on superstitions; others are more acceptable and easy to believe, such as, "it is impossible to cure any cancer." One of the biggest misconceptions in our society today relates to the topic of who is qualified to practice medicine. Thousands of unsuspecting people have little idea of the meaning of "Dr." or "M.D." They assume that these letters refer to specialists of comparable ability. Yet, in some places, almost anyone can hang up a sign in his front yard with "Dr." written on it.

A rather extensive list of harmful misconceptions about health and safety was compiled by Dzenowagis from information given by sixth grade schoolchildren.[23] As in his earlier studies, he points to the needs for health education in a convincing manner. Children in this grade had erroneous beliefs, and they had trouble discriminating between truths, half-truths, and falsehoods. Dzenowagis concluded that certain dangerous misconceptions were prevalent among 28 per cent of the sixth grade children.

Over a 25 year period, Kilander discovered a slight but steady improvement in the level of health information held by children and adults.[24] He also found few individuals to be adequately informed in the various areas of health knowledge to be able to act wisely in their own personal needs. Here are several examples of the more interesting misconceptions selected from several hundred test items:

Approximately one-third of the students in college believe entirely or in part that "a prospective mother can make her child more musical if she listens to good music." Exactly half of a group of 50 mothers in the PTA were similarly misinformed.

About one-third of the public thinks

that water contains calories and is fattening.

About one in five believes that a newborn child's disfiguration may be caused by the mother's fright during pregnancy.

About one out of four students still believe there is some truth to the statement that "fish is brain food." One out of three nonprofessional adults hold this misconception.

The Extremes – Indifference Versus Neurotic Behavior. People seem to vary in their attitude toward health on a scale all the way from a state of indifference with too little concern for health to a state of over-concern to the point of neurotic behavior. Somewhere between the two lies the area of the moderate attitude.

Indifference is closely allied to gullibility and ignorance. It is a negative factor that has always retarded the wheels of progress. It is more common in adults, whose minds are less flexible than in children, who tend to be open-minded. It evaporates slowly when human enlightenment takes hold. Indifference to common health practices is illustrated rather well by the story of the nurse-teacher who called on Mary's mother to tell her about the little girl's long standing case of head lice. After the nurse had spoken to her for several minutes, the mother simply gazed out across the fields, shrugged her shoulders as if to dismiss the whole business and said, "Well, everybody has a few."

Now for the other extreme. This is neurotic behavior. A growing number of children and adults are becoming almost neurotic about their health. In most cases they have been exposed to a little knowledge and have jumped to conclusions. When Pope said that "a little learning is a dangerous thing," he may have had such people in mind. They sometimes join cults, become food faddists, and practice any health fancies which suit them at the mo-

---

[23] Dzenowagis, Joseph G. "Prevalence of Certain Dangerous Safety Misconceptions Among a Group of Sixth-Grade Children," *Journal of School Health,* 33:26-32, January 1963.

[24] Kilander, H. Frederick. "Health Knowledge," *Journal of Health, Physical Education and Recreation,* 32:28-29, May-June 1961.

ment. These people thrive on all the loose bits of information on psychosomatic illnesses that float about in their community. Moreover, their imaginary difficulties sometimes become real, and then their neurotic behavior relates to something more serious.

Citizenship. In the final analysis, citizenship itself is pertinent to both the health status and the health understanding of the citizen. Health education, therefore, may be considered a vital part of education for citizenship. Several decades ago, Professor E. G. Conklin of Yale University said:

> The person who does not believe in vaccination or the so-called "germ theory" of disease, or quarantines, who fights against taxes to improve the water supply or to dispose of sewage or to get rid of malarial mosquitoes, who opposes the appointment of health officers, or the scientific inspection of milk and other foods, or the medical examination of school children, is not only an ignoramus but he is also a bad citizen.[25]

Behind disease control and other health practices is the reasonably good community. And to the "good community," according to Edward Lee Thorndike, is made better in this country primarily and chiefly by getting able and good people as residents — people who, for example, are intelligent, are reasonably happy, do not contract syphilis, or commit murder, or allow others to do so. In short, an enlightened citizenry goes a long way toward building the utopia of tomorrow.

Education Defined

A proper definition of education includes some reference to aims, purposes, or goals. The word "education" comes from the Latin word *edu-*

cere, meaning "to lead forth" or "to lead out." It refers to the drawing out of a person something latent or potential. It suggests a change in some particular direction. Education, therefore, may be defined toward certain preconceived goals. Thus, education is anything but haphazard. There is a well defined purpose expressed through clearly stated aims and objectives.

Educational Aims and Objectives

> Principles, not men — when men desert principles, may they be deserted by the people.
> —COURIER OF NEW HAMPSHIRE 1802

There has always been a high degree of respect in this country for the person with an avowed purpose.[26] One of the most famous remarks used year after year at commencement exercises was made by Leland Stanford who said, "the world stands aside for the man who knows where he is going."

In education, as in other fields of endeavor, one needs to know where he is going. Direction is always important. One must possess a personal philosophy of life that is fundamentally sound. Like Maxwell Garnett, most people believe that human societies should aim toward the fulfillment of some far-reaching purpose.[27] Such a point of view coupled with an interest in education equips the individual with the basic ideas to formulate the aims and objectives of education.

Aims are generally far-reaching purposes, while objectives are usually

---

[25] Conklin, E. G. "Biology and the National Welfare," *Yale Review,* 6 (new series):486, 1917.

[26] For a clear-cut illustration of singleness of purpose, see Abraham Lincoln's straightforward letter to Horace Greeley on the Saving of the Nation. (Willgoose, Carl E. "Health: The Fundamental Objective," *Education,* 68(8):451, April 1948.)
[27] Garnett, J. C. Maxwell. *Education and World Citizenship.* Cambridge, England: The University Press, 1921, p. 315.

near-at-hand goals. The proposition to raise the nation's health 10 per cent would be of such magnitude that it would be considered an aim. A lesser proposition to purify the water supply, however, would be a fair example of an objective.

Most purposes of education make a definite reference to healthful living. In 70 B.C., Cicero proclaimed to his subjects in Rome, "In nothing do men more nearly approach the gods than in giving health to men." Centuries later, in 1550, Rabelais said, "The aim of education is not so much to fill thee with learning as to train both thy mind and thy body. . . . Without health, life is no life." In 1690, John Locke made his much quoted statement: "A sound mind in a sound body is a short but full description of a happy state in this world; he that has these two has little more to wish for; and he that wants either of them, will be but little the better for anything else."

It is quite apparent that the old-timers — Socrates, Plato, Aristotle, Comenius, Rousseau, for example — were just as enthusiastic about healthful living as an objective of education as are the more recent educators.

The essential purposes of education have not varied to any great degree in a century of time. What Herbert Spencer wrote in the 1800's on the question, "What knowledge is of most worth?" does not depart significantly from modern goals.[28] His ends of education were concerned with life and health, earning a living, family rearing, citizenship, and leisure.

The Cardinal Principles of Secondary Education have been recognized since their establishment in 1918. The well-known seven basic objectives were health, command of fundamental

[28] Spencer, Herbert. *Education: Intellectual, Moral and Physical.* New York: D. Appleton & Company, 1860.

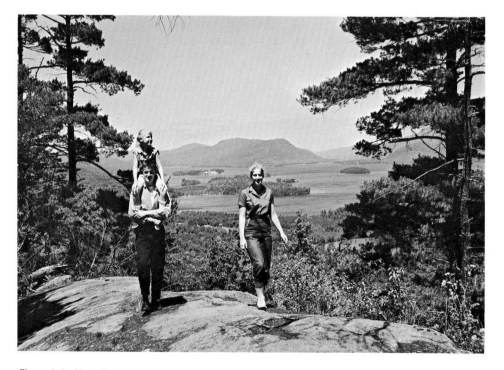

Figure 1–9 The effects of pressure and rapid pace are counteracted through family recreation. (New York State Department of Commerce.)

processes, worthy home membership, vocation, citizenship, worthy use of leisure, and ethical character.[29] It may readily be seen that these aims of education are like those proposed by Spencer. As far as health education is concerned, both sets of purposes stress health as the primary aim. Both point to the need for education for leisure, an item that concerns physical and mental health to a great degree and probably has as much to do with the survival of man as any other aim.

Since 1918, numerous groups of educators have undertaken the formulation of goals and specific objectives in both general and elementary education. The most recent and far-reaching set of educational purposes are these put forth by the Educational Policies Commission.[30] The purposes are:

1. The objectives of *self-realization*. This deals with the fundamental skills such as reading, writing and speaking. It is also concerned with the acquisition of knowledge and habits pertaining to healthful living and the ability to use leisure time in a wholesome manner.

2. The objectives of *human relationship*. This is concerned chiefly with human welfare and man's ability to work harmoniously with his fellow men.

3. The objectives of *economic efficiency*. This deals with man as a producer and consumer and the selection of a vocation.

4. The objectives of *civic responsibility*. This relates to the responsibil-

ities of the citizen in a local, state, national and world community.

The Ultimate Scope of Health Education

It may be seen in the above objectives of education that agreement has been reached by educational philosophers stressing the need for health education in the schools. The ultimate scope of health education is a broad one. Thus, each person, in order to satisfy his own needs and, at the same time, contribute his share to the welfare of society must possess:

1. Optimum organic health consistent with heredity and the application of present health knowledge;

2. Sufficient coordination, strength, and vitality to meet emergencies, as well as the requirements of daily living;

3. Emotional stability to meet the stresses and strains of modern life;

4. Social consciousness and adaptability with respect to the requirements of group living;

5. Sufficient knowledge and insight to make suitable decisions and arrive at feasible solutions to problems;

6. Attitudes, values, and skills which stimulate satisfactory participation in a full range of daily activities;

7. Spiritual and moral qualities which contribute the fullest measure of living in a democratic society.[31]

If we learn anything at all from the present condition of adult mankind, it should be that the problems, diseases, and inadequacies of the moment did not suddenly appear; rather, they emerged gradually, having had their roots established during the early elementary school years. This is to

---

[29] Commission on the Reorganization of Secondary Education. *Cardinal Principles of Secondary Education*. Washington, D.C., Bureau of Education, Bulletin 35, 1918.

[30] Educational Policies Commission. *Policies for Education in American Democracy*. Washington: National Education Association, 1946, p. 189. See also the more recent publication of the Commission, *The Central Purpose of American Education*. National Education Association, 1961.

[31] Statement prepared and approved by the delegates to the American Association for Health, Physical Education, and Recreation Fitness Conference, September 12-15, 1956, Washington, D.C.

say that the backaches, ulcers, gastro-intestinal pains, hypertension, obesity, chronic fatigue, coronary thrombosis, and the neurotic and psychotic behavior related to anxiety, apprehension, worry, fear, hatred, and jealousy are all tied directly to a *pattern* *of living* and level of understanding obtained during the formative years. A sense of values early in life, coupled with the proper skills and knowledge, sets the stage in more ways than one. The part played by health education in this period can be most productive.

Questions for Discussion

1. What is the relationship of physical efficiency to total health?

2. How can we get citizens in the community interested in, concerned with, and involved in school health programs?

3. How can we gain greater cooperation in closing the gap between the objectives of the school health program and what is really being accomplished?

4. How is health related to other objectives of education?

5. What are the values of the Selective Service finding to school health personnel?

6. How has the World Health Organization contributed to child health on an international level?

Suggested Activities

1. Dobzhansky, writing in *Mankind Evolving: The Evolution of the Human Species* (Yale University Press, 1962, pp. 346–347), points out that "nature and nurture" work together. Hoyman writes about the same thing. So does Brightbill. (See references listed at end of the chapter.) Look over an article or two which pertains to human ecology and health. Prepare a written paragraph on what you have read and another one setting forth your comments.

2. Survey a number of persons in health-related professions (public or private) and find out how they feel about education as a means of preventing poor health. Are they concerned about venereal disease or cardiac statistics, or something called "value illness"? Compare your findings with several of your classmates.

3. Compare the views of Plato and Rousseau with those of Oberteuffer and Johns relative to the need for an education for health.

4. Review the list of nine *Imperatives In Education* set forth by the American Association of School Administrators. Indicate ways and means in which health education can contribute to the fulfillment of these points and help meet the needs of the times.

5. Formulate a list of changes which have occurred in American society which might have a bearing on health behavior. Consider such items as cybernation, population explosion, sex behavior of youth, and alcoholism. Is there danger that too many changes coming too fast will tend to cause mankind to overlook certain long-standing truths?

6. In his utopian book, *The Shape of Things To Come*, H. G. Wells assumed that scientific thinking, modern-day engineering, and public education, by their intrinsic worth, would prepare a kind of future that would be approved of by the educated middle-class citizen. Later, when he wrote *Mind at the End of Its Tether*, Wells became dis-

illusioned as he noted that Nazi Germany scored higher on scientific rationalism, engineering, and public education than did any other European nation. Take a moment to examine this observation. Do educational goals and programs need very careful definition as they relate to a civilization? Write out some specific implications for educators and others who build a society "close to the heart's desire."

Selected References

Aristotle. "Pleasure and Happiness," in Randall, John H., Buchler, Justus, and Shirk, Evelyn (eds.). *Readings in Philosophy*. New York: Barnes and Noble, 1946, pp. 356–368.

Boroff, David. *The State of the Nation*. Englewood Cliffs, New Jersey: Prentice-Hall, Inc., 1966.

Brightbill, Charles K. *Man and Leisure*. Englewood Cliffs, New Jersey: Prentice-Hall, Inc., 1961.

Bucher, Charles A., Olsen, Einar A., and Willgoose, Carl E. *The Foundations of Health*. New York: Appleton-Century-Crofts, 1967, Chapters 2, 14, 17.

Calderone, Mary A. "Goodbye to the Birds and Bees: an Approach." *American Education*, November 1966, p. 17.

Carrell, Alexis. *Man the Unknown*. New York: Harper and Brothers, 1936.

Cutler, Robert. *"No Time for Rest."* Boston: Little, Brown and Co., 1966.

Gardner, John W. "The Ever-Renewing Society." *Saturday Review*, January 5, 1963, pp. 92–95.

Hoyman, Howard S. "An Ecologic View of Health and Health Education." *Journal of School Health*, 35:110–123, March 1965.

Kartman, Leo. "Human Ecology and Public Health." *American Journal of Public Health*, 57:737–750, May 1967.

Lake, Alice. "The Pill." *McCall's*, November 1967, p. 96.

Leff, S. V. *From Witchcraft to World Health*. New York: The Macmillan Co., 1957.

Mayshark, Cyrus. "Epidemiology of Health Education." *Journal of Health, Physical Education, and Recreation*, 35:48–50, February 1968.

Millner, Bernard N. "Health Needs of School-Age Children," *Journal of School Health*, 36:276–280, June 1966.

Report: "Is Social Change the Answer to Alcohol Problems?" *The National Observer*, October 16, 1967.

Rosen, George. "Health is a Community Affair." *American Journal of Public Health*, 57:572–583, April 1967.

Schwartz, Jerome L., and Dubitsky, Mildred. "Research in Student Smoking Habits and Smoking Control." *Journal of School Health*, 37:177–182, April 1967.

Shaffer, Thomas. "The Role of the School and the Community in Sex Education and Related Problems." *Journal of American Medical Association*, 195:667–670, February 1966.

Simon, William, and Gagnon, John H. "The Pedagogy of Sex." *Saturday Review*, November 18, 1967.

Vincent, Ronald G. "A Fence or an Ambulance." *Journal of School Health*, 37:369–373, October 1967.

Willgoose, Carl E. "Recreation: An Attitude of Mind." *Education*, 81:42–44, September 1960.

Willgoose, Carl E. "The White House Conference on Health." *Journal of Health, Physical Education, and Recreation*, 37:14, January 1966, p. 14.

The Elementary School Health Program

CHAPTER 2

Health education is a proper goal of elementary education. After a reading of the previous chapter relative to education objectives, the reader should realize that both formal and informal education must emphasize the maintenance and promotion of total health. This is especially true in the elementary school, and it is for this reason that the school health program exists.

Justification for School Health Program

Among the numerous justifications for an elementary school health program are three that stand above the rest. First of all, the immediate health needs of the fast-growing child are specific and ever-present. Nutrition, fresh air, activity, and good eyesight cannot be taken lightly. Secondly, the school health program is a prime mover in preparing the child for the years ahead. Health status in the early years can be a prominent contributing factor in the ultimate achievement of a rich and full life. Finally, a health program is justifiable in terms of the laws of

learning. Thorndike's law of readiness simply means that the individual pupil must be ready to learn. He must be organically sound, mentally alert, and emotionally able to receive the most from the total school curriculum. A pain in the stomach, an earache, or some other such bothersome factor is a distracting stimulus. Whereas an adult can, in effect, say to a stomach ache, pain, or emotional problem, "get thee behind me," the primary grade pupil simply cannot ignore it. His ability to learn is directly impaired, and he will not respond as well as his contemporaries, either in the classroom or anywhere else.

The Educational Policies Commission of the National Education Association has stated repeatedly that an educated person understands the basic facts concerning health and disease; the educated person protects his own health and that of his dependents; and an educated person works to improve the health of his community. If these are some of the characteristics of an educated person, the school program must provide experiences that will impart knowledge about and develop proper attitudes concerning good health and safety practices and physical activity.

When 50 per cent of a balanced sample of adults fail to pass the CBS National Health Test, then one wonders about the knowledge level of schoolchildren. About one-third of the adults tested could not name even one cancer danger signal. More than a third did not know the normal body temperature. Some 60 per cent believed that venereal disease can be caused by contact with unclean toilet seats. One thing that the School Health Study did was to point up the fact that schoolchildren also display a mass ignorance. This "major weakness in the educational system," as it was called by the writers of the School Health Study, prompted them to say that the best place for health instruction is in the school—chiefly because the school is the only agency that can keep pace with the rapid advance of medical science and can give the child the scientific basis of health problems so that he can engage in intelligent health practices.[1] Moreover, the best place to begin is in the lower grades during the habit-forming years of childhood.

History of School Health Movement

The history of public health is as old as the Egyptian and Hebrew civilizations. But the history of school health is much more recent. Certainly, one of the reasons for this is that, in the centuries gone by, man had only a slight regard for the growth and development of youth. It was a man's world; women and children were strictly secondary. Although formal education was fostered in many places, health maintenance and promotion as such were not the concern of the school.

[1] School Health Education Study. *School Health Education: A Call for Action.* Washington, D.C., 1965.

The school health movement has a European heritage. In 1790 Benjamin Thompson, known as Count Rumford, started school lunches for underprivileged children in Bavaria. About this time Johann Peter Frank wrote scientific articles on the topic of school hygiene. Other eminent scientists of the day such as Rudolph Virchow (1821-1902) and Henry P. Bowditch (1840-1911) urged medical examinations of schoolchildren and studies on their growth and development. In England, in 1832, Edwin Chadwick studied child employment conditions and became interested in the schools. Theophile Roussel followed somewhat the same pattern in France. Great writers such as Victor Hugo, Charles Reade, and Charles Dickens were influential in starting a school health movement. It was Hugo, in 1865, who established school lunches for poor children on the Isle of Guernsey. They became so popular that by the early 1900's half the cities in Germany had lunch programs for schoolchildren.

In the United States interest was growing in the areas of school health. In 1842, Horace Mann, Secretary of the Massachusetts Board of Education, wrote in the *Common School Journal,* "So intimately are all parts of the human constitution connected and so vitally do the mental and moral depend upon the physical power, that we can understand either only by studying them in connection with others. For this reason, the knowledge of laws of structure, growth, development, and health of the body is essential to a comprehension of the corresponding particular in the phenomena of the mind." These words carried a great amount of weight. It is not strange, therefore, that by 1885 the American Association for Physical Education was formed. Prominent medical doctors from this group advocated scientific programs of physical activity and hygiene in the schools. By 1894 the Boston schools were ready to begin the first regular medical inspection program in America. Then followed Chicago, New York, Philadelphia, and others. Interest grew and numerous health agencies were born that in turn had a potent effect on school health efforts. Notable among these was the formation in 1912 of the Children's Bureau of the Federal Security Agency, an organization set up to investigate subjects relating to child life and welfare.[2] Shortly thereafter in 1918 the American Child Hygiene Association was formed. This organization grew to become the present American Child Health Association.

From about 1900 to 1915 a continued effort was made in the schools to give medical examinations and control communicable diseases. Public health practices improved in many communities and influenced the promotion of child health. Some schools taught hygiene courses consisting chiefly of anatomy and physiology. At first the teaching emphasis was on health knowledge as pure subject matter. It became apparent after a while, however, that the educator must appraise the quantity and quality of the health information in terms of its effect on attitudes and habits of students. As far back as 1910 men like Luther H. Gulick and R. Tait McKenzie stressed the need for appraisal in school health and hygiene.

Following World War I, school health programs accomplished a great deal. Research was developed illustrating the benefits of properly constituted programs. In 1922, C. E. Turner carried out his now famous Malden, Massachusetts, school health demonstration project. Over a two year period he compared the children of three fourth grades, three fifth grades,

and three sixth grades in two school buildings with a control group of similar grade school children in two other schools.[3] Health education was developed with the experimental group and data were collected concerning growth, health status, and health habits. The demonstration was not only successful, but because it was widely publicized it caused other promoters of school health to "take heart" and begin health instruction in the grades.

The most thorough research into the status of health education and the needs of youth was started in 1961 and brought to a head in 1965 by the School Health Education Study.[4] The findings indicated that health content is repetitious throughout the grades without consideration for the problems of youth; universally neglected content areas of interest to elementary teachers are consumer education, sex education, venereal disease, non-communicable disease, smoking, alcohol and drugs, community health programs, environmental hazards, mental health, and nutrition and weight control. Experimental curriculum materials were later tried out in pilot-study communities to test the conceptual approach to learning.

Today, school health is an integrated phase of the total school program. This has come about chiefly from a rising interest in the welfare of children, an increase in associations dedicated to raising the nation's health, White House Conferences, the monetary funds of philanthropic organizations, and the tireless efforts of pioneers such as Claire Turner, Thomas Wood, Haven Emerson, Mabel Rugen, Mabel Bragg, C. E. Winslow, Oliver Byrd, Raymond Franzen, C. C. Wilson, Sally

---

[2] Van Dalen, Deobold B., Mitchell, Elmer D., and Bennett, Bruce L. A World History of Physical Education. New York: Prentice-Hall, 1953, p. 446.

[3] Turner, Clair E. "Malden Studies in Health Education and Growth," American Journal of Public Health, 18:1217–1230, 1928.

[4] Sliepceuch, Elena M. "Health Education: a Conceptual Approach," Washington, D.C.: School Health Education Study, 1965.

Lucas Jean, Ruth Strang, and Sara Louise Smith.

Legal Foundations for School Health Programs

One of the first laws created for the protection of schoolchildren was passed in 1833 in France. It made public school authorities responsible for the health of schoolchildren. Other European laws followed in Austria, Sweden, Germany, and Russia.

Horace Mann's agitation for the science of health, then termed "physiology and hygiene," resulted in Massachusetts, in 1850, becoming the first state to require hygiene by law as a compulsory subject in all the public schools of the commonwealth. A number of other legal enactments occurred about the turn of the century. Instruction about alcohol and narcotics was required by 1890 in all states. Many states required physical education before 1900. In 1899 teachers in Connecticut were required to test the vision of their pupils. A school dentist was hired in Reading, Pennsylvania, in 1903. Many laws were made soon after this. By 1933 the Nebraska State Supreme Court had decreed that the control of the pupil's health during school hours was the responsibility of the school personnel. This is indeed a big responsibility, and the schools have accepted it in the spirit of service.

Today most states have legal foundations for their school health programs. Many of these are in the form of rules and regulations of state commissions regarding education. The laws in such states as Minnesota, Pennsylvania, and Ohio are particularly clear in setting forth the need for proper attention to health. As an example of the legal control exercised by a state, General Regulation No. 156 of the State of New York appears as follows:

1. All schools under the jurisdiction of the State Education Depart-

ment shall provide a program of health and physical education in an environment conducive to healthful living. This program shall include: . . .[5]

School Health Organization

Paramount to the success of a health program in any school system is the organization of health activities, personnel, facilities and time. With a school population continually growing, it becomes increasingly difficult to meet all the health objectives with ease. Yet, efforts in most places are regularly intensified to improve health through preventive and remedial measures.

Health education is an applied science concerned with relating research findings in health to the lives of people. It narrows the gap between what is known and what is practiced. It is what Will Durant calls "preventive medicine in the classroom." If we say that *health education is the sum of experiences that favorably influence practices, attitudes, and knowledge relating to health,* it is readily seen that we are dealing with something that occurs at all times and in all places in the school.[6] Hence, the entire school personnel and every area of the curriculum have to some degree a part in health education. The organization of these varied efforts into a sound working program is the job of the school administrator.

School health education is essentially a three-pronged process. It consists of health service, healthful school

---

[5] The University of the State of New York. *Regulations of the Commissioner of Education Governing Health and Physical Education.* The State Education Department, January 20, 1950.

[6] This definition of health education is the one agreed upon by the Joint Committee on Health Problems in Education of the National Education Association and the American Medical Association. The report, *Health Education,* 5th ed. (1961), may be obtained from the National Education Association, Washington, D.C.

environment, and health instruction. Definitions of these terms have existed for three decades:[7]

Health service "comprises all those procedures designated to determine the health status of the child, to enlist his cooperation in health protection and maintenance, to inform parents of the defects that may be present, to prevent disease, and to correct remediable defects."

Healthful school living "is a term that designates the provision of a wholesome environment, the organization of a healthful school day, and the establishment of such teacher-pupil relationships as make a safe and sanitary school, favorable to the best development of living of pupils and teachers."

Health instruction "is that organization of learning experiences directed toward the development of favorable health knowledges, attitudes, and practices."

There is a growing point of view that the term "health education" should be reserved for the teaching or instruc-

---

[7] Health Education Section, Committee Report, American Physical Education Association. *Journal of Health and Physical Education,* December 1934.

tional part of the school health program. In this manner the pupil has no difficulty attaching a suitable name to his course; he can call it health education — which indeed it is.

Responsibility of the Classroom Teacher

There is no person in the school system better fitted to make a significant contribution to the health of schoolchildren than the classroom teacher in the elementary school. She alone occupies the key position for improving child health. With her interest, enthusiasm, and understanding, the school health program moves ahead. Without her support, however, the program never really gets started.

The role of the classroom teacher is unique; no other person sees the child as she does. She can readily compare his appearance and actions today with what they were yesterday or a month ago. Or she can compare him with the other 25 children in the classroom who are about the same age. This provides the alert teacher with a vantage point that neither the parent or family physician can match. Thus, every classroom teacher holds a potentially powerful job for building sound health. The

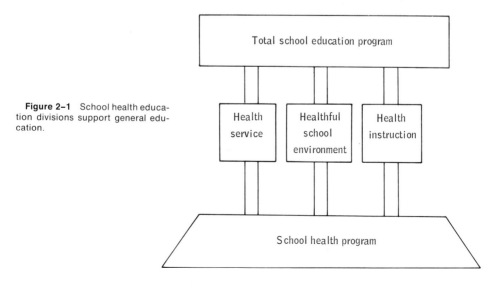

Figure 2-1 School health education divisions support general education.

extent to which she does this will depend upon many things. She will need administrative support. She will need a warm personality and feeling for children, and she will need to use her powers of observation carefully. To use the words of Frederick Mayer, the teacher should also be an optimist with an attitude of encouragement and hopefulness so that the schoolroom may be "an oasis of hope."[8]

How the Classroom Teacher Promotes Health

Specifically, the classroom teacher promotes health in a number of ways:

By Cooperating with the School Health Service Personnel. Children are properly prepared by the teacher for a visit to the school physician or nurse for periodic physical examinations. Teachers take a positive approach to the examinations by saying to their pupils, "The doctor is coming to see how many healthy boys and girls we have." Learning to visit medical personnel and come away happy is an education in itself. Any experience that is satisfying or "feels good" to the child is effective in terms of his future behavior. The nurse, the physician, and the dental hygienist should be their friends.

By Detecting Health Abnormalities and Referring Them to Proper Authorities for Appropriate Follow-Up and Correction. The teacher who uses her "eyes to see' can observe a variety of items related to the onset of poor health. The child with frequent colds and sore throats, who is continually snuffing in class, may have any one of a number of difficulties involving the upper respiratory area. Likewise, the child who squints to see or turns his head to hear simple questions may be in need of medical aid right away. Numerous children appear to be well.

---

[8] Mayer, Frederick. "Education and the Good Life," *Education*, 78(4):497, April 1957.

The child who exhibits signs of emotional upset which may be missed entirely by the parents may be spotted by the teacher as one who behaves differently from the group and needs individual attention. It should be remembered that the younger the person, the more readily he responds to pain or other distracting stimuli. The response may represent a series of incidents leading to poor scholarship. The pupil, for example, who scores well on a test of learning aptitude yet produces work in class that is hardly better than average, is the kind of pupil who bears watching.

By Making the School Environment Pleasant and Desirable for the Pupils. The school, to be at all effective, must be the kind of place a child wants to go to. The classroom is made more inviting by the teacher. She regulates such physical items as temperature, ventilation, lighting, and seating. Her own attitude toward the students has much to do with the health and happiness of the class. There are numerous children who dislike school and show this by coming down with "morning sickness," a disease of the psychosomatic variety that mysteriously disappears on Saturdays, Sundays, and holidays.

By Providing Health Instruction in the Classroom. Teaching is done both formally and informally. In this respect, the teacher seldom misses an opportunity to refer to the child's health and welfare. Health as a topic is also correlated with other materials. The teacher's task is to teach it with the aim of changing habits and attitudes. Health knowledge as such must lead to the kind of understanding that results in changed behavior.

The Teacher's Health

The effective teacher is one who possesses the vitality to do the job expected of her and has left a little reserve at the close of the day for her own enrichment activities. According to reports and opinions, personality maladjustments are responsible for failure in teaching more often than physical disorders. Even the admirable teacher who loves children, is intellectually alert and gets along well with others will be limited in her expression and enthusiasm proportionate to the degree of physical fitness and mental health.

The health status of the teacher has a significant bearing on education in at least two ways. First, and obviously, it pertains to physical, mental, and social efficiency "on the job." Secondly, and every bit as important as the first, it relates to the image the teacher presents to her pupils. The sick teacher with a sour personality can hardly practice what she preaches. Whether we care to admit it or not, teaching has long been a process of making little images of the teacher in the minds of the pupils. Very little effective health education can be expected from the image of a teacher suffering from such complaints as chronic fatigue, gross overweight, nagging headache, low back pain, irregular teeth, and a negative, complaining attitude toward life in general. Thus, in teaching young people, the importance of the example of personal health and well-being cannot be underestimated.

Responsibility of the Elementary School Administrator

Although the alert classroom teacher is worth her weight in gold in any health program, the value of a school administrator who is sympathetic to the goals of school health is highly significant.

The practice of accepting primary responsibility for school health varies in a number of states. Essentially it boils down to the question of whether the school *controls* all health educa-

tion or whether it is the responsibility of the local or county health department. In Florida, for instance, a rather successful program has been in operation for a number of years where the county health department is responsible for school health services. In fact, county school health planning committees are formed and composed of school people, interested citizens, and county health personnel. These committees, meeting with county school superintendents and county health officers, take steps to initiate desirable health programs in the schools. By and large, however, the trend throughout the country is to follow the lead of a number of the eastern states and place full responsibility for school health and health education with the school administrator and board of education.

In the larger cities the administrator may appoint a school health director. Minnesota school regulations, for example, state that "in each school system, regardless of size, the superintendent shall appoint a health director."[9]

The classroom teacher will find the elementary school principal most helpful, especially if he engages in many of the following activities:

1. Provides for health services and "sets the stage" for the work of physicians, dentists, nurses, psychologists, dental hygienists, and teachers of the handicapped.

2. Is concerned with safe and sanitary building construction, and the activities of the school custodial staff.

3. Is interested in the preparation and personal health of teaching personnel.

4. Promotes in-service education for medical personnel and classroom teachers alike.

---

[9] Minnesota Department of Health and State Department of Education. *School Health Manual*, revised 1950, p. 10.

5. Obtains adequate funds for the program.

6. Maintains lines of communication between school and community agencies.

7. Arranges for periodic nurse-teacher conferences and meetings of health councils.

8. Meets with parents to secure adequate treatment for all children.

9. Initiates a total school safety program.

10. Assists classroom teachers in securing necessary facilities, materials, and time for health instruction.

11. Provides leadership to school feeding programs.

12. Carries on studies relative to school absences — health problems and school attendance.

It is interesting to note that in one large city school system, the Los Angeles City Schools, the results of an intensive survey indicated several ways in which school administrators could help improve the existing health education effort. For one thing, in planning and coordinating the health program of the individual school, it was suggested that greater use be made of health councils. It was also felt that more use should be made of the school environment in health teaching experiences. Moreover, administrators were urged to develop teacher guides in health education at each grade level, offer more in-service health education, and do a more thorough job of planning the health instruction program.

The number of administrative activities having a bearing on the health and welfare of elementary school-children would provide material for several chapters. Briefly, and in summary, the administrator accepts the total health viewpoint and, through the medium of a pleasant principal-teacher atmosphere, fashions a health program that produces measurable results in the schoolchildren.

Contributions of Physical Education to the School Health Program

Physical education may be defined as a process of changing behavior toward certain preconceived educational goals, primarily through large muscle activity. Health is advanced by increasing the child's vigor, strength, and endurance. Through a broad and varied program of physical activities in the elementary grades, organic growth is stimulated, fundamental physical skills are developed, social efficiency is promoted, and attitudes toward recreation and leisure time are planted like seedlings in the slowly maturing bodies of young people.

Elementary physical education activities such as games of low organization, sport skills, mimetics and story plays, rhythms and dances, and self-testing stunts are full of meaning to the growing child. When properly taught, their contribution to total health, through the avenue of improved physical efficiency and social emotional behavior, is not insignificant. In fact, physical education with its primary concern for motor activity and physical fitness is more alive today than it has been for almost a century.[10]

In recent years President Eisenhower, President Kennedy and President Johnson have made personal efforts to promote a national awareness of the need for physical fitness. The President's Council on Physical Fitness, through its widely distributed publication, "Suggested Elements of a School-Centered Program," has done much to improve existing programs of physical education.[11] Significantly,

[10] See Chapter I for references to sedentary living. Witness the numerous reports relative to physical fitness of American youth in magazines such as *Saturday Evening Post, U. S. News and World Report, Sports Illustrated, Life, Time,* and *Newsweek.*

[11] President's Council on Youth Fitness. "Youth Physical Fitness: Suggested Elements of a School-Centered Program," revised. Washington: U.S. Government Printing Office, July 1967.

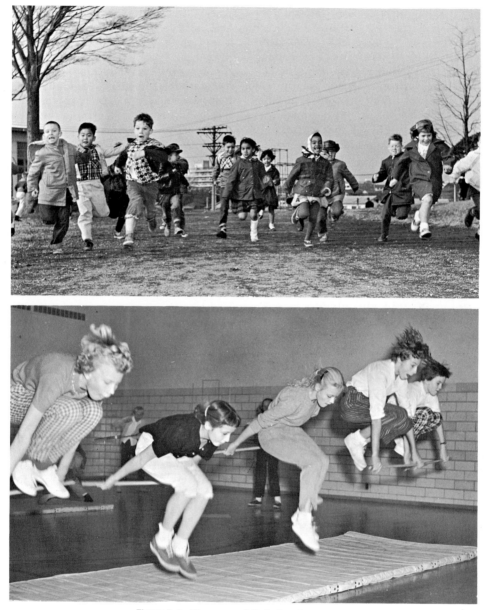

Figure 2-2 Vigorous activity in the elementary school.

where programs have been initiated or improved, levels of individual pupil fitness have risen, resulting in an increase in personal vigor and stamina for the many activities of the school day. Moreover, it is not uncommon to find a corresponding rise in levels of achievement and social accomplishment.

Physical activities, by their very nature, are health teaching activities. They are as much a part of the school health program as food tasting parties or health services. They need to be taught with purpose and understanding. Merely turning children loose on a playground twice a day, day after day, to "blow off steam" is not physical education. In fact, it represents an example of a situation where a unique opportunity is being missed. True, the children will find some relief from the academic activities of the classroom, but they will be denied the chance to learn the skills and develop the attitudes that are so much a part of a good physical education program. This is not to be treated as a haphazard activity, for physical education is not just aimless movement; it is part of the education process. Moreover, physical condition is being increasingly equated with mental efficiency and intellectual productivity rather than with brawn and sports alone.

Elementary teachers who feel somewhat unprepared in the physical education area, who lack the skill and knowledge to carry on even a partial program of purposeful activity, should do one or two of the following things:

1. Visit a class where a good program of suitable activities is being taught and observe how it is done. In most communities there are at least one or two especially successful teachers in this area.

2. Visit the school or community library and search the existing books for appropriate games, dances, and self-testing stunts.

3. Write the nearest elementary teacher preparation institution for program help.

4. Contact the state educational department supervisor of elementary

physical education. Either he will pay a visit, arrange for the teacher to visit a school, or will send written suggestions.

Classroom teachers may feel, therefore, that physical education and health education are cooperative in nature. Both subjects are planned with the purpose of contributing as much as possible to the growth and development of children; total fitness items relating to nutrition, emotional climate, and poor eyesight are the concern of each. In many school classroom teachers work closely with physical educators not only in the improvement of motor skills, but also on individual pupil posture, muscular strength, and remedial exercises.

Present Trends Versus Past Practices in School Health

As education has grown more scientific over the decades, medical and educational workers associated with school health have concerned themselves with the scientific aspects of health status, health knowledge, and health behavior. For example, at one time the teaching emphasis was on health knowledge as pure subject matter. It became apparent after a while, however, that the educator must appraise both the quantity and the quality of the health information in terms of its effect on attitudes and habits of students. This is reflected in the current trends and practices especially when compared with the practices of several decades ago. Some noteworthy examples follow.

Present Trends

1. Physical examinations of schoolchildren are given in less haste and are more thorough. Better use is made of the physician's time.

2. Screening examinations for hearing and vision losses, together with weighing

Past Practices

1. Physical examinations of schoolchildren were incomplete. As many as 60 to 80 children were examined per hour. Improper organization for health appraisal was common.

2. Screening examinations for hearing and vision were carried on haphazardly

Present Trends (continued)

and measuring of pupils, are popular appraisal activities carried on with objective measures.

3. Classroom teachers cooperate with school nurses, dental hygienists, and other medical personnel in an effort to determine the health status of the child. Many teachers have special training to improve their observation of health abnormalities.

4. Schools have effective health service departments designed to evaluate the *total* school health effort.

5. Health councils operate in a democratic way to determine health status and analyze health behavior. Case studies are frequently run on individual children.

6. Provision has been made for facilities for health rooms, nursing service, rest rooms for teachers and pupils and replacement of old-type drinking fountains.

7. The objective is to evaluate the child as accurately as possible and then see that something is done about his needs.

8. Health teaching is done from the viewpoint of a child's needs and interests, and factual information is used to bring about maximum understanding.

9. Tests of health knowledge are improved and there is increased use of tests designed to measure health attitudes and health practices.

10. Health facts are becoming far more prevalent than unfounded opinions.

11. Health education is moving toward a developmental rather than a remedial program.

12. Health education is carried on by concerted action of home, school, and public and private agencies.

13. There is increasing recognition that the emotional health of the teacher influences the emotional tone of the classroom.

As one looks to the future, it becomes quite clear that the impact of such entities as the School Health Education Study and the Joint Committee on Health Problems in Education of the National Education Association and the American Medical Association is such that it will only be a few years before all states implement legislation requiring direct health instruction for all children. There will be a properly *bal-*

Past Practices (continued)

with a good deal of subjective measurement.

3. Schools did not use medical personnel to any great extent. Teachers were not prepared to appraise health status and detect abnormalities but did their best by themselves.

4. Schools used physicians only in a limited way. They were concerned only with giving physical examinations.

5. Health committees or health councils were unheard of.

6. Few rest rooms were provided large enough to relax in. Drinking fountains were often unsanitary and hazardous in terms of mouth hygiene.

7. Examinations that were conducted often revealed defects and abnormalities which were not followed up and corrected.

8. Health facts were given in a formal way and were essentially pure anatomy and physiology.

9. Tests of health knowledge were made to measure health information only.

10. Health opinions and superstitions were more prevalent than health facts.

11. Health education was concerned chiefly with helping those who were ill or deformed.

12. Health education was engaged in by uncoordinated groups and agencies. Often one did not know what the other was doing.

13. The health of the teacher was incidental to learning.

anced curriculum with adequate scope and sequence which does justice to all major health problems rather than singling out any one popular problem for overemphasis. The need will be met for greater numbers of school health coordinators or curriculum specialists to work with classroom teachers and for a continuing in-service program to keep teachers up-to-date with rapidly changing health concepts, and to encourage creative teaching. It is encouraging to note that national health agencies are working together through the National Health Council to strengthen and revitalize school health education. Indeed, health teaching is moving at an accelerated speed from a "do-gooder" activity to a carefully organized and programmed part of the total school curriculum.

Cooperative Planning in School Health Education

The modern school holds fast to certain fundamental principles and knowledge, yet it is flexible and prepared for change. These changes are brought about not by teachers and administrators alone, but by cooperative action among both school *and* community personnel. Every classroom instructor, physician, and community health worker is a health teacher. Said

Alfred North Whitehead: "You may not divide the seamless coat of learning."

The continued need for cooperative action in health education has been stressed by many professional conferences and individuals. Although control of the school health program necessarily rests in the schools, recognition is given to the fact that the school health program is a part of the total program of community health, thus necessitating a close working relationship between the school and community health authorities.

The classroom teacher simply cannot do the job of teaching health alone. Already in some communities she is a health technician, a home visitor, an informal case-finder, a safety expert, and a mental health specialist. In view of these expectations, the teacher needs real assistance from outside the school.

Questions for Discussion

1. In your opinion, how much preparation in the health teaching area should the elementary classroom teacher have? Back up your comments with at least one reference.

2. What is the relationship between physical activity and health instruction in the promotion of health?

3. Try to confer with your local health officer and solicit his opinion on his relationship with the school health personnel.

4. What are three or four of the advantages of county health department control over school health? How do these compare with the advantages of a system where the school administrator controls the program?

5. Discuss the role of the teacher's health in relation to teacher employment and retention practices. Should a teacher object to a physical or mental examination?

Suggested Activities

1. Secure a copy of the National Health Test given over the CBS network in 1966. (See Instructor's Manual for *The Foundations of Health* by C. Bucher, E. Olsen, and C. E. Willgoose, published by Appleton-Century-Crofts, Inc., 1967.) Take the test and see how you compare with the national findings.

2. Look over the nine *Imperatives in Education* set up after a two-year study by the American Association of School Administrators (AASA, Washington: NEA, 1201 16th Street, N. W., 1966). Which of these appear to be implemented the most by improved programs of health instruction in the schools?

3. Find out the health education requirements for your state. Is health instruction required in the elementary or middle schools? If so, how much time has been legislated? If not, is any move being made to bring about a change in state requirements?

Selected References

American Association of School Administrators. *Imperatives in Education.* Washington, D.C., 1966.

Anderson, C. L. *School Health Practice,* 4th ed. St. Louis: C. V. Mosby Co., 1968, Chapter 6.

Conner, Forest E. "Focus on Health." *Journal of School Health,* 37:1–7, January 1967.

Dwork, Ralph E. "Social Innovations and Health Education." *Journal of Health, Physical Education and Recreation,* 38:19–21, April 1967.

Grout, Ruth E. *Health Teaching in Schools,* 5th ed. Philadelphia: W. B. Saunders Co., 1968, Chapters 1 and 2.

Haag, Jesse H. *School Health Program,* 2nd ed., New York: Henry Holt & Co., 1964, Part VIII.

Hoyman, Howard S. "Bottlenecks in Health Education." *American Journal of Public Health,* 56:957–962, June 1966.

Ingraham, Hollis S. "Something Else That Johnny Doesn't Know." *Journal of School Health,* 36:331–336, September 1966.

Irwin, Leslie, Staton, Wesley, and Cornacchia, Harold. *Health in Elementary Schools,* 2nd ed. St. Louis: C. V. Mosby Co., 1966, Chapter 1.

Means, Richard K. *A History of Health Education in the United States.* Philadelphia: Lea and Febiger, 1962.

NEA-AMA. *Health Education.* Washington: National Education Association, 1961, Chapter 12.

Neilson, Elizabeth. "The Team Approach to New Frontiers in Health Education." *Journal of Health, Physical Education and Recreation,* 33:28, March 1962.

Oberteuffer, Delbert, and Beyrer, Mary K. *School Health Education,* 4th ed. New York: Harper & Brothers, 1966, Chapter 2.

Willgoose, Carl E. "Health Education and the Classroom Teacher." *Education,* 78:451–455, April 1958.

Willgoose, Carl E. "Don't Just Turn Them Loose." *NEA Journal,* 49:13–14, April 1960.

Function
and Scope of
School Health Services

CHAPTER 3

Thousands are hacking at the branches of
evil to every one who is striking at the roots.

—THOREAU

Where are the roots to the health problems of children? What are the chief impediments to their happiness? To a great extent the over-all task of school health services is to answer these questions so successfully that the student will realize his fullest expectations in school.

No attempt will be made in this chapter to go into all the details of school health services. But it would be remiss of the author if he failed to give the elementary school teacher an opportunity to understand the function and some of the activities of this operation.

School health services are well defined procedures which are established:

1. To appraise the health status of pupils and school personnel.

2. To counsel pupils, parents and others concerning appraisal findings.

3. To encourage the correction of remediable defects.

4. To assist in the identification and education of handicapped children.

5. To help prevent and control disease.

6. To provide emergency service for injury or sudden sickness.

It may be seen from these precise definitions that school health services embrace a considerable amount of school activity. This is to be expected, for the services are educationally sound and defensible. Not only do they contribute to the realization of educational aims, but they help minimize the hazards of attending school and make it possible to adapt school programs to individual capacities and needs. Also — and this is sometimes unrecognized by many teachers and parents — there are potential educational values inherent in health service activities. Through these activities children become informed of their health assets and liabilities, and develop lasting attitudes toward physicians, dentists, nurses, and other health personnel. They also stand to gain two especially important understandings which may have a bearing on future behavior:

1. The need to establish a lifelong practice of having one's health status evaluated at regular intervals.

2. An appreciation of the value of professional services, methods, and techniques.

Health Appraisal

As in all evaluation processes, the more scientific the appraisal, the sooner the purposes of the program may be reached. Total health status of a child may be appraised in a number of ways. Health histories, teacher and nurse observations, screening tests, medical and dental examinations, and psychological examinations represent the more common appraisal activities. These appraisals serve the medical personnel, the classroom teachers, and the pupils. They help the teachers understand their pupils, and they help the pupils appreciate the findings in relation to themselves. The results of appraisals are also valuable to groups and individuals concerned with health counseling.

Most health appraisal programs are required by law. They function to meet the total health needs of the pupils at the local level and change little over the years. This is evidenced by the aims of the American Association of School Administrators which are nearly two decades old:[1]

1. To identify pupils in need of medical or dental treatment.

2. To identify pupils who have problems relating to nutrition.

3. To identify pupils who are poorly adjusted and in need of special attention at school or treatment by a psychiatrist or a child guidance clinician.

4. To measure the growth of pupils and to assist them in attaining optimal growth.

5. To identify pupils with defects who may require modified programs of education, as, for example, the crippled, partially sighted, hard-of-hearing, mentally retarded, and those with speech defects.

6. To identify pupils who need a more thorough examination than is usually provided at school, for example, x-ray examination, examination by a specialist, or laboratory examinations.

7. To identify pupils who may best be educated apart from the regular school situation, for example, the blind, deaf, and tuberculous.

Some of the more important appraisal activities will be reviewed:

Health Histories. These are of particular concern to both medical personnel and classroom teachers. Just as history usually helps one to understand the present better, so the past diseases and defects of a pupil help everyone to understand his present status. Good teachers generally ask, "What makes Johnny tick?" It helps to know, therefore, what Johnny has had in the way of communicable diseases, immunizations, major operations, or injuries. In some schools today, classroom teachers help maintain health history records by anecdotally noting pupil health behavior items. (See Figure 3–1.)

This kind of record is especially valuable when kept up-to-date and referred to when children behave strangely or appear to be in need of special counseling. It is a functional instrument for the exchange of information concerning the pupil's health between the classroom teacher, the school nurse, and the school physician.

---

[1] American Association of School Administrators. *Health in Schools.* Washington: National Education Association, revised 1951.

		ENTRIES by TEACHER, NURSE and PHYSICIAN				
		CODE—Worker Column: T—Teacher: N—Nurse: Dr.—Physician: T.N.C.—Teacher-Nurse Conference (If no symptoms noted, entry after T.N.C. should be: N.S.N.)				
Date	Worker	Entries With Worker's Signature	Date	Worker	Entries With Worker's Signature	

Figure 3–1   A section of the Cumulative Health Record used by the Department of Health, Board of Education, City of New York.

In California, for example, a particularly useful Health Insert is used with the California Cumulative Record system. It is an integral part of the individual's cumulative record and provides specific information concerning needed adjustments in the school program. It is transferred from school to school and was designed so that a minimum amount of time need be spent in keeping it up-to-date. The health insert is divided into seven categories as follows:

1. Signs observed by teacher
2. Medical history
3. Immunization and test record
4. Growth record and screening data
5. Dental examinations
6. Medical examinations
7. Medical recommendations for needed adjustments in school program

Routine Medical Examinations. The chief purposes of these examinations are to determine health status and solve any problems that arise. Their value is recognized in most states by a law requiring periodic examinations of every child in school. When this is not conducted by the family physician, it must be done by the school physician. The compulsory annual medical examination of all

schoolchildren, however, has not always been effective. For one thing, the schools have ended up performing the "lion's share" of the examinations, thus missing the obvious advantage of having the family physician examine the child. Another factor is that school health service facilities and personnel are over-taxed when annual examinations are compulsory. This, coupled with the shortage of school physicians, suggests a more realistic approach to giving medical examinations.

The routine medical examination should be a thorough one. To be worth the energy put forth, it must allow the physician time enough to see the whole child: his behavior characteristics, nervous reflexes, speech defects, nutritional status, and temperament, as well as the more typical items. For almost two decades the American Public Health Association has had standards calling for a maximum of 12 examinations per hour—at least five minutes per child. This was brought about by findings that showed as many as 70 children being examined per hour. The idea of "processing" a set number of examinations in a certain amount of time cannot be defended. Examinations, to be worth the time and effort involved, need to be complete from head to toe. Thus, a limited number of students should be handled in one year. Thorough examinations every two or three years are becoming more common, with reexaminations of students possessing definite health problems being given wherever necessary.

The American Medical Association, in conjunction with the National Education Association, has suggested a minimum of four medical examinations: one upon entrance to first grade, one in the elementary intermediate school grades, one at the start of adolescence, and one before leaving school. In some places this has not been entirely successful. There is general agreement, however, that all pupils entering school for the first time should have a complete medical examination. Moreover, this should be done early enough to permit an adequate follow-up on recommendations. June has been found to be the most satisfactory month for children who plan to enter school in September.

As previously indicated, there is a definite advantage in having the family physician perform the examination. He knows the family and background of the child. His examination facilities are usually excellent, and he has quick access to laboratory facilities. Moreover a favorable physician-parent-child relationship generally exists. There are a number of communities in the United States that have no school physician for examinations. Everything is effectively handled by local physicians who cooperate fully with the school nurse. In such cases the family physician is completely informed of what the school desires so that there is uniformity in examinations and reporting. Standard examination forms are used. Also, the family physician is advised to use every opportunity to give effective health instruction just as a school physician would do. (See Figures 3–2 and 3–3.) This kind of program has been working well in Connecticut where in a recent year over 25 per cent of schoolchildren were examined by personal physicians. There still remains one big disadvantage in using family physicians; there are always some parents who will not take their child to him, or they employ delaying tactics while the child's health is in question.

A factor that has a bearing on examinations is that private physicians are so busy they frequently do not prefer the paper work involved. For example, the Health Services Branch of the Los Angeles City Schools has tried several times, with parental cooperation, to get private physicians to do pre-school and other physical examinations and send their reports to the

---

HS-3   Department of Health, Physical Education and Recreation
Roslyn Public Schools, Roslyn, New York

Dear Parents: Health Services

We recommend that your child be examined by your doctor before school starts

so that necessary booster injections can be given and any condition requiring attention

can be taken care of before school opens.

Please mail to the school nurse the Annual Medical Examination Form after it

is completed by your doctor, or send it to school with the child on the first day of school.

Figure 3–2 Form suggesting examination by family physician.

```
S-15

   DEPARTMENT OF HEALTH, PHYSICAL EDUCATION & RECREATION
                    Roslyn Public Schools
                      Roslyn, N.Y.
                                              _____
                                                  Date

           NOTICE TO PARENTS - HEALTH CERTIFICATES

Dear Parents:

     Since _____ has not had an annual health examination
by your own personal physician, he/she will be inspected by Dr._____
our school doctor, on_____ .

     Please sign and return this slip to the Health Office.


                                       _____
                                           School Nurse


_____
  Parent's Signature
                                 _____
                                      School Principal
```

Figure 3-3 Form used when family physician has not conducted health examination.

schools. In the end, the school physicians have had to carry the entire assignment of performing physical examinations.[2] In fact, examining pupils has become the school physician's primary duty.

Another very significant item related to physical examinations of schoolchildren is the growth of specialization in medical practice. The general practitioner is disappearing. The family doctor — the man who treated all members of a family, provided continuity of care, and showed concern with the general health of the entire family — is on the way out. In a recent year not a single graduate from three large medical schools in one city went into general practice. They became specialists. It seems likely, therefore, that in the years ahead the health care of the citizen will be a mass cooperative effort in which community physicians

and their several assistants will work together in regional medical centers. In the future such centers will service the schools.

It is a good idea to have the parent or parents on hand during the medical examination to consult with the school physician. This is particularly true in the case of primary schoolchildren. Often during these formative years, when growth processes are fairly rapid, it is imperative that the physician and parent see eye-to-eye in their efforts to remedy the situation. The speed with which discovered defects are remedied has an important bearing on health and happiness in the years ahead. Teeth, for example, do much better when repaired at an early date.

The emphasis in school health practice today is to give the physician time to interpret his findings to teachers and parents and to make workable suggestions in the health matters on hand. This kind of effort sets the stage for teamwork between teachers, parents, nurses, and physicians. *It represents*

[2] Moore, Gilbert S. "The Superintendent Views the Urban Society in Relationship to the School and its Needs," *Journal of School Health,* 37:209–215, May 1967.

one of the finest examples of educational activity within the school system.

Special Medical Examinations. Where the school employs the regular medical examination every two or three years, there will be numerous occasions between examinations when it will be necessary to examine individual youngsters. Children returning to school after an absence due to illness may need a special examination, as will those new to the school system. Those pupils in need of special education may need to be examined from time to time. Since physical education and recreation activities must be adapted to the health condition of pupils, it will be necessary to examine boys and girls who wish to compete on an elementary school team. Also, there will be times in the follow-up and remedial aspects of the program when the physician wants to reexamine a certain pupil. Special examinations have value in that they permit a more careful analysis and diagnosis of the particular child.

Screening Tests. These are measures employed by teachers and health services personnel alike to "screen out" or select those schoolchildren who appear to be in need of further attention. The most effective screening tests over the years have been tests for vision, hearing, tuberculosis, and the appraisal of physical growth by the weighing and measuring of boys and girls. In recent years a number of school systems have attempted to screen children for dental defects, physical fitness, and mental health status. Most of these screening tests can be cooperatively engaged in by teachers and nurses. A broader treatment of how the elementary school classroom teacher can screen children for specific weaknesses appears in Chapter 5.

SCREENING FOR VISION. As a rule, screening tests are not diagnostic tests. They might well be called processes by which school personnel separate those pupils who are most likely to need further examination from those who are less likely to need further examination. Therefore, in vision testing the teacher is not an expert. She is simply a careful observer who helps during the screening period. (Figure 3–4). She knows that first and second graders tend to be farsighted and that nearsightedness in boys and girls develops at about the fourth grade level.

When a pupil is old enough to cooperate in a testing situation, he is ready to be measured. Thus, even a three-year-old child can respond to the symbols on a Snellen E Chart. Proper advance preparation helps improve the response.

The *Snellen Test,* used for a long time in the public schools to test visual acuity, is quite satisfactory as a crude screening instrument when more valid measures are not available.[3] It is useful for noting near-to-far-vision. It will tell the classroom teacher whether or not a certain pupil can see the blackboard or wall chart from either the front or back row of seats. The large Snellen Test chart requires reading test objects (letters, numbers, or symbols) on a chart from a 20-foot distance. The E chart is available for children and illiterates, and the mixed-letter chart is for adults and children above the third-grade level. The largest letters should be read by the normal eye at 200 feet. Because testing is done at 20 feet, this line of large print is designated the 20/200 line. The normal eye should read the 20/20 line at 20 feet; deviation less than normal is recorded 20/200, 20/100, 20/70, 20/60, 20/40, 20/30, and any deviation better than normal is recorded as 20/15 or 20/10. In all probability children below the third grade who cannot read

_____

[3] The necessary testing equipment and detailed instructions can be obtained from the National Society for the Prevention of Blindness, 1790 Broadway, New York, New York.

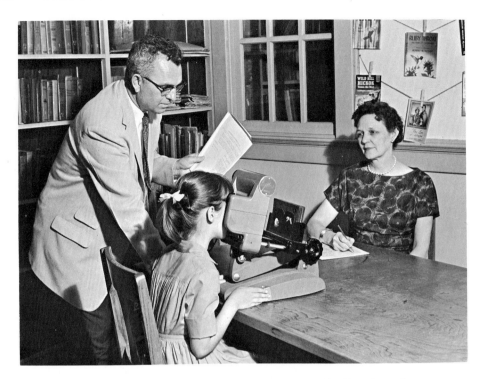

Figure 3-4   Teachers assist with the visual examination (Telebinocular test).

the 20/40 line with each eye should be referred for examination by a specialist.

Although the Snellen Test can be given by a person without medical or nursing training, proper attention must be given to the testing procedure and equipment. Some of the more important items to keep in mind to ensure valid results are the following:

Hang the chart so that the 20-foot line of letters is at the level of the child's eyes.

The heels of the child should touch the line marked on the floor 20 feet away.

Children should be at ease and encouraged to do their best.

Both eyes should be open during the test, the eye not being tested covered with a small card or folded paper resting obliquely across the nose.

Test the child who wears glasses first with them and then without them.

Test the right eye first, then the left, and then both eyes together.

Begin with the 30-foot line and follow with the 20-foot line. If the child fails the 30-foot line, start with the 20-foot line.

Move promptly and rhythmically from one symbol to another at a speed with which the child can keep pace.

Consider a line read satisfactorily if three out of four symbols are read correctly.

Record results immediately in fraction form.

Look for eyestrain, such signs as excessive blinking, frowning, scowling, tilting of the head, and watering of the eyes.

Correlate Snellen Test results with classroom observations.

Needless to say there are several more complicated tests of vision that are recommended when a more complete screening examination is de-

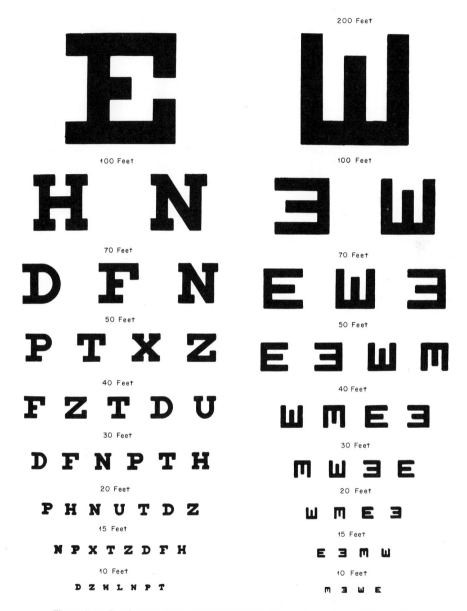

Figure 3–5 The Snellen Charts (National Society for the Prevention of Blindness).

sired. These include the Keystone View Company Telebinocular, the Massachusetts Vision Test, the Atlantic City Vision Test, the Titmus School Vision Tester, and the Ortho-Rater.

In recent years considerable attention has been focused on *pre-school vision screening* and the importance of visual readiness for learning. Studies show that large numbers of chilren require professional eye care. In New York City, for example, pre-school screening examinations discovered that seven per cent of the children had visual defects at 20/50 or worse in one eye. In a study carried on in Minneapolis, Minnesota with a sample of 633 first grade pupils from eight public elementary schools, it was found that over 16 per cent of the pupils required professional eye care.[4] In most communities, therefore, it is advisable to begin the vision screening in nursery schools where the young children are already congregated.

SCREENING FOR HEARING. Early and repeated hearing tests are important. Accurate screening is necessary, especially when one considers that an average of two children in every classroom have a hearing problem, that many cases of incorrect speech supposedly due to poor mentality are actually caused by poor hearing, and that there are needless grade repetitions among hard-of-hearing children.

Although whisper tests have been used for years, group audiometers are far more reliable. Six or ten children can be handled very nicely in a pure-tone-audiometer test. Here, each subject has a set of earphones. Sound intensity is regulated by a knob up to maximum intensity. Different pitches in tone are given (frequency range) by turning another knob. One hundred

pupils a day can be tested easily, and it can be used with children of all ages. In Figure 3–6 the raised hands of the children indicate that all of them have been able to hear the first tone produced by the audiometer. Some of the children may not be fortunate enough to hear succeeding tones as the tester lowers the volume on the audiometer. Hearing tests for small children are especially important, because of the fact that early discovery of hearing loss and follow-up can frequently prevent permanent loss of hearing.

SCREENING FOR PHYSICAL GROWTH. There is a close relationship between pupil health status, personal growth characteristics, and academic achievement. Learning, in its many forms, depends upon sound health. Very often a simple sign of retardation in growth, discovered by nurses or teachers, is significant. Yet the growth period of boys and girls cannot be neatly divided and subdivided into set periods. There is too much individual variation in pupil size, shape, and form due to such factors as heredity, constitutional endowment (body build), and physiological maturation.

A number of screening devices to evaluate over-all physical growth have been developed for school use. These involve age-height-weight measures and are usually handled through the health service department. Frequently teachers weigh and measure their own pupils. The children remove hats, coats, jackets, sweaters, and shoes. Weight is recorded in pounds and half pounds. Height is recorded in inches and quarter inches.

Interestingly enough, the child who fails to gain in height and weight in a four-month period frequently has some degree of ill health. This may be due to a physical defect, an organic strain, a prolonged emotional problem, or perhaps a number of unhygienic health habits. Turner points

[4] Rosen, Carl L. "A Modified Clinic Technique in a Visual Survey of a First Grade Population," *Journal of School Health*, 36:448–450, November 1966.

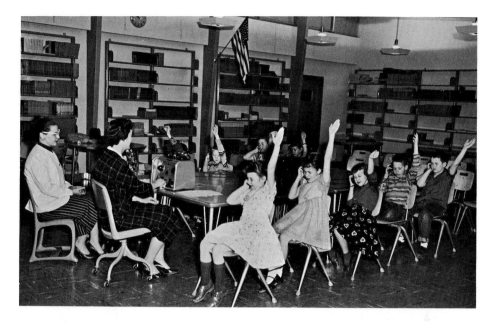

Figure 3–6   A group test using the pure tone audiometer. (Courtesy Oregon State Board of Health.)

out that height and weight should be screened every month because practically all elementary schoolchildren (98.4 per cent of 4200 observed) fail to show a gain on at least one monthly weighing during the school year.[5]

An easy-to-read and use graph for teachers is the *Meredith Physical Growth Record.* There is a record for each sex, divided into zones (Figures 3–7 and 3–8). For height there are five zones: tall, moderately tall, average, moderately short, and short. For weight the zones are heavy, moderately heavy, average, moderately light, and light. The graphs cover ages four to 18.

The child's measurements are plotted on the graph for any one period. Successive measurements permit the observer to note whenever the points do not fall in *like zones* (that is, tall and heavy, short and light). In such instances the pupil is referred to the

[5] Turner, Clair E., Sellery, C. Morely, and Smith, Sarah L. School Health and Health Education, 5th ed. St. Louis: C. V. Mosby Co., 1966, p. 54.

physician for examination. It may be that the child is perfectly healthy but of a particular body build. On the other hand, he may have some infection, need an improved diet, or require changes in daily living habits.

Health Maintenance and Control

Certainly one of the big tasks of school services has to do with the prevention of illness. This is accomplished through a program of control of personal and environmental factors. Such factors as communicable disease, emergency care and first aid, accident prevention, and school sanitation are major items.

Communicable disease control involves both the school and the community. The school health services department is generally aware of the sickness rates in the area and is prepared to control disease in the school population through widespread use of vaccination, immunization, prophylactic therapy, and isolation of ill

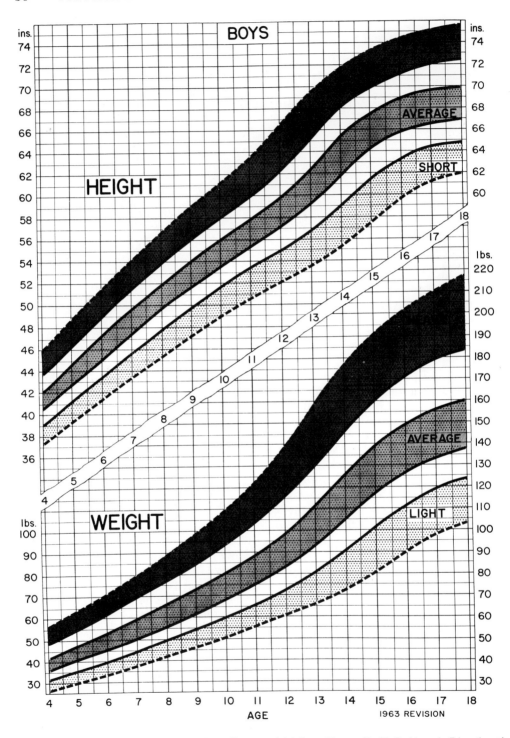

Figure 3-7 Physical growth record for boys. (Courtesy Joint Committee on Health Problems in Education of the NEA and AMA.)

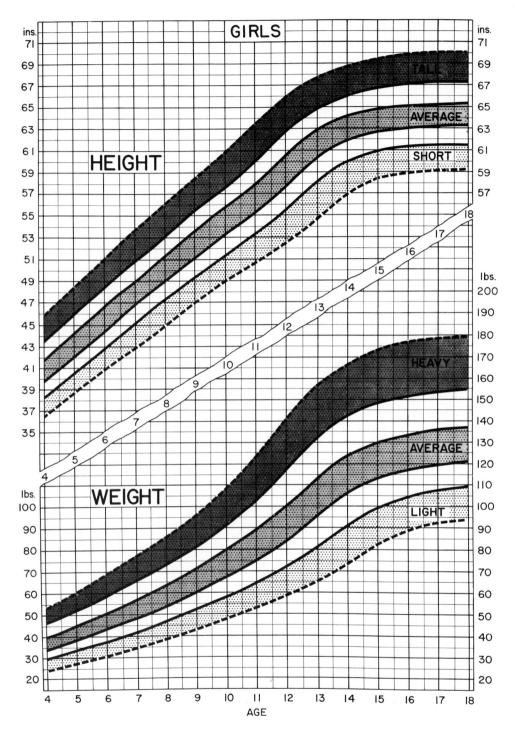

Figure 3-8 Physical growth record for girls. (Courtesy Joint Committee on Health Problems in Education of the NEA and AMA.)

SCHOOL HEALTH SERVICE

Syracuse, N. Y.

NOTICE TO PARENT OR GUARDIAN

....19.........

A recent physical examination of your child

....

attending...School

indicates an abnormal condition of the

....

....

....

It is urged that this condition be given immediate attention. If, for any reason, you are unable to do this, please
consult the nurse or teacher who may be able to assist you.

TAKE THIS CARD WITH YOU

....
School Physician

WILLIAM E. AYLING, M.D.
Health Director

DEPARTMENT OF HEALTH

- -

(Tear off and return this part to School)

Name ....

Grade.. Has been taken to

Dr. ....

for ....

Date..................19...... ....

K-132 20M 1-48 Parent or Guardian

Figure 3–9 Form used to notify parents in Syracuse Public Schools, Syracuse, N.Y. (Used by permission.)

pupils. While children are in school, they must be protected from other children who may be ill. The gathering of pupils in the classroom may set the stage for the transmission of disease. Here, the classroom teacher can be most helpful by observing carefully and reporting quickly those pupils who appear to be ill. (For details see Chapter 5.)

Because of its place in the community, the school is in a position to prevent disease. Measles epidemics, for example, can be wiped out completely in the United States if parents have their kindergarten, first, and second grade children vaccinated. About four million cases of measles a year occurred before measles vaccine became widely available in 1964. Over 500 children a year died, and hundreds were left with lasting handicaps including hearing disorders and mental retardation. Since young children can spread epidemics rapidly, the school health service personnel must always be alert. Following the introduction of measles into a classroom, all unprotected children are usually infected. Because of this the U.S. Public Health Service made a concerted effort in late 1967 to vaccinate 25 million children and rid the country of this communicable disease.

Emergency care procedures for children who become ill or injured while attending school are also the responsibility of school personnel. The school administrator and his staff must always act *in loco parentis*, i.e. in place of the parents; not just any parents, but the wisest and most enlightened type of parents. This can be a sizable job because the figures collected by the National Safety Council indicate that some 60 per cent of the accidents to children of school age occur on the school grounds, in the buildings, or going to and from school. It becomes necessary, therefore, for the health services personnel to cooperate with the teacher and school principal in the event of an emergency.

Children who appear to be ill should be segregated right away. Sometimes an emergency rest room is used. At other times it may be necessary to transport the child to his home. In either case the school physician or nurse should make the decision as to how the sick child will be handled. In the absence of either of these people, the principal and teacher will have to use their best judgment. When the child is sent home, the parents should be contacted so that appropriate action may be taken with the family physician. And when he returns to school after an illness, he should report directly to the health service office for clearance to the classroom. Most local school boards have established a definite policy of readmissions.

The question of *first aid* in an emergency is something that requires careful planning by all school personnel. Ideally, only medical personnel should render emergency care. There will be times, however, when only the classroom teacher is available.[6] What should she do? How far should she go in giving temporary treatment at the site of the emergency? Each teacher should have some knowledge of first aid procedures. She may be able to relieve suffering and prevent shock, or prevent a disability, or even save a life. It is effective school health practice, therefore, to have the school physician discuss this topic at the start of each school year in order that all school personnel will be prepared for the emergency when it occurs.

No attempt will be made here to go into the many details relative to the various conditions of illness, injury, and suffering which may require first aid attention. Familiarization with the standard first aid course material of the American Red Cross would be most beneficial. However, there are several points that classroom teachers should keep in mind relative to helping during an emergency:

1. It is important to note whether the child is having trouble breathing, or is bleeding profusely.

2. Note also whether the child is in a state of shock. Here the skin is damp and cold, and may be ashen or pale in color. Breathing may be shallow; the pulse rapid and weak, and there may be a vacant, glassy stare in the eyes. The child should be made comfortable, wrapped in a blanket with his head lower than his feet. No liquids or stimulants should be given by the teacher.

3. If the face is flushed, lay the child down on his back with the head raised; if he vomits turn his head to the side.

---

[6] Practically every major group of educators has recommended that teachers have training in first aid. This includes the American Association of School Administrators, Elementary School Principals, National Education Association, American Public Health Association, and American Association for Health, Physical Education, and Recreation.

4. Do not move the child who has had an accident until medical assistance arrives.

5. Always comfort and reassure a child. It is encouraging to know that he will be all right.

6. Do not give food or liquid to ill children. It may cause nausea, vomiting, or strangulation.

7. First aid is always rendered to reduce suffering and discomfort. Remaining with the child until assistance arrives, or until he is with his parents, may frequently be quite essential to his welfare.

Every elementary school should have a well stocked and strategically located first aid cabinet. This should be in the office of the nurse, or if necessary in the office of the principal. The accompanying list of supplies would be considered essential for first aid practice. No antiseptics or medicines are included.[7]

---

[7] Adapted from a list developed by C. L. Anderson in *School Health Practice*, 3rd ed. St. Louis: C. V. Mosby Co., 1964, p. 239.

Accident prevention is another health control item that requires some organization. It is closely related to the content of the elementary school curriculum, and it is one that teachers can discuss at length in the classroom. It is also related to the administrator for he sees that steps are taken to prevent accidents, engages in research projects to determine the causes of accidents, and prepares plans to use in case of fires, hurricanes, and other disasters.

School sanitation is a responsibility in health maintenance and control that rests primarily with the school physician. He cooperates with the local board of health to see that such school items as water supplies, dishwashing facilities, food service areas, and locker and shower rooms are safe and pleasant to use. Occasionally an unsanitary drinking fountain — something that all primary school children seem to like to put their mouths over — will spread a definite disease. The design and installation of fountains,

---

First Aid Cabinet Supplies

Items	Use
Absorbent cotton roll	For large pads or dressings
Adhesive tape, roll (widths ½″ to 2″)	To fasten splints and dressings
Aromatic spirits of ammonia	Stimulant
Blades, wood (500)	For depressors and small splints
Eye droppers (6)	To apply oil
Forceps (3″ tweezer type)	For grasping small objects
Glass jars (2)	To hold wood blades
Hot water bottle and cover	Pain relief
Ice bags (2)	Relief of swelling
Mineral oil or petroleum jelly	Relief of irritation
Paper cups (100)	As containers
Roller bandage, 1″ (12 rolls)	For dressings
Roller badange, 2″ (12 rolls)	For dressings
Roller bandage, 4″ (12 rolls)	For dressings
Safety pins (24)	For triangular bandage
Scissors (blunt)	To cut dressings
Splints (10)	For support
Sterile gauze, 3″ x 3″ squares (100)	To protect injuries
Sterile gauze, 2″ x 2″ squares (100)	To protect injuries
Tincture of green soap	For washing injuries
Toothpicks (500)	To remove particles
Tourniquet (3 ft. ¼″ rubber tube)	To control excessive bleeding
Triangle bandage (4)	For sling
Wooden applicators (1000)	For swabbing and removing particles

therefore, is of interest to teachers as well as sanitation experts.

School Absences

In a number of school systems 15 per cent of all pupils are absent daily. Illness is the major cause. It is also the greatest factor in non-promotion because of the high correlation between illness and poor scholastic achievement.

Respiratory difficulties are by far the largest single group of acute conditions reported nationally. Independent studies in New York and California indicate that close to 50 per cent of all absences are due to respiratory disease, with the common cold leading the list. Accidents also contribute to school absenteeism—about 2,200,000 school days are lost annually due to accidents.

Good patterns of attendance are cooperatively developed between school, parents, community physicians, and welfare agencies. Both parents and teachers should realize that stressing "perfect attendance" is frequently detrimental to proper school health practice. According to Dr. Carl S. Shultz, chief of the School Health Section of the U.S. Public Health Service, the usually healthy child should stay home from school: if he is feverish; if his symptoms (headaches, drowsiness, runny nose, nausea, or diarrhea) are sufficiently severe to be disabling; if he is likely to be disturbing to the class; or if it is improbable, due to his general condition, that he will profit from school. Moreover, the child who is permitted to go to school with a slight fever will probably have more fever later in the day; and the child returning early to school while recovering from an upper respiratory infection may pick up from his classmates other organisms that could produce serious secondary complications.

Remedial or Follow-Up Program

Healing is a matter of time; it is also a matter of opportunity. — HIPPOCRATES

To have an effective school health organization the medical and teaching personnel must do much more than carry out a program of detection and discovery. They must have the time, facilities, staff, and know-how to implement effective follow-up procedures.

The efficient follow-up program begins with careful planning. Once a defect is discovered, one might ask whose job it is to contact the parents. In the small elementary school this may be done by the physician, nurse, or classroom teacher. Notices sent to the parents, notifying them of the suspected difficulty, are generally respected when signed by the school physician. There is considerable logic, however, in having the classroom teacher sign the notice. This is especially true at the primary grade level. Here, the judgment and concern of the teacher are appreciated by most parents, perhaps more than at any other period in the school years to follow. If the teacher says, "Your John needs glasses now," there is a very good possibility something will be done about it right away. Parents, like most people, tend to procrastinate and put off what they know should be done soon. Sometimes they fail to realize the seriousness of the situation. They say to themselves, "After all, John isn't blind, he doesn't walk into the side of the barn." As true as this may be, he still could fail to read the printed page.

Formal notices of medical examinations sent to parents are often like report cards. They are easy to send home but difficult to get back with an indication that something has been done. The larger and better organized elementary schools send out notices that provide space for an answer. Parents have the opportunity to check off whether they have taken their child to a physician or dentist, plan to do so, or need help in doing so. Other school systems use a form with a detachable section to permit parents to acknowledge receipt of the notification. (See Figure 3–9.)

The success of a follow-up system depends upon the kind of contact school personnel have with parents, the availability of needed services, and the seriousness with which parents view the health abnormality. Cauffman, working in 48 Los Angeles City Schools with 458 fourth grade children, discovered several significant parental factors favorably influencing proper follow-up. Among these were higher social status, small families, parents' national background, an education beyond high school, and non-working mothers. Also, follow-up was more likely when parents received more than one notification, and by more than one person.[8] As part of the same study Cauffman found that children from families carrying health insurance were more likely to receive care for their defects than were children from non-insured families.[9]

If the school nurse or the teacher in the small elementary school has some method of suspense date record keeping, practically all notifications to parents will be accounted for. It will then be possible to keep in close contact with delinquent parents and see that they proceed with the necessary remedial work for their child. In this way the same children with the same defects will not appear year after year

in succeeding classrooms with a handicap that might have been corrected.

Duties of Health Services Personnel

The list of duties and responsibilities of personnel connected with the health services department is an extensive one. Some of the outstanding functions are as follows:

The School Physician. Ideally he is a general practitioner or pediatrician interested in children and their problems and in public health. He helps the administrator coordinate the health services with other parts of the school program. He diagnoses diseases and defects of children but is not responsible for the medical care of individual children. He is familiar with the methods of integrating school health services with health teaching, physical education, special education, recreation, and lunchroom service. He is responsible for control of disease, sanitation, emergency cases, and safety within the school. He practices the techniques of group work and directs health service as a cooperative enterprise within the school.

Across the country a large number of school systems are unable to employ a full-time physician. In such instances the part-time physician is concerned primarily with basic health services. In 1967 the Committee on School Physicians of the American School Health Association formulated a manual relative to the duties of school physicians. The minimum duties set forth for the part-time physician are as follows:[10]

1. Consults and assists in the direction and implementation of health screening programs. Examines all can-

[8] Cauffman, Joy G., et al. "Medical Care of School Children: Factors Influencing Outcome Of Referral from a School Health Program," *American Journal of Public Health*, 57:60–73, January 1967.

[9] Cauffman, Joy G., Roemer, Milton I., and Shultz, Carl S. "The Impact of Health Insurance Coverage on Health Care of School Children," *Public Health Reports*, Vol. 82, No. 4, April 1967, pp. 323–328.

[10] Report of the Committee on School Physicians of the American School Health Association. "A Manual for School Physicians," *Journal of School Health*, 37:395–399, October 1967.

didates for interscholastic athletics prior to each season and periodically thereafter. Implements state labor laws in those states requiring boards of education to provide medical examinations for employment certificates.

2. Assists in the coordination of the school immunization programs conducted by family physicians and health departments.

3. Advises on the control of communicable disease within the school.

4. Obtains from family physicians and interprets medical information pertinent to the appropriate classroom management of the child with a physical or emotional handicap.

5. Assumes responsibility for establishing and supervising school emergency facilities and first aid training programs for school personnel. Arranges for emergency care of pupils injured or ill at school when the parent and family physician cannot be reached.

6. Arranges for meetings with groups of community physicians, at which time procedures and communication are discussed to resolve problems to the mutual satisfaction of the school and the physicians.

7. Assists with the planning of parent-education meetings concerning school health problems.

8. Arranges for medical appraisal of pupils who show signs of health problems and whose parents are unable to pay for such service.

9. Compiles reports of the services rendered by the school medical program and of the health problems identified.

Since physicians spend more time in schools than ever before, they need to develop, not a bedside manner, but a "schoolside manner" which is demonstrated by a genuine interest and technique for working with teachers and other school-community personnel.

The Nurse-Teacher. She is more than a nurse; she is a respected member of the teaching faculty, and, as such, participates with other teachers in school affairs. She interprets the school health program in the home and assists in the planning of learning experiences in the classroom. She cooperates with the health agencies in the community that are interested in child health. She assists in first aid and home nursing courses. She assists the physician, organizes teacher-nurse conferences, and follows up with parent-nurse conferences.[11]

The relationship of the nurse to the classroom teacher is of major importance. The success of a nurse's work in school is directly related to the closeness, continuity, and harmony of her association with the teacher. This was brought out in the findings of the extensive seven-year health program evaluation study conducted in the Los Angeles City Schools. Some idea of the extent of the nurse's duties is reflected in these additional findings:[12]

1. There was a high degree of joint planning of the school health program by the principal and the school nurse.

2. There was agreement among schools concerning the utilization of the school nurse as resource person in health education.

3. There was wide participation in group health conferences.

4. There was extensive individual health consultations.

5. In the follow-up program of the nurse the individuals most commonly contacted were administrators, other school personnel, parents,

---

[11] In some states, public or county health nurses will be assigned to town and city schools. Some of their duties will be the same as those of the nurse-teacher, yet in many respects experience indicates that they do not become as much a part of the school "team" as nurses employed by and responsible to the school administrator. This is due, in part, to the fact that their loyalties are divided between school needs and the public health needs of the community.

[12] Los Angeles City Schools. *Evaluation of the Health Program in the Los Angeles City Schools, 1954-1961.* Los Angeles City Schools, School Publication No. 673, 1962.

and pupils. The most popular method of contact was the conference.

6. The prevention and control of disease by the nurse was considered most satisfactory.

7. The nurse had an important day to day role in promoting healthful living in and about the school.

The School Dentist. Dental health services are under the control of the school dentist. Surveys show, unfortunately, that only about one school in 20 has a dentist that visits the school and participates in the education program.

The effective school dentist likes children well enough to perform dental examinations on each child periodically. He supervises preventive dental work and oral prophylaxis done by dental hygienists. He may take part in a school-sponsored dental clinic. (See Figure 3–10.) He also aids classroom teachers and nurse-teachers in the preparation of curriculum materials in dental hygiene.

The dental health "inspection" indicates a cursory observation of the mouth and teeth of each child. It includes clinical observation using a mouth mirror and explorer in good light. This is not a diagnostic examination such as would be carried out in the office of the family dentist. It does, however, have certain benefits: it is a fact-finding instrument which serves as a basis for the school dental health education effort; it helps build a positive attitude toward the dentist and dental care; and the child and his parents are motivated to seek and to accept dental treatment as a part of their total health protection. Moreover, such efforts are effective. In Gary, Indiana, for example, the dental health program yielded a dramatic improvement in dental health in the first four grades of schoolchildren; there

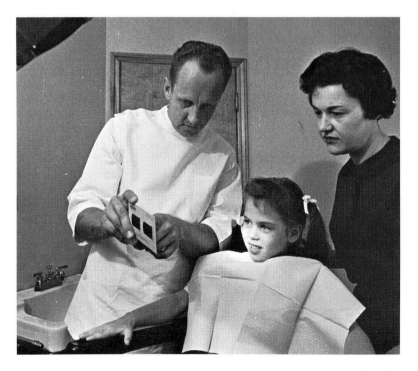

Figure 3–10 Examining the x-ray is an educational adventure. (Reprinted by permission of the American Dental Association.)

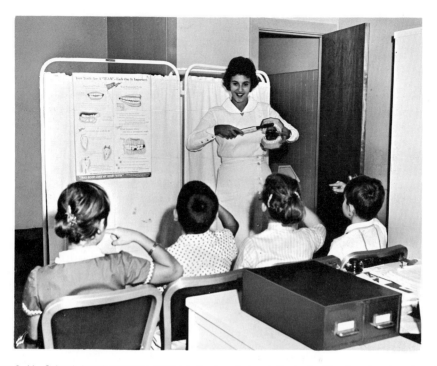

Figure 3–11 School dental hygienist demonstrates how to brush the teeth. (Courtesy American Association for Health, Physical Education and Recreation.)

was also an improvement in the continuation of periodic visits to the family dentist in grades four through six.[13]

Few school administrators realize that the local dental society, with the blessings of the American Dental Association, will gladly conduct a dental survey to determine dental health. The information obtained may be used as a basis for stimulating dental health education. Societies will also provide teaching materials, sponsor in-service education programs for teachers, and assist with the development of teaching guides.

The Dental Hygienist. Despite the efforts in some of the larger states such as New York and California, the dental hygienist as a member of the school teaching staff is still rare.

[13] Pierson, Howard W., Jr., "Dental Health Program of the School, City of Gary, Indiana," *Journal of School Health,* 36:183–184, April 1966.

The dental hygienist may periodically clean teeth, and assist the dentist or school physician in the examination of the teeth. She may make topical application of sodium or stannous fluoride where state law permits her to do this. She interprets dental defects to parents, and helps parents make plans for dental corrections. An increasing number of dental hygienists have a degree in education and are prepared to assist elementary schoolteachers in the area of health instruction.

Coordinating Personnel

There are a number of people in the school who have a rather special function to perform which touches upon the area of health services. These specialists are a part of the total school health effort. Their day to day activities may rightly be called health coordinating activities. Moreover, their work comes so close to involving the classroom teacher that brief mention will be made of their duties:

The Health Supervisor or Coordinator. The elementary school health supervisor or health coordinator is a trained school health educator who works with teachers to develop an organized health education curriculum. He coordinates health service activities with classroom activities. He is familiar with the techniques of instructional supervision. He meets with the school health council to harmonize all school activities.

The Physical Educator. The physical education teacher is one of the most popular teachers with elementary schoolchildren. He is concerned with building health, primarily through large muscle activity. He helps the grade teacher develop physical activity programs to meet the needs and interests of her children. He is interested in health safeguards on the playgrounds and in the gymnasium. He cooperates with health services in providing a remedial exercise program for children with postural defects, orthopedic difficulties, and a low level of physical fitness. He provides leadership in recreation for both pupils and teachers. He promotes total health—physical, mental and emotional—through a broad program of individual and group experiences.

The School Nutritionist. She is a trained person in nutrition and home economics. She supervises the school lunch program, cooperates with the kitchen staff, and helps in promoting health primarily through nutrition education.

The School Custodian. The unknown hero in many elementary schools is the man behind the physical environment—the custodian. He is one of the most important health promoters in the school. He is concerned with sanitation, ventilation, heating, cleanliness, and safety conditions in corridors, on floors, walks and exits.

He is one of the best friends a classroom teacher can have. Without his help the teacher may have a difficult time with young children.

In a study put out by the United States Department of Health, Education and Welfare, it is pointed out that the schools need trained custodians who, by the satisfactory performance of many duties and tasks, can contribute to the educational objectives of the school.

Mental Health Consultants. Ordinarily the guidance specialist will be interested in helping children overcome adjustment difficulties in school. He will help children understand themselves better and guide them in the solution of their immediate problems.

Schools are employing psychologists, social workers, and psychiatrists to give more specialized help than guidance counselors can provide. The psychologist is able to diagnose individual abilities and personalities. The social worker is the contact between the school and the home and is familiar with available community resources. The psychiatrist, in the few school systems fortunate enough to have one, generally does consultative work with school personnel, and may do diagnostic and therapeutic work with individual boys and girls. A fairly unique characteristic of the Los Angeles program is the wide use of psychiatrists throughout the school health service departments.[14]

The Health Council

Health counseling follows health appraisals. The child's health needs can often be served best by combining the thoughts of several interested people. Sometimes a person designated as health counselor plans a meeting

[14] See review by Harry R. Brickmen and Marcia Meeker, "Mental Health Consultation in Schools," *Journal of School Health*, 37:79–85, February 1967.

where a number of people sit down together to discuss a particular child. In many places the health coordinator is the logical person to head such a committee or council. This type of group in the elementary school may consist of the school nurse, health supervisor or coordinator, the classroom teacher of the child being discussed, the parent, and possibly another person. Working groups such as these are able to make a real contribution to the over-all health program of the school. They solve many difficulties and permit the school to give more than "lip service" to the problem of meeting individual needs.

There is also another type of school health council which is broader in scope and embraces much more in the way of school-community health than the committee already referred to. Such a council affords opportunities for widespread discussion of health problems in a whole system; it consists of teachers, administrators, parents, medical and dental personnel from the community, and representatives of health and welfare agencies. This health council in itself does not assure an adequate health program. It is still necessary that leadership and resources be available in the school or community to carry out the recommended programs.

The Classroom Teacher Cooperates with Health Services

Without the help of the sympathetic teacher, the health services personnel would indeed be handicapped. Some of her significant contributions involve the following:

Detection and Referral. The limitations of the routine medical examination of schoolchildren make it desirable to use the classroom more fully in the detection of pupil health problems. To the teacher who is trained to observe children carefully will come many significant signs and symptoms of poor health. Although the teacher is in no position to diagnose, she can certainly detect changes in behavior and refer those to the health services department.[15] It is of interest to note, in connection with these detection and referral activities of teachers, that a great deal of this kind of observation is done across the country in isolated areas where physicians are not plentiful. New York state, for example, is rich in physicians. It has one-sixth of all the country's physicians and one-fifth of all pediatricians. The figures are quite different in New Mexico or Montana. Yet, even in New York state, the vast majority of the physicians are concentrated in big cities, and upstate counties sometimes have difficulty obtaining one for school examinations. The health observation role of the classroom teacher is further emphasized by the report that many small cities have no school nursing service. And in many places a health examination is merely a brief inspection by the classroom teacher.

Following-up Deviations from Normal Health. The value of an appropriate follow-up program in a school has already been pointed out. The teacher's unique contribution here cannot be overstressed. In this country there are great numbers of children who come from homes where they do not have adequate preparation for school. They lack the sleep, food, or emotional climate that make for satisfactory schoolwork. Poverty, ignorance, and parental indifference are behind this. In the classroom the child falls short of what is expected of him; he may appear listless or lazy, easily discouraged, and show poor scholarship. The alert teacher may be able to notice his dry scalp, sallow skin, poor posture, lack of energy in physical activities, restlessness, and general ir-

---

[15] Chapter 5 will show more clearly what the teacher may observe and screen out in the way of disease, growth abnormalities, and behavior changes.

ritability. It is important that something be done quickly. This situation is not different from one where a child is in need of glasses because he cannot see the blackboard. Expert medical judgment is needed. Follow-up to see that something is done is vital. Here, parents and teachers need to cooperate, but it is the teacher who is in a position of *control*. She actually controls the situation from the classroom, where she has a day by day check on the pupils concerned. Nevertheless, boys and girls still appear year after year with the same defects or difficulties despite the efforts of school personnel.

The following case report from a teacher in Florida represents a practical approach to a problem of malnutrition. It is more difficult than most cases, but is the type of case that is present in almost every community. It clearly demonstrates the role of the classroom teacher as a *prime mover* in following up basic health abnormalities. The classroom teacher speaks:

Melvin was ten and a half years old in my third grade. There were three younger children in his family. He repeated the second grade where he was considered to be a slow student. He was thin and small for his age and showed other signs which made me suspect that he was malnourished. He was very pale and his skin had a sallow look; his hair was dry, stringy and dull looking; he had dark circles under his eyes and had a pinched look on his face.

Melvin came to school barefooted. His skin was so dirty it looked rusty in spots. He looked as if no one had ever seen that he had a bath. He was absent from school quite often. Sometimes his excuse was that he had a cold or didn't feel good or that he had to stay home and look after his baby brothers. Often he complained of being tired or sleepy.

I talked to Mrs. Irvin, our school nurse, and she told me to bring him around so that she could see him. She examined the mucous membranes of his eyes. She looked at his teeth and found several small cavi-

ties. She talked to him for some time and found that quite often he came to school without breakfast. His mother's health was bad. Often he would get up too late to fix breakfast for himself and his other little brother who was in the second grade. He said he never drank milk at home because it was needed for the babies.

Mrs. Irvin had both the boys checked for hookworm, and when the report came back negative, she decided to visit Melvin's home. From this visit she found that Melvin's father made fair wages but was a heavy drinker and often used the grocery money for buying whiskey, leaving barely enough for food. She said that many times Melvin sat up rather late at night to keep his mother company when the father was out. Mrs. Irvin impressed upon the mother how important it was for the children to get the proper amount of rest. The mother needed medical attention but could not afford it, so Mrs. Irvin made an appointment for her and the children to see the county health physician. She consulted the Welfare Department regarding the family situation.

After her visit we talked to the school principal and the lunch room supervisor. We made arrangements for Melvin and his brother to have milk each morning when they arrived at school. The children had been going home for lunch so we arranged for them to have free lunches.

Within two month's time Melvin improved considerably, both in his contacts with fellow pupils and in his scholastic achievement. He was simply a different boy.

Sometimes the part of the country makes little difference in what teachers find in their classes. Here is a case from upstate New York:

John was an 11 year old boy who lived in a trailer camp. His family consisted of father, stepmother and two stepbrothers, ages one and two years old.

He came to school with dirty clothes, unkempt hair and had been classified for two years as a problem child.

The fourth grade teacher noticed that he was listless, complained of headaches and was retarded in his schoolwork. Then some of the children who brought lunches to school complained that a sandwich, apple, orange, or cooky was missing from their lunches. On inquiry, it was discovered that John was guilty of the misdemeanor. What was the cause? The teacher took John to the school nurse. A conference of nurse, teacher, and John brought out the fact that he was coming to school without breakfast and going without a noonday lunch.

Since the stepmother couldn't leave her small sons, the nurse arranged for a visit to the trailer. The nurse and stepmother discussed John's physical condition and his meals, but the stepmother displayed disinterest. She said that the milkman didn't come until after John's school bus had gone and that the milk on hand in the trailer had to be used for the babies' cereal. She didn't have time to give John toast or egg or to make him a lunch to take to school.

The nurse contacted the father at the factory where he worked and tried to make an appointment to talk to him. His wife had already mentioned the nurse's visit to the trailer, so his reply to the nurse was, "The wife takes care of the food and the feeding of our family." No satisfaction was gained from him.

The nurse reported the results of the investigations to the principal. The principal, nurse, and school cafeteria manager discussed the case and came to the following decision:

Each morning when John's bus arrived, he went to the cafeteria to perform some little task for the cafeteria manager. In return she offered him juice, a slice of bread and butter, and a glass of milk. He didn't realize that this had previously been decided by the conference.

At noon, tickets were given to the children who purchased school lunches. John had been going without lunch or taking hand-outs from the other children, and was now given a ticket each day with the explanation it was given for doing errands for the principal. This was all arranged without humiliating John.

In June, John had shown a year's growth in achievement over the previous year. This was the greatest achievement he had shown in three years. He was a much happier boy in June than the previous September. Cooperative effort of principal, nurse, teacher, and cafeteria manager improved John's nutritional condition and gave him a new outlook on life.

Assisting in Screening Measures. The grade teacher in most school systems works with the nurse to screen pupils for a number of health difficulties. There are numerous places where screening is done entirely by the teacher; if she does not do it, it will not be done.

In addition to helping with vision and hearing measures, teachers also screen children to determine rate of growth. Growth is usually steady over a long enough period, so teachers weigh and measure their pupils periodically. Sometimes this is done with the aid of the school nurse so that some kind of further appraisal may be made on the spot.

Children are screened for characteristics of poor mental health in some of the more progressive schools. A program, carried out by the teacher, is set up for administering and scoring selected tests and recording the data obtained. Tests measuring the attitude of the child toward school and toward other children, and tests measuring his general behavior are especially useful in combating items of maladjustment.

It should be pointed out that "screening" tests used by teachers are not intended to diagnose. They serve only to select those pupils who appear in need of a diagnosis by a physician.

Carrying Out a Daily Inspection. For years classroom teachers have been employing the "morning inspection" to single out those boys and girls in need of health counseling or special examination. In fact, in some New England schools today, one might almost set a watch by the punctuality with which certain teachers check over their pupils.

The principle of observing hands, fingernails, faces, skin, eyes, hair, teeth, and glands, is a good one. The question often asked deals with whether such a daily inspection should be a formal one or an informal one. Certainly the formal inspection is an orderly approach—one which the pupils soon learn to accept, and one that lends itself to various competitive activities. Rows of classroom students have for years competed against each other for various gold and silver paper stars and the special praises of the teacher. In this manner primary grade children have been motivated to "do something" about their dirty hands or uncombed hair. When teachers are careful not to place *too much* emphasis on these health items, the interest of the pupils is just enough to permit valuable learning to take place. Highly competitive morning inspections, however, sometimes force the pupils to be a part of the group "at any cost," even to the extent of being dishonest and re-porting that they brushed their teeth when they did not.

Probably the daily inspection can best be carried out on an informal basis. Sometimes during the morning activities the teacher moves about the classroom observing the boys and girls. She obviously will be more interested in noting the appearance of those pupils who had poor health habits the day before. She can still post a record of her observations as a motivation technique for health education. In fact, several companies print daily inspection charts that may be obtained by request.[16] Some teachers, instead of keeping the charts at school, send them home with the children. They

---

[16] Proctor and Gamble Co., the makers of Ivory Soap, make charts available to elementary schoolteachers. (See Chapter 11, Sources of Free and Inexpensive Materials.)

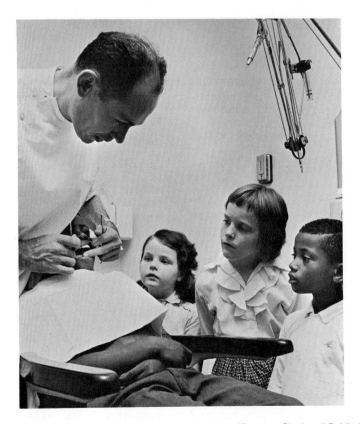

Figure 3–12 Health education is not limited to the classroom. (Courtesy Cincinnati Public Schools.)

are taped to the back of the bathroom door so that the child may keep his own record. This can be very effective for it also serves to keep the parents aware of what is going on.

Health Counseling. Either individually or as a member of a school health council the classroom teacher follows up appraisals by discussing the findings with her pupils. This is most generally planned for, but carried out informally. With younger children the parents are involved right away in the counseling procedure. Some of the finest counseling is done just like good teaching—"as if you taught them not."

Opportunities for Health Teaching. As already suggested in Chapter 2, the classroom teacher has a wonderful chance to educate for health every time the class is scheduled to visit the school physician. If this job is well done, the boys and girls will look forward to going to the physician's office with true delight. Furthermore, having a medical examination can be a most rewarding experience for the youngster in the early grades. These children are curious and, as a rule, they need little external motivation to prepare them for the day when they are looked over by the doctor. The teacher with a pleasant and positive outlook can discuss the why, the what, and the how of such a visit.

Why are we going to have the examination? Will it hurt?

What will the doctor find?

How will all this affect me?

These are good questions. If the pupils are allowed to work on this topic awhile they will come up with a number of other things that have been bothering them—questions relating to the instruments carried in the black bag, or why doctors do not seem to catch the measles or mumps when they visit sick children.

In some classrooms or nurses' offices children have a chance to handle a real stethoscope before the examination, and listen to the beat of their own hearts. Questions are asked and answered so that by the time of the examination the class is practically bouncing with enthusiasm to get started. This kind of approach almost guarantees a *satisfying experience.*[17] Such positive health teaching may be briefly summarized by referring to a story told by a pioneer in health teaching, Mabel Bragg. In a Newton, Massachusetts, school one day, Dr. Emmett Holt stopped a group of children who were skipping merrily down a corridor. "Where are you going?" he asked. "We're going to see the doctor," said a little girl. "Why?" asked Dr. Holt. "Are you sick?" "Oh, no," she replied, "We're going to see how well we are."

The In-Service Program

Orienting teachers and keeping them up to date is the responsibility of the local administration. School health is promoted this way through the in-service program.

A number of school programs have been completely reorganized from time to time because teachers have sat down together to talk about the health of their children. In Indiana, for example, the in-service training of teachers in health education has been successfully carried on for many years. Weekly conferences, under state education department guidance and promotion, have prompted many principals and classroom teachers to modify their existing health efforts. Moreover, in a number of the larger cities, notably Columbus, Ohio, the nurse-teachers speak to all school personnel each year about the health services available in the school and the community. Surveys have indicated that in a number of elementary schools there are numerous teachers who are quite un-

---

[17] An expression used by William James to convey the idea of something that gives deep gratification to the individual, and will be apt to be repeated again because of this.

familiar with the health services available for their immediate use within a few miles or minutes of the school. It cannot be pointed out too often that school health education involves more than the school—it concerns the whole community in practically all of its aspects.

Teamwork in School Health

It must be obvious from the preceding sections of this chapter that in seeking solutions to health problems, and particularly to one so complex as the problem of health in schools, the teamwork approach is the most effective. With all persons in the school fully aware of the objectives, and with some one person appointed to be responsible for coordinating health activities, the load may be made light through the combined efforts of many.

Parents, too, are a part of the team— even the ones who are difficult to approach. Most parents are very cooperative, and with their help and encouragement children profit from instruction given at school. In a dental health unit, for example, the parents in one particular community helped their children keep a record of toothbrushing habits. They become so interested in the activity that they got together and supplied the teacher with toothpaste and brushes so that the children, under the teacher's supervision, could brush their teeth following the midday lunch. This is the kind of education that does more than impart knowledge. It satisfies immediate and long term needs of boys and girls because the parents and teachers are working together.

Questions for Discussion

1. What part should the social worker in the community have in the school health program?

2. Does it appear to you, because of the number of specialists that may be assigned to health services, that the school is bordering on socialized medicine? Explain.

3. To what extent do teachers of your acquaintance engage in "detection and referral" activities?

4. How would you as a teacher feel about keeping anecdotal records on the health behavior of your children? Would it be a chore or something you believe would be useful to other teachers?

5. Are school psychiatrists necessary? Is it not possible that a guidance counselor or school psychologist might be a reasonable substitute?

6. It has been hypothesized by Gabrielson and others (see *Selected References*) that there is a positive relationship between "increased parental perception of seriousness and parent action in school follow-up recommendations." How would you comment on this statement?

7. What can you discover about the duties of dental hygienists that go beyond those referred to in the chapter?

Suggested Activities

1. Find out what kind of duties school nurses actually perform. Do they do everything this chapter says they do? How do they relate to crippled children? To drop outs? To children who may take advantage of illness? To children who miss classes? To the social worker or health center?

2. According to the Brookings Institution, the medical manpower for the 1970's will be in short supply. To meet this situation it is urged that there be an expansion of group practice and a training program for auxiliary medical personnel. What can you discover from talking with practicing physicians about the truth of this statement? How do you think the United States will cope with this growing demand for physicians? What bearing will this have on the schools?

3. Interview a school nurse, preferably one in a large city and another in a small town, in order to discuss factors affecting school health follow-up practices. This may be organized as a committee project to discover some of the difficulties involved in following up and in improving the health conditions of schoolchildren. Write out your comments following the interview.

Selected References

American School Health Association. "The Nurse in the School Health Program." *Journal of School Health,* 37:1–40, No. 2a, February 1967.

Anderson, C. L. *School Health Practice,* 4th ed. St. Louis: C. V. Mosby Co., 1968, Part 3.

Fein, Rashi. *The Doctor Shortage: an Economic Diagnosis.* Washington, D. C.: Bookings Institution, 1967.

Fricke, Irma B. "The Illinois Study of School Nurse Practice." *Journal of School Health,* 37:24–28, January 1967.

Gabrielson, Ira W., et al. "Factors Affecting School Health Follow-Up." *American Journal of Public Health,* 57:48–59, January 1967.

Gair, Catherine. "What Is School Nursing?" *Journal of School Health,* 36:401–402, November 1966.

Haag, J. H. *School Health Program,* 2nd ed. New York: Holt, Rinehart, and Winston, 1965.

Millner, Bernard. "Health Needs of School-Age Children." *Journal of School Health,* 36:276–280, June 1966.

National Education Association-American Medical Association. *Health Appraisal of School Children,* 4th ed. Washington, D. C.: National Education Association, 1968.

National Education Association-American Medical Association. *Suggested School Health Policies,* 4th ed. Washington, D. C.: National Education Association, 1966.

National Education Association-American Medical Association Joint Committee. *School Health Services,* 2nd ed. Chicago: American Medical Association, 1964.

Randall, Harriet B. "Strengths and Limitations of the Cumulative Health Period." *Journal of School Health,* 37:86–99, February 1967.

Randall, Harriet B. "Use of the School Physician's Time." *Journal of School Health,* 38:116–119, February 1968.

Turner, C. E., Sellery, C. M., and Smith, S. L. *School Health and Health Education,* 5th ed. St. Louis: C. V. Mosby Co., 1966.

Aspects
of Healthful and

CHAPTER 4

Safe School Environment

Education, formal or otherwise, is a continuous process, and as such it becomes involved with negative influences as well as favorable ones. These negative influences retard progress toward educational goals. Educational philosophers and classroom teachers, for example, spend a great deal of time making elaborate plans for the youth of the community; yet it takes only a few seemingly small items in the school environment to disrupt them.

If it were possible to hold the environment constant, i.e., be sure that school facilities, physical surroundings, and classroom atmosphere were optimum, we could practically guarantee that the professionally trained teacher, using the appropriate curriculum, could effect a kind of learning that would astound pedagogues and parents alike. Such is not the case, however, and it never will be because we cannot exercise as much control as we would like over the school environment.

Importance of Healthful Living to the School Program

The healthful school environment is one which provides for healthful living throughout the school day. It is not a haphazard setup; there is organization to bring this about. The administrator, the physician, and the custodian work together to provide safe and sanitary facilities and such pupil-teacher relationships as are favorable to the best growth and development, optimum learning, and welfare of all.

Concern for the living conditions of students is not new. Most civilizations have given it some attention. Spartan educators realized the importance of favorable surroundings dominated by teachers with strong personalities. Through the years in American schools there have been numerous distractions such as lack of heat in the winter months, poor lighting, inadequate ventilation, unadjustable desks and chairs, unattractive walls, and poor acoustics.

Parents sometimes made themselves heard. So did medical doctors who were interested in the schools. At the founding meeting of the American Association for the Advancement of Physical Education, held in Brooklyn, New York, in 1885, Dr. W. L. Savage spoke about "ill ventilated school houses and weary children and of the relief which open windows and physical exercise would bring."[1] Overcrowded classrooms and poor school construction in the late 1800's resulted in several tragic fires which stimulated the populace to look more closely at the school environment. In 1892 William H. Burnham, one of the better known school health pioneers, wrote extensively on "school hygiene" and presented evidence to show the necessity for greater attention to school furniture, cleanliness, growth, schoolhouse architecture, reading, writing, fatigue, and aspects of school health neglected at that time.[2] Gradually, more attention was given to child health, and today educational buildings and programs are continually being modified to provide healthful school living.

No one, however, should be misled into believing that most of the schools are "up to date" just because new buildings are being erected. The problems of the backward areas of this country, coupled with the tremendous burden on school facilities of a fast growing school population, point to many current needs. Teachers still register complaints relative to inadequate drinking fountains, overcrowded classrooms and playrooms, noisy environment, and insufficient janitorial services. In a great number of schools it is possible to discover inadequacies

in basic safety measures. School bus transportation is a good example. Despite an increase in new equipment and improved bus regulations, there were in 1967 still only 18 out of 50 states forbidding pupils to stand in moving buses.

Not to be overlooked are the variety of potentially hazardous by-products of population growth and prosperity. For instance, approximately 70 per cent of the population is crowded into urban areas representing only 10 per cent of the total land. It was just such a statistic that caused René Dubos of the Rockefeller Institute to state that:

> You can go to anyone of the thoughtful architects or urban planners . . . none of them knows what it does to the child to have a certain kind of environment, as against other kinds of environments.
> The whole process of mental development, as affected by physical development of cities, has never been investigated.[3]

The Internal Environment— The School Building

Whether or not the elementary school contributes to the over-all purposes of health education depends in the first instance upon the thinking and planning of members of the Board of Education. Where is the building to be located? Is it to be near main highways, busy streets, noisy factories, or active train yards? Of what is it to be constructed? How will it face? Is there play space within the structure? Are the corridors soundproofed? Are the stairs moderately inclined? What kind of windows does it have? Are the classrooms attractive? Is the health

[1] Proceedings of the Association for the Advancement of Physical Education. Brooklyn: Rome Brothers, 1885.

[2] Means, Richard K. A History of Health Education in the United States. Philadelphia: Lea and Febiger, 1962, p. 62.

[3] Report of Task Force on Environmental Health and Related Problems. A Strategy for a Livable Environment. U.S. Department of Health, Education, and Welfare, June 1967, p. 19.

examination room adequate in size? Are there locker room and shower facilities? How satisfactory are the lunchroom facilities? These and a dozen more pertinent questions must be discussed by the board members, architects, sanitary engineers and others before the building is constructed. Moreover, it is not uncommon today for teachers' committees to sit down and plan the facilities that to them seem desirable for the maintenance of good health and the promotion of a reasonable degree of individual pupil achievement.

The importance of the internal school environment to the elementary school teacher should not be underestimated. The finest health teaching is done by example. Where there are no facilities for handwashing, for instance, it is pretty difficult to discuss visiting the toilet and washing the hands before eating. There are numerous schools that fit this category. Until recent years the city schools were usually better equipped than the rural schools, but with the closing of many old-time rural schoolhouses and the opening of thousands of consolidated and centralized schools serving large areas of the population, the trend for superior facilities is moving away from the large cities.

No matter how poor the facilities are, the classroom teacher owes it to her pupils to strive personally for improvements. She should know that:

1. The water supply must meet the minimum standards for chemical bacterial purity established by the state and local health departments.

2. The common drinking cup is prohibited.

3. The sanitary drinking fountain should be installed in the classroom, or at least one on each floor to serve a minimum of 50 pupils; the height of the nozzle should range from 23 inches for kindergarten to 29 inches for intermediate grade school pupils.[4] The fountain should be of the modern, slanting type with self-closing valve and mouth guard. Adequate water pressure must be maintained at all drinking fountains.

4. The drinking fountain water should be cool, less than 75° F.

5. The rural schools without running water should use sanitary privies, either the pit privy or septic privy type, or chemical toilets.

6. In the absence of a garbage grinder, food and refuse from the school cafeteria should be disposed of by local collection, burning, burying, or other methods approved by sanitation authorities.

7. Toilet facilities — clean, ventilated, bright, well-kept, and properly lighted — encourage pupils to maintain these conditions. The dark toilet room, without paper towels and liquid soap, poorly kept, encourages a lack of respect for standards of sanitation. There should be a minimum of one urinal for 30 boys and a split-seat toilet for 25-30 girls.

8. The handwashing basins should range in height from 20 inches for kindergarten to 25 inches for intermediate grade school pupils. There should be one for every 30 children.

9. School cafeteria sanitation must meet the standards of any public or community eating establishment. The cafeteria should also be an attractive place to eat.

10. The school swimming pools and shower room facilities must meet sanitary standards. The use of pupil footbaths is not recommended; instead, individuals are encouraged to practice proper foot hygiene. This involves drying the foot and using foot powder if necessary. Hygiene also includes periodic inspection of the pupil's feet for

---

[4] National Education Association, American Medical Association. *School Health Services,* revised 1964. Washington: National Education Association, p. 71.

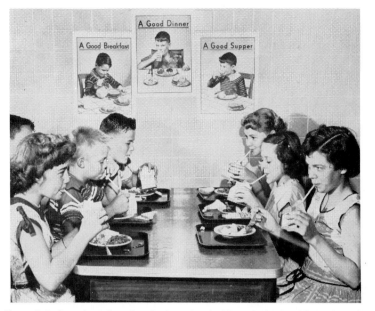

Figure 4–1 Learning takes place in the cafeteria. (Courtesy National Dairy Council.)

athlete's foot and other skin infections. Floors should be hosed and washed daily.

11. The teachers' rest rooms should be attractive and functional.

12. The school custodian is the teacher's friend and needs the concrete help of the teacher and her pupils.

13. The gymnasium must be well lighted and ventilated and have protective wiring over exposed lights.

14. The halls, stairways, classrooms, and auditorium must be checked for accident hazards.

15. The playground should be clean and level and preferably have an asphalt (blacktop) surface.

16. The school area should be relatively free of disturbing noises, obnoxious odors, and other distractions.

17. School personnel must be constantly alert to observe buildings, grounds, and equipment for possible hazardous conditions:

Broken or splintered furniture or playground equipment
Defective stair rails
Broken sidewalks
Protruding objects anywhere, such as nails
Holes in blacktop surfaces
Sandboxes not properly maintained
Blocked or obstructed exits
Slippery floors
Gas leaks

18. Fire prevention equipment must be conveniently located and inspected at regular intervals.

Aspects of Classroom Environment

The classroom is the teacher's domain. Here are influences too subtle to measure, and here also are influences of major proportion that may contribute to or detract from learning and pupil achievement. These influences, or environmental elements, may be divided into physical factors and human factors. They touch upon all phases of healthful school living, from physical and emotional climate to classroom safety.

Physical Factors in the Classroom. Other things being equal, if the classroom is a pleasant place to live in, the student will find many opportunities for a satisfying experience.

The teacher should know that the physical aspects of the classroom may have as much to do with her success as the motivation techniques and educational methods employed. She should know that:

1. An air temperature not in excess of 68° F. represents an optimal condition for comfort, with a slightly higher temperature of about 70° F. desirable in the primary grades.

2. Such items as humidity, air movement, and children's clothing must also be considered when comfortable room temperatures are being discussed.

3. It is good education for health to have pupils read and record room thermometers at set intervals.

4. Ventilation is as important to comfort as room temperatures; windows should be opened from the bottom to permit incoming cold fresh air to mix with the warm air rising from the radiator, and combined air moves toward the exhaust.

5. Standards of classroom lighting are steadily being revised, both for artificial and natural light. The lighting must be soft, even, properly distributed, and bright enough for eye comfort.

6. The responsibility for checking the operation of window shades and lights is the classroom teacher's.

7. To obtain the best working light from natural sources within the pupil's field of vision and with a minimum of shadows, individual pupil consideration should be given to seating arrangements. The 50° rotation of classroom furniture (in schools with movable desks and chairs) allows for maximum utilization of natural lighting by permitting the light to fall upon the work surface of each child's desk, unobstructed by body shadows.

8. The eyesight of schoolchildren is influenced by differences in brightness. This involves natural lighting, artificial illumination, and the color used to finish the interior surfaces of the classroom. Excessive brightness, which is glare, can be avoided by the type and color of paint used. Upper walls should reflect more light than lower walls and floors. But floors should reflect about 30 per cent of the light; they should not be dark and oiled. Desks should be light enough to reflect 40 per cent of the light, while the chalkboard should not reflect more than 15 per cent. Furniture, chalkboards, and other fixtures should have non-glossy finishes.

9. Uncontrolled sunlight is a fatiguing element that detracts from the total learning process.

10. The classroom should be free from acoustic difficulties.

11. The location and size of desks and chairs should be suited to the pupils using them. Fatigue and tension are often caused by ill fitting classroom furniture.

12. The writing surface of the desk should be at a height which permits the student to write while squarely seated so that there will be no need to elevate one shoulder out of line with the other when writing.

13. The ability of any one pupil to see or hear should be the major point in determining where he sits in the room.

14. Eyestrain may be relieved by alternating instruction involving close eye work with learning activities that are visually less fatiguing.

15. Clean teaching materials, such as maps and books, are desirable. Too often soiled materials are employed on which there is poor contrast between the paper and the print.

Healthful school living is in itself a health teaching item. All pupils must share the load of keeping the school clean and pleasant. By so doing they gain an understanding of the proper use of school property, the rights and feelings of others, and an appreciation for healthful surroundings. It is of interest to note that on many occasions this kind of pupil appreciation carries over into the home environment rather quickly, and is manifested by such actions as cleaning kitchen floors, hanging bright curtains, and helping parents wash windows and paint interior walls.

There are, in addition to the physical factors already referred to, a number of other classroom items that have a bearing upon healthful living. The scheduling of activities and the allotment of time, for example, may be done in such a way that the interest of the class members is kept to a high level throughout the day. This may be ascertained by experimenting with the difficult activities at various hours of the school day. Keeping a rigid time schedule, particularly in the lower grades, does not allow for individual and group variations in capacities and interest. Other classroom environment elements that are of concern here include such things as the length of the school day, the spacing and duration of rest and recess periods, class load,

and programs and surroundings adapted to individual needs.

Human Factors in the Classroom. It seems to be a rather common practice to relate all the elements of human behavior, on the part of both pupils and the teacher, to one general category — classroom climate or atmosphere. To be sure, classroom climate does embrace physical surroundings, but it probably is influenced more by individual human factors such as human peculiarities, idiosyncracies, attitudes, prejudices, likes and dislikes, and health status of the moment.[5]

Just as the general circulation of the atmosphere over the earth is the cause of the climate and weather behavior we have, so also is the classroom atmosphere related to classroom behavior. There is no mystery about it, but there is difficulty in putting what is known into practice. For one thing,

---

[5] For a full discussion of classroom climate see M. Karl Openshaw, *Development of a Taxonomy for the Classification of Teacher Classroom Behavior.* Columbus, Ohio: the Ohio State University Research Foundation, 1966.

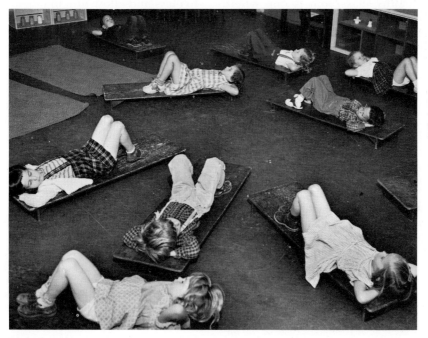

Figure 4–2   A relaxation period fosters healthful school living (Courtesy Los Angeles Schools.)

few laymen have any idea of the complicated juggling of forces and personalities that is the everyday job of the classroom teacher; it is like trying to stage an important show while trying to keep a dozen billiard balls, knives and forks in the air all at once without dropping or forgetting one.

The role of the teacher is to attempt to maintain an environment for good health, which in turn creates the optimum atmosphere for learning. She must be realistic and deal objectively with pupil relationships. She must think in terms of individuals while operating in the medium of masses of children. She must exercise leadership and be firm with pupils, while at the same time demonstrate cooperation and sympathy for children with personal problems of adjustment.

Human factors are more difficult to control than physical factors. The elementary schoolteacher is faced at the beginning of each school year with the task of building a mentally healthy environment. She must understand child behavior and recognize that the mentally healthy classroom is one where the children have a high level of self-esteem, are relaxed and at ease, are challenged by the situation to want to learn, are confident they can succeed and receive a personal satisfaction from such success. Furthermore, the teacher must recognize that in adjusting to school the child is making three of the fundamental adjustments to life. First of all, he is making a social adjustment, i.e., to his classmates. In the second place, he is making an adjustment to authority. This is an adjustment made to teachers and principals, "not as a blind force to which he must submit, not as a hostile one, cruel and unfair, against which he secretly or openly rebels, but as a force which is just and friendly, essential for happy group living,"[6] In the

    [6] Department of Child Guidance of the City of Newark, New Jersey. *Mental Hygiene in the Classroom.* New York: National Committee for Mental Hygiene, Inc., 1949, p. 5.

third place, the child learns in school to adjust to his own limitations. This, in itself, places the teacher in a unique position, for every child wants to be the best, the brightest and the most productive; the teacher must help him discover his own strong points and live with his limitations.

The teacher does more than recognize these factors. She works to create a school environment that is mentally hygienic. Such activity on her part is a first-rate example of proper health education. Some of the more specific tasks she can engage in to foster feelings of acceptance, affection and achievement include:

1. Making the classroom a friendly place. "Big Brothers" and "Big Sisters" can be assigned to help newcomers feel at home. Look for the child without a friend and see that he has a chance to sit with an especially friendly person.

2. Showing concern for each pupil. Celebrate birthdays. Telephone the home of the sick child to inquire about him. Welcome him back on his return to class and allow him to talk about his illness to the group.

3. Permitting boys and girls to have a part in planning the class activities.

4. Treating all pupils kindly. Avoid constant nagging, scolding, or correcting. Let children know, without saying in so many words, that you like them, and if they have trouble with something you will try to see their side of the problem.

5. Accepting children's feelings of the moment. Angry children have their difficulties, but these may be overcome to some extent by directing their attention to some constructive form of expression such as helping the teacher, painting a picture, or talking over the trouble with an older person.

6. Providing for success experiences. Each pupil needs to feel success in at least one area of effort, whether it be sport skills, music, reading, or in picking up paper from the floor! At the same time it should be

noted that children learn by their failures. Thus they shouldn't be protected from their failures but should understand them clearly in terms of their successes.

7. Praising individuals and groups for their fine efforts. Praise, properly administered, acts as an effective tonic which spurs pupils on to greater accomplishments.

8. Making provisions for specific student weakness and deficiencies through avenues of adapted instruction and program modification.

9. Helping parents develop a wholesome attitude toward ability and success in the classroom.

10. Recognizing that academic and social pressures may be somewhat offset by "low pressure" teaching and flexible pupil scheduling.

It would be an error to dismiss human factors in the environment of the classroom without briefly mentioning the school custodian. Use of germicidal sprays for trash, nonskid wax, noiseless grass cutters, ability and willingness to adjust school furniture for optimum comfort and hygiene, fall to the custodial and maintenance crews. The physical and mental health and the open-mindedness of these workers is an important item.

Teacher's Personal Health Status. The most favorable physical and human factors brought to bear in the classroom may mean very little if the teacher's own health status is below par. Yet various surveys of the mental and physical condition of teachers have produced evidence that a good many of them are ill in one way or another.

Not all teachers will be well. Because of this, many communities require periodic health examinations. Hypertensive individuals showing some irritability and fatigue and teachers with a history of severe mental illness probably should not teach school. Unfortunately a very small number of teachers are kept from teaching because of poor health. Studies are needed to show more clearly the re-

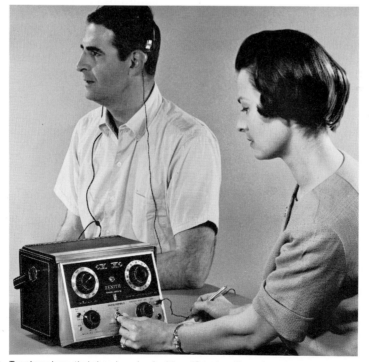

Figure 4–3 Teachers have their hearing checked too. (Courtesy Bausch and Lomb, Inc., Rochester, N.Y.)

lationship between classroom-pupil efficiency and teacher health defects and illness. Certainly no one likes a grouchy teacher. How can she create happiness? Said Ben Franklin in his *Almanac*:

> If you would have others merry with cheer, be so yourself or so appear.

It should go without saying that the physical health status of the classroom teacher is related largely to her personal health practices. Teaching is considered one of the vigorous occupations, on a level with medicine, military life, and police duty, and, as such, demands much of the vigor and enthusiasm of the individual. Habits involving good nutrition, dental care, recreation, moderate exercise, and rest are therefore important if one is to sustain an active constitution for effective teaching.

Every day there are untold circumstances that challenge the strength, ingenuity and adaptability of the teacher. Some of these exert pressure on a conscientious teacher and tend to warp her attitude so that she is a little less friendly and appears not to enjoy her job quite as well as before. Teachers need time for enrichment. Just as other people show signs of psychological stress and fatigue from their efforts to make a living, teachers too need relaxation, diversion, and play. Art, music, golf, fishing, photography, and other hobbies provide "just what the doctor ordered" for harrassed teachers. The teacher who understands this basic point of view is far ahead of the one with great zest who "pushes" herself until she becomes unbearable to her class.

Aspects of School Safety

The topic of safety and safety education is an area of study in itself. Actually, safety falls within the school heath education domain. It cuts across all fields and involves all personnel that have anything at all to do with the schools. Children learn about safe living through programs of instruction and by well defined school safety practices that are engaged in by all pupils and teachers.

Needless to say, the school building has its share of hazards to guard against. There are stairways, corridors, lavatories, classrooms, shower rooms, swimming pools, gymnasiums, cafeterias, auditorium stages, and industrial arts shops to worry about. And there are programs associated with these facilities that require constant attention on the part of teachers lest accidents occur that might have been prevented. The same reasoning applies to the external environment. Safety on the playgrounds and playing fields, on the school buses, at the crossings adjacent to the school, and on field trips into the community all relate to healthful school living.

Accidents constitute the major hazard to the lives of children. They account for about half of the deaths among boys and for one fourth among girls. For boys especially, the accident hazard increases rapidly as they reach their late teens. A great many of these accidents occur in the school area.

Research reported by the National

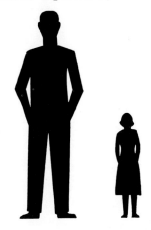

Figure 4–4 Boys have approximately twice as many accidents as girls. (Reproduced by permission of Gerald J. Hase and the New York State Education Department.)

Safety Council indicates that 800,000 injuries occur each year to boys and girls.[7] According to the U.S. Public Health Service, this figure may be closer to three million accidental injuries per year, half of which are due to falls and bumping.[8] In the first six grades the frequency of accidents is highest in the unorganized activities. Serious accidents, as determined by the average number of days lost from school, occur at the bicycle rack area, stairways, athletic fields, doorways, and school sidewalks, in that order.

Obviously there is a need for safety precautions in every school. Administrators, working with teachers, must formulate school safety procedures and establish local regulations. In numerous large city systems such as Boston, Los Angeles, New York, Cincinnati, and Boulder, special policies relative to accident prevention and environmental health have been set forth in administrative handbooks. A particularly useful publication which illustrates the contents of two handbooks is available from the National Safety Council.[9]

An appraisal instrument designed to help teachers and administrators improve their school safety efforts is available from the National Commission on Safety.[10] It is a checklist that encourages action on school safety problems relative to facilities and other environmental considerations, and educational programs.

With over 7200 fires a year in schools, the fire departments carry out inspections, and boards of educa-

tion are required to implement fire department suggestions with respect to remedying hazardous situations. Police departments frequently study school traffic safety and erect special traffic signals and signs, and order appropriate crosswalk markings. Local civil defense groups also have a genuine interest in school health and safety activities.

Accident Prevention. There are at least four major considerations worth reviewing when an effort is being made to promote school safety. The first of these, which has already been discussed at some length, is the *determination of pupil health status*. The sick child is a hazard to his own safety. His reflexes and responses are slower; he is not as alert; and he lacks the physical capacity that his personal safety demands. Even children convalescing from disease and getting over colds probably should have a modified school program, for it is conceivable that their interaction with children could have some bearing on the safety of others. The second consideration is *concern for equipment and facilities*. Activities in the classroom, on the playground, in the gymnasium, and in the shops involve the use of special equipment. It is the teacher's responsibility to see that this equipment is in proper repair and safe to use. Very often when a jungle gym frame is loose, or a sliver of wood breaks off a teeter board, or a stone under the swings works up out of the ground, the classroom teacher will complain that it is the duty of the school custodian to do something about it. But in most instances constructive action will be taken in the way of repair only when the teacher personally discusses the situation with the custodian.

The third program safeguard has to do with the *development of activity skills*. In every subject matter area there are specific skills to be mastered. Proficiency in these skills — in the

[7] Estimated Pupil Accidental Injuries in U.S. Elementary and Secondary Schools. Chicago: National Safety Council, 1967.

[8] Parrish, Henry M., et al. "Epidemiological Approach to Preventing School Accidents", *Journal of School Health*, 37:236–239, May 1967.

[9] *School Safety Handbook*. Chicago: National Safety Council, 1965.

[10] *School Safety Education Checklist: Administration, Instruction, Protection.* Washington, D.C.: National Commission on Safety Education, National Education Association, revised 1967.

classrooms and laboratories and on the playgrounds—makes the difference between a low and high accident rate. It would be improper for schools to remove every dangerous piece of equipment or condemn all hazardous activities. Children need the experience of meeting challenging situations by developing satisfactory skills. Electric jig saws are not removed from the shops because they can cut off a wayward finger; playground equipment is not dismantled for fear that some child may fall off; and automobiles are not outlawed because of automobile accidents. We learn to live with these things. There is no substitute for skill. The child, for example, who possesses the skill for operating the jig saw, is far better off than the one who has little ability but is closely supervised. This leads directly to the fourth and final consideration, namely, *adequate supervision.* The stairways,

corridors, halls, playgrounds, and classrooms need constant supervision, not only because teachers are liable, but also because youngsters are often too busy to look after their own safety. Satisfactory accident prevention involves a combination of all four considerations, especially personal skills and adequate supervision. For example, children boarding school buses, riding bicycles, crossing streets, and taking part in fire drills need to practice well identified skills in the presence of capable teacher supervision.

The prevention of school accidents has become one of the major interests of board members, teachers, and administrators. A few of the more significant *accident prevention activities* are worth listing, for they have more than a slight influence on school health:

In the classroom:

1. Put sharp objects away.

2. Cover exposed projections such as plant boxes and table corners.

3. Cover exposed lights, radiators and electric fixtures.

4. Play games that are safe for the particular classroom.

5. Move about the classroom in an orderly manner, neither pushing nor running.

6. Use tools at workbench or desk.

7. Keep furniture in proper place.

8. Encourage children to keep feet out of aisle and under the desk.

In the halls, corridors and stairways:

1. Do not leave locker doors ajar.

2. Avoid running and pushing, especially on stairs.

3. Exercise care at drinking fountains.

4. Use care in passing closed doors; they may be opened suddenly and cause serious injury.

5. Report slippery surfaces and worn or broken stairs.

6. Appraise the hall traffic in terms of congestion; rerouting may be advisable.

DEATHS AMONG RIDERS OF PEDAL CYCLES

By Age. United States, 1965

Ages	Number of Deaths*	Death Rate per Million Population
All Ages	706	3.6
Under 1	—	—
1-4	7	0.4
5-9	209	10.2
10-14	296	15.6
15-19	97	5.7
20-24	11	0.8
25-34	11	0.5
35-44	22	0.9
45-54	13	0.6
55-64	11	0.6
65-74	19	1.7
75 and over	10	1.5

*Excluding deaths in railroad crossing collisions with trains; data, not available.

Source of basic data: Reports of the Division of Vital Statistics, National Center for Health Statistics.

Figure 4–5 Violation of safety rules is the major factor in four out of five cycling fatalities. (Courtesy *Statistical Bulletin,* Metropolitan Life Insurance Co., July, 1967.)

In the shops and laboratories:

1. Keep floors clean of litter.

2. Look for "shop sloppies" who wave boards wildly around in the air and leave nails sticking up for others to step on.

3. Check and repair equipment each day.

4. Post and discuss safety rules for using laboratory or shop tools and equipment.

5. Provide a minimum of first aid supplies, especially for burns and bleeding.

6. See that gas, water, and electricity are turned off when no longer needed.

7. Stress the importance of good footing and safe clothing. Sleeves should be rolled and ties removed.

8. Use color to denote parts of machinery or chemicals that are particularly hazardous.

In the gymnasium, locker, and shower rooms:

1. Encourage safe play through personal example and discussion with pupils.

2. Stress the rules of the game, point out the boundaries and penalize for infringements.

3. Do not overcrowd the play space. There is danger when groups practice their skills in adjacent areas.

4. Select activities within the physiological and skill limits of the pupils.

5. Seek out the hazards of each game and plan to counteract them.

6. Check exposed projections, gymnasium equipment, lighting, and floor surfaces. Lights should be protected with a heavy wire mesh.

7. Insist that pupils dress in proper uniform with sneakers for all gymnasium activities.

8. Regulate showers from master control panel.

9. Prohibit pushing, wrestling, and fooling around in locker and shower rooms.

On the playgrounds:

1. Enclose the entire playground area with a five or six foot fence.

2. Provide adequate space between pieces of equipment.

3. Mark well and properly space all courts for outside games.

4. Check apparatus for repair items and terrain for foreign objects, such as tree roots or stones.

5. Encourage safe play. Teach the correct use of each piece of apparatus.

6. Carry on team games such as soccer, speedball, and softball in an area away from the apparatus and small children.

7. Reserve one section of the playground that is protected and near the school for kindergarten and first graders.

8. Encourage courtesy, patience, and fair play: they breed a degree of respect for the other fellow and reduce accidents.

Going to and from school:

1. Discuss with children the routes they take home.

2. Encourage parental interest in the safety program, particularly as it concerns going to and from school.

3. Remind children to stay on the walks and in crosswalk lanes, to obey rules, signs, and the traffic directors.

4. Encourage children to report hazardous obstructions along school routes.

5. Cooperate with school bus drivers in the aspects of bus safety.

6. Provide supervision of school traffic patrols.[11]

What has been said here applies primarily to the classroom teacher. If

---

[11] Standard rules governing the operation of school safety patrols have been adopted by states and on a national level by representatives of the National Safety Council, National Congress of Parents and Teachers, National Education Association, American Automobile Association, National Association of Chiefs of Police, and the U.S. Office of Education. Standard rules have been published by the National Safety Council.

school living is at all healthful, it will be due in part to the teacher's convictions and alertness relative to hazardous conditions. She will need to stress directly and indirectly what Abraham Lincoln accentuated more than a century ago, i.e., every man has a personal duty to protect himself and those associated with him, from accidents which may result in injury or death. Thus, learning to protect oneself is a function of the school. The schools have done a splendid job so far not by submerging life's challenging situations, but by teaching that successful living in our modern world requires a degree of intelligence and courage, and that there are certain risks in everyday living that must be faced with determination and bravery.

Questions for Discussion

1.   Should apparatus such as swings, slides, and teeter boards be eliminated from the school playground because of the possibility of accidents?
2.   Does the expression "healthful living" mean more or less to you than "healthful school environment"? Explain.
3.   What are some of the outcomes of democratic human relations in the classroom that relate to healthful living?
4.   Suppose the teacher's personal health influences learning in a negative way. What should be done in a school system to prevent this situation? To remedy it?
5.   Discuss the construction of a check list of items designed to screen the environmental conditions of a school from the viewpoint of health and safety.

Suggested Activities

1. Using more than one source, obtain a list of the desirable qualities of the good teacher. Compare your list with those of your classmates. Would it appear that characteristics of sound mental health are significant? Comment on your findings.

2. Formulate a committee to survey a local school for environmental inadequacies that relate primarily to *safe* living. If possible, obtain and use the *School Safety Education Checklist* (revised, 1967) distributed by the National Committee on Safety Education, National Education Association, Washington, D. C., 20036.

3. Talk with a school physician regarding environmental health problems as they have a bearing on children.

4. Consult the literature of such organizations as the National Safety Council, the National Commission on Safety, and the U. S. Public Health Service, and compare accident statistics for children in the first six grades. Comment on the significance of your findings.

Selected References

A *School Safety Education Program.* Washington, D. C.: National Commission on Safety Education, National Education Association, 1966.
Bidwell, Corrine. "The Teacher as a Listener—an Approach to Mental Health." *Journal of School Health,* 37:373–383, October 1967.

Florio, A. E., and Stafford, G. T. *Safety Education*, 2nd ed. New York: McGraw-Hill Book Company, Inc., 1962, Chapter 5.

Irwin, Leslie W., Cornacchia, Harold J., and Staton, Wesley M. *Health In Elementary Schools*, 2nd ed. St. Louis: C. V. Mosby Co., 1966, Chapter 3.

Mand, Charles L. "The School Environment and Emotional Health." *Journal of School Health*, 32:375–378, November 1962.

Randall, Harriett B. "The Teacher's Responsibility for Mental Health in the Classroom." *Journal of School Health*, 37:448–451, November 1967.

Stack, Herbert J., and Elkow, J. Duke. *Education for Safe Living*. Englewood Cliffs, New Jersey: Prentice-Hall, Inc., 1966.

Normal Growth and Deviations From Normal

The human body is the organ of the will. It is the machine through which the mind works and social behavior is expressed. Every exhibition of mental activity is accompanied by some physical activity and the quantity and quality of mental work depend as certainly upon the conditions of the machine by which it is exhibited as do the quantity and quality of work produced by any less complex man-made mechanism.

These "mind-body machines of ours," says Rogers, "vary greatly in their original capacity for work, just as one type of automobile differs from another; but it would be foolish to expect either a passenger car or a truck to do its best with a flat tire or when supplied with little oil and inferior fuel, and it is just as absurd for a teacher to expect his best school work from a child who has defective sense organs, who is badly fed, insufficiently rested, or who is depressed by other faulty

conditions. There are children who are normally bright and those who are naturally dull, but both the bright and the dull do finer and more persistent mental work when they are physically fit."[1] Certainly, therefore, it is a waste of time and money not to see that "every little human machine is given an overhauling" upon its entrance to school, put in the best possible condition, and looked upon from day to day thereafter to make certain that it does not lapse from that condition or, because of the development of acute disease, become unfit for work or a possible menace to its fellows. It is the teacher's business to carefully observe and spot the abnormal child in a classroom of essentially normal children.

---

[1] Rogers, James F. "What Every Teacher Should Know About the Physical Condition of Her Pupils," Washington: U.S. Government Printing Office, Pamphlet No. 68, 1955, p. 1.

THE CONCEPT OF NORMAL

In discussing normal growth it might be well to refer to a well known quotation from William Shakespeare's *The Merchant of Venice:*

I am a Jew. Hath not a Jew eyes? Hath not a Jew hands, organs, dimensions, senses, affections, passion? . . . fed with the same food, hunt with the same weapons, subject to the same diseases, healed by the same means, warmed and cooled by the same winter and summer, as a Christian is? If you prick us, do we not bleed? If you tickle us, do we not laugh? If you poison us, do we not die? And if you wrong us, shall we not revenge? If we are like you in the rest, we will resemble you in that.

This quotation is intended to reflect the certain fundamental likenesses which all people' have in common. People are never so different that they are not recognizable as human beings, differing only within the limits that human ranges allow. Yet every person differs enough that no two are alike.

What is normal? This question is often disturbing, for in every direction there abounds a multitude of persons and things that are not as they are "supposed to be." A man shuffling along wearing size 13 shoes catches our attention not when he towers well over six feet in height, but when he is only five feet tall. His health may be perfectly normal, but his feet are not; they are too long for a man of his limited height. An appropriate norm table would show this, for a norm is no more than a standard point of reference. It is a kind of average of all extremes of existing characteristics. This may be good or bad, for the norm is in no way an ideal.

A normal characteristic is simply a typical one. It is built around some specific factor or phenomenon and is based solely on generalizations. It considers typical cases and typical behavior and is used for purposes of comparison. If several thousand 12 year old girls have freckles, then freckles are typical and to be expected. If a thousand 12 year old girls, 62 inches tall, generally weigh 90 pounds, then 90 pounds is typical and becomes the norm. We have generalized so that the girls at either extreme, whose weights were part of the several thousand cases, would be below or above normal in weight; they would be labeled "abnormal," "atypical," or "deviants." Yet, there are so many of these deviants in a given sample that they might well represent a large segment of the population.

When an individual is a long way from the norm and is classed atypical, although he is in perfect health, it becomes rather obvious that he is profoundly different and should be treated so if he is to be fully understood. Thus, sociologists, anthropologists, and educators alike think and speak in terms of individual differences for a very good reason. Furthermore, there is almost no such thing as a "normal" human being. Two individuals may compare alike (almost alike) in a certain characteristic, but they may vary immensely in another. It is difficult, then, to say who is normal. Roger Williams, former President of the American Chemical Society, has said that "if 95 per cent of people are normal with respect to one comparable item, only 90 per cent would be normal with respect to two items, 60 per cent would be normal with respect to ten items, and only a little better than half of 1 per cent when we include 100 items."[2] Thus, practically every human being is a deviate in some respect.

To proceed to the question of what is normal health, it must be admitted that it is quite normal to see people with bad teeth, digestive upsets, near-

[2] Williams, Roger J. "Chemistry Makes the Man," *The Saturday Review,* April 6, 1957, p. 42.

sightedness, baldness, aching feet, advanced obesity, or mental instability. It even seems normal for close to a million people to succumb to heart disease each year, but these items can hardly be accepted as desirable even if they come close to being within the normal range of what might be found in a cross section of the population. It is imperative, therefore, that we do not generalize all health characteristics and behavior and be blind to the distinctions which make each of us an individual. Healthy people are different. Healthy children are different. Sheldon admirably points this out in his monumental work on the study of body build and constitutional behavior.[3] Sheldon's findings have been related to educational practice in an article in which it is pointed out that *if children fail to act as we think they should, it is probably because we have not learned to tell them apart.*[4] Williams illustrates it by quoting the Russian novelist, Ivan Turgenev.[5] Turgenev pokes fun at scientists and educators by saying that "a man's capable of understanding anything — how the ether vibrates and what's going on in the sun — but how any other man can blow his nose differently from him, that he's incapable of understanding."

THE NORMALLY HEALTHY CHILD

Educators usually think of the healthy child as one who is well-adjusted to his surroundings, is free from physical defects and organic drains, and demonstrates emotional

stability. He is not necessarily perfect, but he is well. There are other children who are almost as well, but they are not quite up to average when it comes to some special function such as heart efficiency or hearing. In this respect they are considered atypical and abnormal. If, however, they were extremely tall, they would certainly not be typical, yet they could not rightfully be called abnormal from the viewpoint of health; health is not as directly related to height as it is to hearing and heart efficiency. Children with obvious individual differences in body build, physical and mental capacities, behavior, and interests may be completely healthy. But *it will take a teacher who is trained to observe children carefully to be able to select from such a group of individually different children those who deviate too far and appear to need medical or psychiatric help.*

Determining whether a pupil is normally healthy can at times be a most difficult job. Some diseases are carried for a long while and are only slightly noticeable in the early stages. A pupil with tuberculosis, for example, may do nothing more serious than cough occasionally for months, thus behaving not too differently from his compatriots in the class. General behavior is a complex process at best and involves an interrelationship of physical, mental, emotional, and social activity. The body operates as a whole; both *psyche* and *soma* are part of the same constitution. A disease or attitude that affects one has a measurable bearing on the other. Thus a malnourished pupil might be irritable and bite his fingernails in class and be mistaken by the teacher for a pupil with an emotional problem. Or a child might actually have a stomach upset because he was concerned over his inability to recite before the class. This might easily be interpreted to indicate that he ate too many green apples during the noon

---

[3] Sheldon, William H. *The Varieties of Human Temperament.* New York: Harper & Brothers, 1942.

[4] Willgoose, Carl E. "Educational Implications of Constitutional Psychology," *Education,* 73(4):225, December 1952.

[5] Williams, Roger J. *Biochemical Individuality.* New York: John Wiley & Sons, 1957.

hour when in reality it was probably associated with a defense mechanism wherein he became "psychologically" ill, even psychosomatically ill, because he did not know his lesson and was not prepared to recite before the class.

DEVIATIONS FROM NORMAL HEALTH

To understand thoroughly the concept of normal health and its deviations it is necessary that the beginning teacher have a knowledge of the growth and development of boys and girls. (See Chapter 6.) The extremes of early and late maturation may appear to indicate deviations from normal health when such is not the case. Children do not grow according to a rigid, set schedule; there is no growth pattern to which every child must conform. One must be aware of the fact that mental and social growth may be retarded due to genuine physical difficulties. Inadequate hearing, for instance, may result in poor speech or a reluctance to speak. And because social growth in children is more abstract than physical growth, it will again be difficult to note behavior deviations from normal.

It is worth repeating that the elementary school classroom teacher is in a unique position to be of service to the child and his family by detecting abnormalities and referring them to the health service personnel. This teacher also has the opportunity to advance the health instruction program through the method of selecting pupils in need of health counseling and working with them on an individual basis.

One can learn the characteristics of optimum child health and can also become familiar with the common deviations. Since most people are more familiar with the marks of good health, this chapter will call attention chiefly to the signs and departures.[6]

Teachers may see what is often missed by parents who are too close to their children, and what would be of interest to physicians and nurses if they had access to the child on a daily basis. They may be puzzled if a hitherto cooperative child becomes inattentive, or the otherwise bright child is unusually slow in learning to read, or the ordinarily happy and enthusiastic youngster develops a case of extreme docility. They may wonder about pimples around the mouth, swollen glands in the neck, low shoulders, underweight and malnutrition, or excessive snuffing or coughing. It is when teachers *are* this much concerned with what they have seen that pupils may be helped early and at a time when the greatest good can be accomplished in remedying the situation.

What are the signs and characteristics of general poor health, specific physical and mental defects and conditions which can be readily detected in day-to-day contact with boys and girls? Following are some that relate to long-standing defects, chronic illness, neurological disturbances, improper nutrition, and poor health habits.

IMPORTANT POINTS FOR OBSERVATION
Height and Weight

Numerous misconceptions exist regarding weight changes and health status. Maturation and growth are influential variables. Bulk weight is not in itself a sign of health. A pupil of

---

[6] The treatment of the topic will be brief for no attempt is made here to embrace the area of health abnormalities of schoolchildren. Such a topic is broad enough to fill a book. It is referred to here only because observing pupil deviations is a part of the total school health program and is one method of health instruction useful in the grades.

normal height and weight may be suffering from some hidden abnormality or disease. Probably less than 4 per cent of obese or thin children have any glandular disturbances. White and Negro pupils are larger than Mexican and Japanese. Extremes of body build, although somewhat related to nutrition and activity, are quite apt to reflect constitutional patterns passed along from parents or families. The better norm tables allow for individual variations in structure.

Evidence of the wide variation of weight for age was clearly demonstrated by Falkner for white North American children in an extensive study of physical growth. At age ten, for example, boys varied in height (between the fifth and ninety-fifth percentiles) by as much as nine inches and in weight by as much as 40 pounds. Girls at age ten varied six and one-half inches in height and 47 pounds in weight.[7]

Since there is a relationship between the quality of growth and the rate of learning, it is appropriate to weigh and measure boys and girls. Moreover, this is a first-class health instruction activity.

Children should be weighed wearing as little clothing as practicable and without shoes. Although the frequency of measurement varies in different schools, the most effective screening combines monthly weighing with height measurements two or three times a year. This procedure screens out the approximately 10 per cent of elementary schoolchildren who fail to gain weight for three successive months between September and May. Failure to realize a weight gain in three to four months is nearly always a sign that something is wrong, either because of poor health habits, disease, or conditions which call for medical examination.

A simple record for each child is suitable for classroom use. Individual growth records are available for each pupil; the Meredith Tables are useful. So is the Wetzel Grid for revealing trends in growth [8]

Deviations in Appearance and Behavior.

Failure to gain in height and weight over a three to six month period

Excessive overweight

Small and underweight for age

Fluctuating weight changes

Skin

The skin shows a great deal to the observing teacher. Pale pupils who appear flushed, and rosy cheeked pupils who appear pale, are usually not up to par. Skin eruptions such as impetigo are very contagious. A number of communicable childhood diseases begin with a flushed or spotted skin. Vesicles appear in chickenpox, red rash in measles, and pallor in malnutrition. Skin deviations are often accompanied by fever, chills, headache, and loss of appetite.

From the pupil's viewpoint skin eruptions are serious in terms of personal appearance; social health seems more important than physical health.

Deviations in Appearance and Behavior.

Pale or sallow

Flushed appearance

Eczematous condition with rashes, scales, and crusts

Persistent sores

Pimples

Acne on face

Boils, warts

Cuts, scratches, bruises, burns

Blueness or pallor of lips

Common skin disease such as ringworm, impetigo, scabies ("itch"), and pink eye

Sensitivity to several substances; allergy

---

[7] See report, together with growth tables, in *Obesity and Health*. Washington, D.C.: U.S. Public Health Service, 1966, p. 11.

[8] The Wetzel Grid is published by National Education Association Service Inc., 1200 W. Third Street, Cleveland, Ohio.

Easily bruised
Itching or burning skin
Fever

Teeth and Mouth

The pupil with a foul odor on the breath day after day probably has a mouth, tooth, nose, or alimentary disorder. Decayed teeth and diseased tonsils are often accompanied by enlarged glands. Total body infection, over-all fatigue, and poor appetite may be caused by grossly decayed teeth. Diseased teeth and tonsils set the stage for sore throats, inner ear disturbances, speech disorders, and the more serious viral and bacterial infections. Dental defects occur among children about six times as rapidly as the rate at which they are being corrected.

Deviations in Appearance and Behavior.

Bad breath
Cavities in teeth
Excessive tartar at necks of teeth
Toothache
Malocclusion
Irregular spacing of teeth
Protruding and broken teeth
Speech difficulty
Inflamed or bleeding gums
Sores in mouth
Cracked lips, especially in corners of mouth

Neck

Swollen lymph glands are visible as lumps on the side of the neck and below the ears. They are readily seen in mumps and other systemic infections. Glands appearing as small lumps may be large when examined by touch. Swollen and tender glands demand immediate attention.

Enlargement of the thyroid gland is usually accompanied by rapid heart rate, more than normal sweating, and irritability and distractibility in the classroom.

Deviations in Appearance and Behavior.

Enlarged lymph glands
Enlarged thyroid glands on either side of windpipe
Position of neck out of alignment with spine

Hair and Scalp

Dirty children with dirty underclothes often have unclean hair and scalp. The white eggs (nits) of head lice (pediculi) cling to hair while female gray-backs move about. Pubic lice invade the groin area and cause much scratching. Micro-organism infections may follow lice and ringworm; both are highly communicable.

Brittle hair and dry scalp often accompany cases of malnutrition. Pride in oneself begins with combed hair.

Deviations in Appearance and Behavior.

Uncombed, uncontrolled hair
Dirty, dry scalp
Signs of vermin and ringworm
Brittle, stringy, and lusterless hair
Small bald spots
Crusty sores on scalp
Excessive dandruff
Frequent head scratching

Upper Respiratory Tract (Nose, Throat, Sinuses)

Nasal and throat abnormalities affect the quality of the voice. Speech improvement comes about when the nasal passage is clear and mouth breathing ceases.

Sinuses and the middle ear may be acutely infected in colds, measles, scarlet fever, diphtheria, influenza, typhoid, and infected teeth. Diseased tonsils and adenoid tissue are deleterious to the whole upper respiratory tract.

Enlarged mucous membranes (hypersecretion) are present with severe head cold and hay fever. Mucous membranes are continuous within eyes, nose, mouth, throat, inner ears, bronchial tubes, and lungs.

Deviations in Appearance and Behavior.

Speech thick or muffled
Mouth breathing
Frequent sore throats
Persistent nasal discharge
Excessive colds
Frequent school absences
Difficulty in swallowing
Sore or scratchy throat
Discharge from ears
Frequent snuffing and coughing
Face or forehead pain (sinusitis)
Fever and bad breath
Sudden sneezing spells associated with allergies

Nutrition

Good nutritional status means much in terms of appearance, vigor, and personal enthusiasm for school activities. The classroom teacher is more effective here than any other person; behavior is so general that one must notice several of the accompanying signs before suspecting malnutrition.

Deviations in Appearance and Behavior.

General fatigue; tires easily
Poor, sloppy postural attitude; postural defects
Frequent and prolonged infections
Restlessness and irritability
Fingernail biting
Difficulty going to sleep
Restlessness during sleep
Lack of ambition
Dark circles or puffiness under eyes
Flabby musculature; possible muscle and joint pain
Poor teeth
Lack of appetite
Dry, scaly scalp, hair, and skin
History of sore mouth, tongue, or gums
Abnormal intolerance of light

Posture and Body Mechanics

Posture is a functional item and involves total body movement especially standing and sitting, and attitude and gait in walking.

Functional difficulties due to weak musculature, uneven length of the legs, or one's temporary mental attitude may be corrected by exercises and activities assigned by the physician and physical educator, and reinforced by the encouraging words of the classroom teacher. Structural defects (immobile bumps or enlarged joints) need special medical attention.

Even minor postural defects need to be discovered and remedied early in order to obtain the greatest body efficiency in later years.

Many times postural abnormalities are indicative of poor nutrition, organic strains, hidden disease, low physical fitness, sedentary living, chronic fatigue, hearing defects, emotional disturbance, and asthma.

Other things being equal, the way the schoolchild feels at any one moment is often reflected in his posture.

Deviations in Appearance and Behavior.

Flabby musculature
Chronic fatigue
Round shoulders (kyphosis)
Head forward
One shoulder lower than the other
Protruding shoulder blades (winged scapulae)
Pigeon or funnel chest (rickets)
Lateral curvature of spine (scoliosis)
Unequal height of hips
Irregular gait in walking
Arches of feet are flat
Feet toe-out too far in standing and walking
Tendon above heel bone is bowed inward when standing
Heels of shoes wear down on inside borders
Pain in joints of body
Pain in bones of foot

Eyes

The list of deviations is rich in items that the classroom teacher can observe easily, especially in terms of reading difficulties. Some 80 per cent of the work a child does in elementary school is built around visual acuity within arm's reach; it is most important that visual difficulties be corrected just as early in the grades as possible.

Seeing is a process both of eye optics and brain development. Young children are normally far-sighted and see large objects, large print, and pictures, quite well. In most schools students are screened for difficulties involving visual accommodation. Three fourths of all study activities in the elementary school require reading ability. Promotion from first to second grades is often on the basis of reading ability. Yet four out of five retarded readers have normal intelligence. The teacher may notice that the retarded reader often achieves considerable success in those activities where reading skills are not of primary importance.

School surveys show that less than half the children who need glasses actually have them. School follow-up programs need more attention and control.

Early and repeated examinations are important. Good lighting, frequent rest periods, and the avoidance of prolonged sewing, drawing, painting, or reading by primary grade pupils are recommended.

Instruction should be given in how to view television and how to protect eyesight in the home and community. Some 20 to 25 per cent of all schoolchildren have eye defects.

Deviations in Appearance and Behavior.

Complaints of dizziness, headache, nausea

Crusts on lids among lashes

Red rims on lids

Watery eyes; styes

Swollen eyelids

Reading difficulties:

Holds book far away from face when reading

Holds body tense or thrusts head forward at distant objects

Holds face close to page when reading

Inattentive in wall chart, blackboard, or map lesson

Reads but brief periods without stopping

Screws up face when reading or looking at distant objects

Shuts or covers one eye when reading

Tilts head to one side when reading

Tends to look cross-eyed when reading

Tends to make frequent changes in distance at which book is held

Confusion in reading and spelling *o* and *a; e* and *c; n* and *c; h, n* and *r; f* and *t*

Apparently guesses from quick recognition of parts of the word in easy reading material

Rubs eyes frequently

Poor alignment in writing

Reversal tendencies in reading

Attempts to brush away a blur

Irritation over work or some emotional display

Strabismus or "squint"

Ear

Children with hearing loss in the classroom account for a sizeable proportion of all people with hearing loss. Two children in every classroom have a hearing problem. Early detection through screening tests permits the parent to obtain treatment reasonably quickly for the child. Pure tone audiometer testing permits quick sweep checks up to the 8000 frequency level. Some pupils fail the 4000 to 8000 high range, others fail the range below 500; but it is important for them to hear in the middle range. With middle range loss the child is experiencing much difficulty. Also, 35 per cent of the failures are in both ears.

Hearing loss varies, indicating a need for constant teacher observation and annual screening tests.

Deviations in Appearance and Behavior.

Discharge or odor from ears

Earache

Failure to answer and misunderstandings

Habit of saying "what?"

Turning head to one side when spoken to

Facial expressions indicating a lack of awareness of all that is going on

Heart

Children with heart defects total about 1 per cent of the school-age population. Most of these children can take part in the normal classroom program. With some degree of restriction, most of these pupils may engage in modified or adapted physical education activities.

Rheumatic fever is declining in incidence and severity, but there are still many children whose heart valves are impaired due to this disease or other chronic infections such as scarlet fever, pneumonia, streptococcus sore throat, measles, mumps, and tonsillitis.

Heart disease in children is prevented by observing and acting on prolonged infections (sore throats or persistent fatigue) and by making sure the child engages in stimulating physical activity, eats nutritious foods, partakes of recreation, and obtains adequate sleep.

Deviations in Appearance and Behavior.

Fainting and dizzy spells

Rapid heart beat

Irregular pulse

Frequent complaints of pain in joints, arms, legs

Repeated nose bleeds

Clubbed fingers

Shortness of breath and sudden flushing of the face on exertion

Early fatigue

Failure to gain weight

Blueness of lips (cyanosis)

Social-Emotional Adjustment

Every young child needs from his teacher a degree of love, warmth, praise, and consistency. He needs gentle and firm guidance and someone interested in his welfare. With these factors he becomes secure, sticks to his tasks, sees himself in relation to his class, is tolerant and creative, possesses an outgoing attitude toward others, profits from his mistakes as well as successes, and, above all else, is a happy pupil equipped to live life with zest, enthusiasm, and hope.

The signs indicating deviations from normal social-emotional behavior are all about. To the observing teacher they are as evident as pimples on the face, and, like many physical ailments, they are best controlled or remedied through early detection and treatment.

Deviations in Appearance and Behavior.

Infantile speech

Unestablished toilet habits

Restlessness, nail-biting, stammering or lip-sucking not due to any discoverable physical cause

Frequent accidents or near-accidents

Over-timidity; seclusiveness

Over-aggressiveness; constant quarreling with others

Suspicion and fearfulness

Excessive day dreaming; inattentiveness not due to any discoverable physical cause

Extreme sensitiveness to criticism; feelings hurt easily; cries easily

Failure to advance in school work at a normal rate in spite of adequate physical health and satisfactory intellectual capacity

Extreme docility or anxiety to please

Excessive boasting, showing off, attracting undue attention

Resistance to authority, constant complaints of being discriminated against or "picked on"

Poor sportsmanship, some unwillingness to engage in group activities which might result in losing or in loss of face; playing unfairly or cheating in group games

A Health Manual for the Classroom Teacher

As she lacks medical training, the classroom teacher feels the need of professional guidance to help her face many of the everyday health problems that she meets in the classroom and on the school grounds. A manual gives the teacher in non-medical terms the knowledge she should have about accidents, emergencies, and responsibilities. It also sets forth in detail many of the health deviations in appearance and behavior as well as the symptoms of communicable diseases, which may be seen in and about the school.

A useful health manual for teachers is one which summarizes the symptoms and signs of diseases. The summary on pages 92–95 illustrates the nature of this kind of teacher's guide and should be of value to the reader of this chapter.

Suggested Activities

1. Visit a large elementary school and ask the school nurse how many cases there are of serious allergies, heart defects, epilepsy, diabetes, and orthopedic defects. Having determined this, find out how many of these children have restricted programs and to what extent. How do you feel about the adequacies of restricted programs?

2. Compile a list of the health characteristics of schoolchildren; keep the mental and physical items separate. Having done this, visit a school nurse or physician and inquire about the frequency with which these characteristics appear in a given school situation.

3. Arrange for several individuals to solicit from several different school departments copies of health manuals or written instructions to teachers relative to health observations and practices in the school system.

Questions for Discussion

1. What evidence is there to show that mentally healthy elementary schoolchildren show greater achievement in schoolwork?
2. From your reading and experience, where does the detection and referral program fall down?
3. What are the general characteristics of appearance and behavior associated with good physical health?
4. Consider the signs of good social-emotional behavior. What are several ways these signs may be developed within the limits of classroom activity? Playground activity?
5. Discuss the proposition that "the observation of normal growth, coupled with deviations from normal, provides a usable method of health instruction."
6. What can be done to help children of indigent parents receive glasses or hearing aids if they need them?

SUMMARY

Disease	Recognition	Prevention	Incubation	Control	General
Common cold	Sniffles, sneezing. Feels poor. Coughing common.	General good health helps.	1-2 days.	Isolate fresh cases for 3 days. Encourage parents to keep child home. Teach proper use of tissues.	Most frequent reason for absenteeism. Potentially dangerous because of ear, lung, throat, complications.
Influenza	Cold symptoms, but child is sick, feverish and weak.	Vaccine, particularly effective, protection only 6-12 months.	1-3 days.	Isolate fresh cases for 5 days from onset.	More serious, "grippy" cold with high fever. Occurs sporadically each winter.
Chickenpox (varicella)	Small spots and blisters on body and at hairline. Often fever. Itching.	None.	12-21 days; usually 13-17 days.	Isolate and exclude for 6 days after rash.	Common, minor illness, highly contagious among susceptibles.
Diphtheria	Sore throat with white patches; fever.	Effective with 3 doses of toxoid. Boosters every 3 to 5 years.	2-5 days.	Isolate in hospital. May not return until Health Department approves. Classmates and other close contacts receive immunization.	Very dangerous disease—now almost eradicated through mass immunization.
German measles (rubella)	Mildly ill, if at all. Pinkish spots on body, arms, *not* on face.	None, for disease.	14-21 days; usually 18 days.	Exclude case 3 days from appearance of rash.	A common, highly contagious but mild disease.
Measles (rubeola)	Cough, red eyes, fever, followed by blotchy rash on face and body.	Measles vaccine.	10 days to first symptoms. 14 days to rash.	Exclude for 7 days following appearance of rash.	A common, highly contagious acute illness. Most common complications: ear infection, pneumonia.

Mumps (infectious parotitis)	Swelling of cheeks or 1 or more salivary glands; fever.	None effective.	12-26 days; usually 18 days.	Exclude until swelling disappears, or 1 week from onset.	A relatively common and usually mild disease in children, not very contagious.
Streptococcal infections including scarlet fever	Sore throat with fever. Hurts to swallow. Diffuse red rash with tiny spots in scarlet fever.	Antibiotics given promptly.	2-5 days.	Exclude according to pre-arranged school plan. Observe classmates for one week.	A common disease which can be complicated by rheumatic fever, heart disease, or nephritis. "Scarlatina" is the same disease.
Whooping cough	Characteristic cough, with choking, redness of face, and "whoop" on drawing breath.	Vaccine usually given with diphtheria and tetanus to infants. Not desirable for older children.	7-10 days.	Exclude for three weeks after onset of typical cough.	An increasingly rare disease especially among pre-school children.
Athlete's foot	Peeling, cracking redness and occasionally oozing between toes or soles of foot.	Scrupulous foot hygiene. Rigid cleaning of locker and shower rooms.	10-14 days.	Exclude from physical education, locker and shower rooms. Check custodial job.	Mild, very common fungus infection of feet, especially feet which perspire easily; occurring wherever people go barefoot frequently.
Impetigo	Moist patches on skin around mouth, on hands with brown yellow crusts.	Good hygiene.	2-5 days.	Exclude until treatment is started and lesions dry.	Common bacterial infection of skin, mostly in younger children with poor hygiene.
Lice	"Nits" seen; itching scalp, "mobile dandruff."	Good hygiene.	1-2 days.	Exclude until treated. Check classmates' heads at discovery and 2 weeks later.	Parasitic infestations of hair, mostly girls, directly related to poor hygiene.

Ringworm of scalp	Patchy baldness with stubble left.	Good hygiene.	10-14 days.	Exclude until treatment started. Must wear cap, but not take physical education.	Hard to clear up fungus infection of scalp. Rare after puberty.
Pinworms	Itching behind, crankiness, vague stomach pains.	Good hygiene.	4-8 days.	No exclusion necessary, little chance of spread in school. Enforce handwashing.	A common, mild, worm infection, with more unrecognized cases than known.
"Pinkeye" (conjunctivitis)	Reddened, irritated, weepy eyes. Often whitish discharge with sticky eyelids.	None.	1-3 days.	Exclude only in grades K-3. Observe classmates one week.	May accompany cold; more often a mild virus infection.
Poliomyelitis (infantile paralysis)	Headache, stiff neck, fever.	Either series of polio shots or oral vaccine. Consult physician.	7-21 days; usually 12 days.	Exclude 2 weeks. Observe classmates and give booster vaccinations.	A potentially crippling disease coming in about 7 year waves.
Tuberculosis	By tuberculin test and x-ray.	Early detection.	6-8 weeks; occasionally month.	Routine mass testing. Test and x-ray of classmates.	Usually very mild and often unrecognized in school age children. Source is an adult.
Meningitis	Fever, violent headache, stiff neck.	None available. Contacts can be protected by drugs.	Variable, but seldom over 10 days.	Isolate in hospital. If meningococcal exclude from family until treatment starts.	A group of diseases, caused by many agents—some serious, others not.
Tetanus (lockjaw)	Stiffness of face muscles, neck and back.	Mass immunization. Booster doses whenever child is cut or wounded.	4-21 days.	Booster dose for child with dirty cuts or wounds.	Poison from germ in dirty wounds affects nervous system; highly fatal. Not contagious.

Infectious mononucleosis	Persistent fatigue, low grade fever, sore throat.	None known.	4-14 days.	Exclude from school until fever is gone.	A not very contagious virus disease that may take a week to get over.
Infectious hepatitis	Jaundice, fever, vomiting.	Clean water and food. Can be prevented in contacts by gammaglobulin.	10-60 days; usually 25 days.	Exclude 2 weeks; or until well.	A virus disease affecting the liver —long recovery period needed.
Cat-scratch fever	Sore at site of scratch, with swollen glands, accompanied by fever.	Avoid cat scratches.	2-8 days.	Exclude until child feels well.	Virus disease from cats. Mild. Not contagious.

Selected References

Anderson, C. L. *School Health Practice,* 3rd ed. St. Louis: C. V. Mosby Co., 1964, Chapters 2, 3 and 5.

Hein, Fred. "School Days Should be Healthy Days." *Today's Health,* 62:90, September 1964.

Sheldon, William H. *The Varieties of Human Physique.* New York: Harper & Brothers, 1940.

Stuart, Harold C., and Brugh, D. G. *The Healthy Child, His Physical, Psychological, and Social Development.* Cambridge, Mass.: Harvard University Press, 1960.

Turner, C. E., Sellery, C. M., and Smith, S. L. *School Health and Health Education,* 5th ed. St. Louis: C. V. Mosby Co., 1966, Chapter 5.

Wetzel, Norman C. "New Dimensions in the Simultaneous Screening and Assessment of School Children." *Journal of Health, Physical Education and Recreation,* 37:33–35, May 1966.

Willgoose, Carl E. "Body Types and Physical Fitness." *Journal of Health, Physical Education and Recreation,* 27:26–28, September 1956.

The Health Instruction Program

CHAPTER 6

*We need education in the obvious
more than in investigation of the
obscure.*

—OLIVER WENDELL HOLMES

The entire elementary school staff has a responsibility for the school health program. At some time or other all of them will find themselves teaching some aspect of physical, mental, emotional, or social health. But for the most part, it is the classroom teacher who carries on the health instruction. This is no longer done haphazardly as in the past. Today it is a planned program. Health education is a basic area of the curriculum along with arithmetic, science, language, physical 'education, music, art, social studies, and other areas. In a sense health instruction programs have "come of age." This has occurred chiefly because of the current needs of children and adults in a civilization that is becoming more and more complex. And amid the complexities are health problems that cannot be solved by leaving them to chance.

The validity of the Holmes quotation which introduces this chapter is strikingly sound. Indeed, the vitality of a people is firmly linked to a knowledge of the obvious. In the long run individual health status has more to do with understanding the advances of medical science than with creating remedies and corrective devices for human inadequacies. Dr. Albert Starr, cobuilder of a highly successful artificial heart valve, reinforces this viewpoint when he says, ". . . Our job is not to design a valve identical to nature's, not to see how close we can come to duplicating a natural phenomenon, but to overcome the clinical problems of the diseased heart valve." Hopefully, therefore, the next step in the evolution of mankind will be a self-conscious striving to *prevent* destructive illnesses and maladjustments through a carefully developed curri-

97

culum—one that will help close the wide gap between the advent of medical discoveries and the application of medical findings.

THE NATURE OF HEALTH INSTRUCTION

Instructional programs are geared to the principles of learning and carried on in the light of individual pupil differences. These programs are good chiefly because of good teachers. When classroom teachers understand the purposes of health instruction, the program becomes a significant part of the total school health effort.

The broad topic of health instruction in the elementary grades is related to a large number of factors which include program objectives, pupil needs, pupil interests, capacities, and other psychological considerations. Also included are teacher qualifications, educational methods, material sources and aids, and evaluation. Needless to say, instruction becomes a complicated topic, one that must be approached with patience and understanding.

The general objectives of the health instruction program are about the same for all the elementary grades.[1] But the specific objectives for the primary area will differ from those for the intermediate area. Essentially, this difference is due to the varying capacities and needs associated with chronological age and growth.

Health instruction may be defined as the organization of learning ex-periences directed toward the development of favorable health knowledges, attitudes, and practices. Although the fundamental purpose of instruction is to impart knowledge, there should always be a greater emphasis on the formation of desirable practices and attitudes resulting from instruction. Knowledge of mere facts and mechanical skills is of doubtful value; no knowledge is complete until it is understood enough to be applied. The age-old expression, "understanding passeth knowledge," is most appropriate, for, despite the truth that knowledge is at the base of all understanding, it is understanding that is behind man's most effective actions.

The desired outcome of health instruction is a change in the behavior of the pupils. This is revealed through daily habits of school and community living, the expression of positive health attitudes, and the grasp of a body of scientific knowledge which provides a basis for intelligent self-direction. To accomplish these outcomes is quite a difficult task. It is relatively easy to impart knowledge in the classroom. Children, for example, will readily learn the names of the vitamins or the rules of bicycle safety without having it affect their pattern of living in any way. Moreover, it is even conceivable that the same children may have no particular feeling or attitude toward the previously discussed vitamins or bicycle riding. In such a case the knowledge has been "book knowledge" or "test knowledge." It has not been understood and acted upon. The school health instruction program, therefore, must be concerned with certain elements that will *effectively* educate for health.

THE ESSENCE OF UNDERSTANDING

The term "understanding" is both a psychological process and an educational outcome. To possess it is to have

---

[1] Oberteuffer points out that school health instruction is offered to secure behavior favorable to a high quality of living; to assist in the development of a well-integrated personality; to clarify thinking about personal and public health matters, to remove superstitions, false beliefs, and ignorance; to facilitate the development of security through the acquisition of scientific knowledge; to enrich the life of the community; and to establish the ability in students to see cause and effect. See Oberteuffer, Delbert, and Beyrer, Mary K. *School Health Education*, 4th ed. New York: Harper & Brothers, 1966, Chapter 2.

more than a knowledge of particulars. A pupil does not begin to understand until he is able to react to factual information by moving, feeling, or thinking intelligently with respect to a given situation. Activity is the key word—the kind of activity discussed at length by educational philosophers of the John Dewey era, i.e., "pupils learn by doing." The more activity engaged in, the more senses . . . stimulated, the greater the retention and recall of information to be learned.

In recent years it has been emphasized that the way to successful instruction and eventual understanding is to take heed of the following:

1. Factual information must have meaning for the individual if it is to be translated into proper health practices. How a child perceives an item is significant. This is substantiated by the Committee of the Association for Supervision and Curriculum Development in their publication *Perceiving, Behaving, Becoming,* in which it is pointed out that learning is the exploration and discovery of personal meaning in a process that must be a highly personal one.[2] To structure personal experiences in a curriculum is difficult, for the schools are part of the society that has made a fetish of the elements of objectivity—facts, figures, and phenomena.

2. Life in school must be stimulating and rewarding. In the early school years it is more important that pupils develop a liking for learning and for the school environment than that specific subject matter be remembered.

3. Relationships and principles are more important than scattered and rote information. In perceiving what they are learning, children may respond more to specific questions involving personal discovery than to the traditional questions so frequently used to initiate a unit of work. In short, it is not uncommon to ask children the wrong questions.

Jerome Bruner has written at length on the importance of discovery. He has said:

---

[2] Association for Supervision and Curriculum Development. *Perceiving, Behaving, Becoming —A New Focus on Education.* Washington, D.C.: National Education Association, 1962.

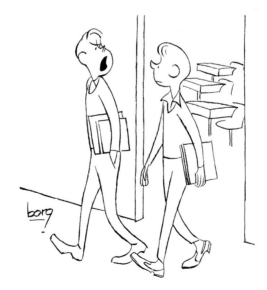

"What gets me is when someone comes up with the answer before I understand the question."

The virtues of encouraging discovery are of two kinds. In the first place the child will make what he learns his own, will fit his discovery into the interior world of culture that he creates for himself. Equally important, discovery and the sense of confidence it provides is the proper reward for learning. It is a reward that, moreover, strengthens the very process that is the heart of education — disciplined inquiry.[3]

4. Although verbalization has weaknesses, most understandings should be verbalized.

Symbols such as words, numbers, or formulas are examples of verbalized understandings. In all areas of instruction they have to be used sooner or later. "Vitamin A" is symbolic of a body of information, but it is meaningless unless it is associated with the realities for which it stands. In health education there may be many empty verbalizations that are recited parrot-like by children in dozens of classrooms around the country. Children are taught too often by rote learning. They sing "My country *tears* of thee," and recite that "the circulatory system is composed of arteries, veins, and *artilleries.*" Why does this happen? It seems that there is too much emphasis on isolated items rather than upon wholes and relationships; too much memorization of what has been brought to one's attention, and undue attention given to individual recitations as contrasted with cooperative group activity. Also, there is at times in all classrooms the tendency to make instruction and artificial item by divorcing it from the ordinary activities of life.

5. The student's understanding is inferred from observing what he says and does with respect to his needs.

What the pupil says and does, or fails to say and do, about health situations confronting him, determines the

amount and kind of understanding he has developed as a result of a particular program of health instruction. The child who fails to register any particular attitude is sometimes as bad as the child who takes on a negative one. In fact, the child who fails to react to all may be much worse off. Teachers of health, therefore, should continuously appraise their instructional programs. This is especially necessary in the elementary grades where children are not yet mature enough to put distractions aside and fare well under the lecture method.

In addition to what has been said about understanding, there are other guiding concepts which should be considered when health instruction is being examined. Some of these concepts are so sound that they border on being principles. They apply not only to the health area but to all subject matter areas. For example, the laws of learning apply to health instruction, and readiness to learn is a highly prized characteristic when a new topic is brought to the attention of the pupils; motivation influences behavior and sets the stage for optimum learning; interests and needs influence learning, and they may be cultivated; children are taught positively what to do, not what not to do; provisions for individual and group differences improve instruction; drill is effective if related to pupil goals; rewards are superior to punishment in promotion of learning; interest in the activity provides the drive to engage in it; attitudes manifested in several situations become real — "wide use favors habit"; socializing the activity promotes retention and recall; and success in a subject matter item breeds security in a subject matter area. Needless to say, this is only a partial list of generally recognized concepts relative to learning and understanding. Health instruction can never quite succeed where psychological factors such as these are ignored or treated haphazardly.

---

[3] Bruner, Jerome S. *On Knowing.* Cambridge: Harvard University Press, 1963, p. 124.

FACTORS THAT DETERMINE WHAT TO TEACH

There is only one subject matter for education, and that is life in all its manifestations.[4]
— ALFRED NORTH WHITEHEAD

This statement should discourage once and for all the people who are disturbed over the fact that the schools seem to be in the business of teaching something about everything. Certainly if life is to be lived realistically, at the moment within the school environment and after one's formal education terminates, then there is truth to the statement. Yet everything cannot be brought to the attention of school-children. There simply is not enough time. How then does one determine what to teach? Where does a teacher begin?

Determining Pupil Needs in General

What children need to receive from the elementary school is pretty much what society wants children to have. Since the child grows up in an American culture, the culture molds him and influences the nature of his needs.

The basic needs of elementary schoolchildren have been set forth in five categories by the Bureau of Elementary Curriculum Development in New York State as follows:[5]

A Child Needs:

1. Interpersonal and intergroup relations.

2. Understanding of the world and people and things.

3. Self-development.

4. Control of the communicative arts and skills.

5. Moral and spiritual values.

Society Wants Every Child:

1. To understand and practice desirable social relationships toward individuals and groups, and within the many varied groups of which he is a member. To be a good neighbor and good citizen of the world.
2. To appreciate and participate in worthwhile activities with others at home and abroad.
3. To discover and develop desirable individual aptitudes, interests, and abilities.
   To develop powers of creative expression.
   To have sound physical and mental health.
4. To cultivate the habit of constructive, careful thinking.
   To gain command of common integrating knowledge and skills.
5. To develop sound emotional attitudes and habits.
   To appreciate and accept for himself moral and spiritual values.

[4] Whitehead, Alfred North. *The Aims of Education and Other Essays.* New York: The Macmillan Co., 1929.

[5] The Bureau of Elementary Curriculum Development. *The Elementary School Curriculum.* Albany: New York State Education Department, 1954, p. 13.

To determine what to teach, Rath and Metcalf studied the needs of children and set up eight groups of needs:

1. A feeling of belonging
2. A sense of achievement
3. Economic security
4. Freedom from fear
5. Love and affection
6. Freedom from guilt
7. A share in making decisions
8. Integration in attitudes, beliefs, and values[6]

Whatever phase of health is taught must be done in the light of these needs for these are bona fide feelings that children have — even if they are not aware of them at the time. The interrelationship of these needs is impressive. Layman makes this clear in reviewing psychogenic and psychosomatic research. She points out:

> Studies of infants have shown quite strikingly how a single type of experience can contribute toward organic health, intellectual development, emotional security, and socialization. For example, a common sight in children's hospitals and institutions is that of babies who are undersized and emaciated, with the wizened features of little old men. These babies may have somatic symptoms, such as chronic diarrhea or cyclic vomiting. Invariably, they are retarded in development of skills in all areas. Usually they do not smile when spoken to, and their reaction to people is one of withdrawal. Often the baby lies quietly with thumb in mouth, seemingly unaware of what goes on around him, or stares at the bars of his crib.
>
> The histories of these babies show that usually they have been fed according to a formula prescribed by a pediatrician and have been adequately cared for in terms of attention to physiological needs. What they have lacked has been warmth and love from the mother. If this type of deprivation continues, they become

mentally retarded children, socially unrelated, and physically underdeveloped. Nearly 40 per cent of such children die before reaching school age.

On the other hand, if these babies receive tender loving care from a mothering person before this process has gone too far, they can develop into strong, husky, intelligent, happy individuals. Thus, we see how what we would regard as an emotional need is related to physiological functioning and intelligence as well as to emotional and social development.[7]

Determining Pupil Health Needs

Prior to setting up the health curriculum it is necessary to ascertain the child's characteristics for a certain age, his health needs, and his health interests. Children vary in constitution, growth and development, health status, and background of experience. Some have health problems that others know relatively little about. If, however, there are enough children with a particular health problem, then there is a need in the curriculum for instruction in this area. Sometimes a problem is school-wide. Hookworm and intestinal parasites, for instances, are always of concern in certain southern states and have to be discussed regularly.

It is safe to say that there has been considerable difference of opinion as to the amount of emphasis that one should place on different types of needs. All are important to some degree, but in the interest of economy, some needs must be considered more vital than others. Furthermore, there is a strong point of view that it is not the school's responsibility to meet all of the needs. There are numerous agencies, institutions, and individuals which share this responsibility. The home, the church, scout organizations,

---

[6] Rath, Louise, and Metcalf, Lawrence. "An Instrument for Identifying Some Needs of Children," *Educational Research Bulletin*, 24:169, October 1945.

[7] Layman, Emma McCloy. "Emotional Health," *Journal of Health, Physical Education, and Recreation*, 28(3):22, March 1957.

4-H clubs, libraries, recreation centers, radio, television, and summer camps all play a part in meeting the needs of children. The school must do its share, but not attempt to carry the whole burden by itself. Dispensing health information is an example of a shared responsibility, for other community organizations do it too. Many schools cooperate in 4-H and scout work and set aside time for religious instruction.

It is quite easy to say that most growing children have about the same health needs. They all need good nutrition and proper eating habits, protection against illness and disease, avoidance of accidents, sleep and rest, regular elimination of body wastes, continuous care of eyes, ears and teeth, good body mechanics and posture, good emotional adjustment, the right attitude toward the opposite sex, and an understanding of themselves. It is not uncommon to find states and larger cities that have excellent courses of study in health which have been carefully prepared over a long period of time to meet the health needs, interests, and capacities of children. Such courses of study are made available to classroom teachers as a basis on which the program can be planned. No one will quarrel with this. But, as good as these courses of study are, they should be used only as guides, for much of the material contained therein will amplification or adjustment in some way to fit the needs of the local community and the particular pupils.

When one considers the whole child in a society that is continually changing, it is readily seen that needs are something more than psychological, social, intellectual, and emotional; they are also individual, moral, and spiritual. Thus the conscientious teacher has quite a task ahead of her as each school year begins. It will be necessary to seek the answers to some of these questions on needs before arranging the course of instruction in final form:

Question 1. What are the characteristics of my children at specific age levels? In short, what are the signs of growth and development in terms of physical, intellectual, social, and emotional behavior?

Characteristics and Needs of the Elementary School Child

General Characteristics	Needs
1. *Physical Characteristics* Large muscles are better developed than small ones. Can run, jump, skip, climb; enjoy simple tag games, group singing and singing games. May frequently be clumsy and awkward, and continuous activity brings on early fatigue. Eye and hand coordination not well established. Farsightedness prevails.	To experience basic body movements involving the arms, legs and trunk, with and without music and rhythms. To participate in games with simple rules and boundaries. To have quiet periods of activity; to have rest periods. To have large pictures and large print to read.
2. *Health Characteristics* Usually healthy except for occasional colds, digestive upsets, and "children's diseases." Accidents are the leading cause of death. Burns off considerable energy in short periods of time.	To be aware of colds and sore throats and how to act with them. To understand how to safely use school equipment indoors and outdoors; to know fire drill procedures; to know about the existence of poisons and neighborhood hazards. To eat mid-morning food, milk or juice.
3. *Mental-Emotional Development* Shows curiosity over a short period of time. Proud of possessions, proud of clothes.	To have experiences beyond the home. To gain confidence in himself as a person.

Often brags to others, likes to hear stories.
Capable of self criticism (Gesell).
Active imagination with shifting of ideas as he paints.
High interest in dramatizations. Speaks and acts spontaneously.
Amazingly ignorant of many facts of life.
Very vulnerable and sensitive, quick to feel hurt or humiliated.
Naturally "mother-centered" and self centered.

To have freedom to scrawl and scribble and figure paint.
To engage in rich, stimulating activities.
To learn what is right and wrong, permitted and forbidden.
To love a warm, friendly, reassuring teacher who understands them.

Primary School Age (Early childhood, Ages 6 to 8 years)

General Characteristics	Needs

1. *Physical Characteristics*

Growth is relatively slow during this period as compared to the early period. Large muscles of the trunk, legs and arms are more developed than the smaller muscles.

Hand-eye coordinations are incomplete, but developing. Eyes slow to focus and usually far-sighted at start of this period.

Bones are hardening. Heart and lungs are small in proportion to body weight and height.

The loss of temporary teeth begins at five to six years and continues up to eleven or twelve years of age.

To experience many kinds of vigorous activities involving many parts of the body. This will increase heart action and respiration and help build endurance. It will also improve skills of body control.

To have instruction in habits of personal hygiene, such as using the handkerchief, covering coughs and sneezes, the selection of clothing appropriate to weather, etc.

Relaxation periods to follow periods of physical activity. Continued emphasis on posture in all activities.

2. *Health Characteristics*

Quite susceptible to infectious diseases at beginning of this age period. Respiratory difficulties common in winter. Toxins and bacteria may damage heart, especially if protection is not afforded during convalescent stages of contagious diseases of childhood.

Alimentary tract difficulties common in summer and fall.

Endurance may be poor. Fatigue is "enemy of childhood," but recuperation from fatigue is usually good.

Accidents are leading causes of death, especially for boys.

The healthy 5 to 8 year old has bright eyes, color in his face, great vitality, is happy and radiates enthusiasm and an exuberance for most activities.

To be checked regularly for signs of disease and defects.

To have twelve hours sleep a night.

To have constant teacher supervision to reduce risks of accidents and to have proper instruction in the hazards of home and school.

To have the chance to express himself through many activities that stimulate physical, social, and mental-emotional growth.

3. *Mental-Emotional Development*

Short span of attention.

Individualistic and possessive, egocentric after age six.

Dramatic, imaginative, and highly imitative. Curious about things in general.

To engage in a number of health activities all of short duration.

To learn to share with others, to play alone and with small groups, and to play as an individual in larger groups. Needs recognition for his personal abilities and to shift gradually to more group activities.

To create and explore, and identify himself with persons and things. Primary grade health stories appeal to the imagination.

Wide variety of emotional reactions.
Enjoys rhythm and rhythmic sounds.

Reasoning ability present, but with little experience upon which to base judgment. Concern for sex differences made known by pertinent questions.

Increase in vocabulary. Language grows with experience.

When approaching age eight he wants his chances to act on his own and is sometimes annoyed at conformity. More sensitive to judgment of peers together with a decrease in concern for adult opinion.
A group most eager to learn and most eager to please the teacher.
Interests are now, not later; will accept things on "faith," less interested in explanations and reasons.
Somewhat self-dependent toward end of this period. Brushes own teeth and hair, dresses self and ties shoes; cleans table, dries dishes, empties wastebaskets, sweeps floors, watches younger children for parents.

To receive guidance in social development.
To respond to rhythmic sounds such as drums, rattles, voice, etc.
To have a chance to discuss and relate personal experiences in classroom health topics.
To receive just enough information on sex as is necessary to answer questions of the moment. Best handled at home.
To visit new places, discuss health implications and stimulate growth in vocabulary of words with a health meaning.
To make own choice in selection of health projects, films, plays, and to help evaluate results of activities.

To see own work displayed.

To cooperate at home and at school in play and other group activities.

To taste some success, carefully sprinkled with enough defeats to provide a stimulus for greater effort and sound adjustments.

Intermediate School Age (Middle childhood, Ages 9 to 11 years)

General Characteristics	Needs

1. *Physical Characteristics*
A noticeable growth spurt at end of period which continues into adolescence. This differs with individual levels of maturation.
Sex differences appear, with girls more mature and taller. Sex antagonism gradually appears. Sexual modesty is seen.
Rough and tumble activities highly enjoyed, often by the girls.

A few girls begin menstruation by ages eleven and twelve.
Muscular strength is behind physical growth, postural habits vary.

Some girls may be more developed in motor skills than some boys.
Coordinations are good. Many physical skills are now automatic. Reaction time is improved.

2. *Health Characteristics*
Eyes function well but nearsightedness (myopia) may develop at ages 8 or 9.

Resistance to contagious and infectious diseases is much better than in primary grades. Tuberculosis is a threat.
Endurance is improved. More rest is needed for the more mature child.

To engage in strenuous activity that taxes the muscles, heart, lungs and other organs to the limits of healthy fatigue.
To engage in wholesome corecreation and coeducational relationships both in the classroom and on the playing fields.
To participate in those physical skills which properly utilize elements of roughness to build motor skills and physical fitness.
To be recognized as different individuals.

To have instruction in body mechanics, fatigue, nutrition and factors influencing growth in height and weight.
To have chance to appraise self through self-testing activities. To relate success in motor skills to personal health habits.

To have periodic eye screening tests to determine need for eyeglasses. This should be coupled with health instruction in this area.
To learn about personal and community health practices which have direct bearing on their welfare.
To get as nearly as possible eleven hours sleep a night and not to play beyond the point

Permanent dentition continues with incisors and lower bicuspids appearing. Bad teeth begin to appear in large numbers.

Accidents are on the increase for this age group, with burns, automobiles and bicycles heading the list.

Increased interest in foods together with improved appetite. Fewer food refusals and a wider range of preferences.

Girls interested in appearance; boys in developing strong bodies.

3. Mental-Emotional Development

They like a wide variety of activities, have a longer span of attention and greater interests.

Strong sense of rivalry and noticeable craving for recognition.

An increasing attitude of independence coupled with a desire to help.

Strong sense of loyalty to groups, teams, or "gangs." Some children are now in a period to be influenced unfavorably. Greater concern over group approval than teacher approval.

Enjoys competition, whether physical or essentially mental, but may become angry when tired, or easily discouraged.

Interest in opposite sex indicated by teasing, hitting, chasing, etc. Girls are more interested in older boys.

Broadening intellectual horizons. Interest shifting from the immediate environment to the wider world.

Strong interest in collecting things. Love of pets.

More critical, need to be shown why. Adventuresome; interested in all kinds of experimentation.

Girls are clearly superior to boys in language development, especially toward end of this period.

of great fatigue. Girls tire more readily than boys, and because they are usually more mature, they require more rest and food.

To have attention directed to dental care. This is a period when many children's teeth are neglected.

To understand the nature of personal accidents at school, en route to school, and in the community.

To discuss nutrition and the role of the four basic foods in maintaining optimum health.

To talk about personal grooming and nature of physical fitness.

To participate in a wide range of health activities involving several methods of teaching and material aids.

To succeed often in a variety of health areas, and to do so through some degree of cooperative effort which affords individual satisfaction.

To have a chance to formally plan, lead, and execute certain projects and to check the progress made. To assist the teacher in the preparation of health exhibits, specimens, posters, etc.

To participate in those activities in which achievement is recognized in the eyes of their group. To gain respect and approval of others.

To compete fairly with others, obtaining an understanding of the place of personal cooperation in the process.

To work coeducationally in those health activities which broaden social relationships and obtain answers to questions involving the opposite sex.

To study world health conditions and what they mean in terms of personal, everyday existence.

To be given a chance to seek detail in a wide variety of health activities.

To stimulate improvement of the health vocabulary, a number of meaningful field trips, projects, or dramatizations may be engaged in.

Growth is a continuous process — an unfolding as children move toward adulthood. It is difficult to subdivide the growth period into specific age levels, for the child never abruptly completes a particular stage of development and begins the next. Moreover, there is never a time when all children in a class are at the same growth stage. Chronological age and physiological age (maturation level) may be quite a distance apart.

The following chart, depicting some of the growth and development characteristics of elementary schoolchildren, is a simple device to help answer the question of characteristics of children at specific age levels. The subdivisions used serve only as convenient labels for periods of growth.

Each child is an individual. He has his own path to follow; he may behave more like the child a year or more younger or the one somewhat older. Yet, his general capacities and needs at any age level aid the teacher materially in the organization and content of a program of health instruction.

Question 2. What am I able to observe in the way of the health and safety practices of my children in specific situations? How do the children behave in respect to food handling, play and rest, handwashing and toilet activities? What do they eat? What kind of a lunch do they bring to school? Is the home health teaching in keeping with accepted health practices? The observing teacher can tell a great deal about what her children need, and these needs are different. Children, for example, in rural communities sometimes lack health information that may be quite familiar to city children. The teacher, in such a case, who moves from the city to the rural area will often be surprised at the needs that are evident on the local scene. In one first grade class a teacher found one of the boys drinking from the urinal. The boy came from a part of the town where outside privy toilets were used and water was hauled by bucket from a nearby property. School needs, therefore, relate to home needs.

The direct statements of classroom teachers who have observed children over the years are very useful in gaining an understanding of health needs together with implication for what to teach. Some of the pertinent statements, recorded just as they were made, are as follows:[8]

Nutrition:

"Frequently children must get their own meals."

---

[8] From a report by The Cooperative Committee on School Health Education. *Health Needs of School Children.* Oneonta, N.Y.; The American Association of Colleges for Teacher Education, 1955, pp. 18–25.

"Many children come to school improperly fed. Results in early fatigue and loss of energy."

"Some of my children have been drinking coffee since they were old enough to hold a cup."

"Occasionally we have attempted programs for mothers on nutrition but we have been discouraged. We feel that mothers who need it do not come to our meetings. We do not know how to reach them."

"Inadequate lunch. Child brings money for full lunch and buys only soup, saving rest for candy. Hastily made, poorly balanced lunches. Gulping food to get out to play earlier."

Emotional Health:

"Many of our children lack emotional security because working mothers have no time for them."

"We have so many disturbed children . . . in trying to analyze the causes for this we have discussed the economic level of the families of this neighborhood and the resultant insecurity in the home; the high percentage of broken homes; . . . the physical surrounding our children live in; our transient population; the the irregular home life of many of our children. We feel we are achieving stability as a group in our classrooms, but we are unable to help individual children achieve stability."

"In our school, we have problems of emotional malnutrition such as a child's hunger for affection, status with his peers, and hunger for success."

Disease — Prevention and Control:

"Parents send children to school when they are ill . . . parents are working or too busy to have them 'underfoot'."

"Overcrowded classrooms contribute to spread of infections such as ringworm, colds."

"Dripping noses: How to care for the common cold? . . . Certain children will not blow their noses often enough or will not wipe them when necessary. I keep Kleenex available to all, but still some have to be told, 'Blow your nose before we can go on with our work.'"

"Head lice—We have had difficulty in controlling the spread of pediculosis."

"Ignorance—If a child is sent home from school by the school nurse with the mumps, a strep throat, or such, that evening, he will be seen at the motion picture theater spreading the infection and endangering his own health."

Rest and Recreation:

"Not enough sleep . . . The three R's seem to take precedence over the play period."

"Sleep—Television—child acquires spectator attitude—child over-stimulated comes to school sleepy."

"Insufficient outdoor exercise. The individual health habits include staying up late at night."

"Lack of proper sleep and rest at home . . . waiting for mother to come home from working on second shift at the mill, or sleep being interrupted by a parent going to work on the second shift."

". . . We would like to cite a boy in the fourth grade who sits up until 11:00 or 11:30 P.M. watching wrestling matches and other television or radio programs. This boy is unable to concentrate individually or with the class on a subject, unable to contribute to the class discussion, his grades are poor, and he is too tired to play with the group at recess."

Cleanliness:

"Too many children exhibit a lack of personal cleanliness; offensive odors, soiled clothing, dirty hands and face, unclean finger nails, uncombed hair and unbrushed teeth are far too common."

"Some of our children live in run-down, rat-infested, cold water flats. Nothing about this environment in which they live is conducive to good health. This overcrowding often makes it necessary for children to sleep near a kerosene stove, the only source of heat. Such children come to school with a strong odor of oil . . ."

"Lack of pupil interest in personal hygiene . . . Some children never take a bath and often wear the same clothes for weeks. Lice and itch are common among a few families."

"Poor habits of sanitation, due to ignorance and carelessness at home . . . We dare not provide shower bath periods for girls because the parents would be shocked at the idea of girls undressing in the presence of anyone else. Symptoms of this problem are lice, skin infections, pink eye, spitting anywhere and careless use of drinking fountains."

"Body odor . . . This odor is more evident during the winter months when heavier clothing is not changed when necessary."

". . . older children have to sleep with others who wet the bed . . . The odor is carried on the clothing of the older children."

Dental Health:

"Need for dental care is especially serious. Toothache is a frequent cause of absence . . . There were a few who did not even recognize the article (toothbrush) when it was shown to them in a magazine."

"Our greatest cause of absence is toothache . . . Ninety per cent of the primary children have never been to a dentist."

"General fear of dentists that results in harmful neglect of teeth."

". . . About 20 per cent of the children in my school did not own toothbrushes at the beginning of the year."

"The nearest dentist is 20 miles."

Vision and Hearing:

"Problems prevalent—auditory and visual defects."

"One teacher in the first grade informed a mother that her child was doing failing work because he was unable to hear, and that he should be given a hearing test. The mother said, 'John is not deaf; he is just naughty, and does not want to listen' . . ."

"A child in kindergarten was very hard of hearing. Not until an examination by the school nurse was it known that he had infected tonsils. The tonsils were removed and the child's hearing was much improved. The loss of hearing had affected the child's speech so that it was hardly understandable."

It is hard to believe in this day and age that home living conditions can be so different. Unless the teacher actually tours the countryside, seeks the out-of-the-way places, gets into the apartment buildings and sizes up the community health situations, she is apt to have little real knowledge of pupil health needs. Where a child in one home has his own room and bed, another child in another home sleeps with three others in the same bed; and it may be in a one room dwelling. Numerous places exist where a family of eight, ten, or more live under one roof in one room. Here they eat, sleep, play, and exist in unclean surroundings and without respect for personal privacy. Even today public health workers find it necessary to visit homes on the outskirts of a number of communities in Florida and Georgia, attempting to get the people to build outside privy toilets. One inquires in amazement as to what they have been using all these years, only to find that these adults and their children have simply been going further and further back into the woods.[9] Attitudes and

---

[9] Two thousand years ago in the days of the ancient Hebrews, personal health practices were better than this. The Bible says, "Thou shalt have a place within the camp . . . and it shall be, when thou wilt ease thyself abroad, thou shalt dig therewith, and shalt turn back and cover that which cometh from thee." (Deut. 23:12–13.)

habits formed in this kind of environment can hardly be modified overnight, and they are most difficult to change right away in the schoolroom.

Question 3. What are the health and safety hazards in the local community? What are the special health problems? Are there hazardous obstacles such as rivers, waterfalls, open sandpits, or automobile traffic, and are there hazardous activities being carried on near by?

These questions are partially related to the previous question dealing with the observed health and safety practices of the children in school. The questions go together because local conditions *do* affect classroom behavior and point to the necessity for certain kinds of health instruction to meet existing needs.

Local statistics relative to the prevalence of certain communicable diseases, the purity of drinking water, the cleanliness of local eating establishments, and the safety of milk are fundamental considerations that should be understood by the teacher. If, for example, a community is bothered by black flies or mosquitoes, this should become one of the health topics covered during the year. Moreover, such a topic is probably somewhat familiar to all pupils in the class, and very little preliminary motivation work will be required to provoke discussion and get some action. Several years ago in one Georgia community the sixth grade class became so interested in malaria mosquito breeding that they set out to personally initiate a mosquito control program. They drained small ponds and put oil on stagnant waters. In fact, they became so active with enthusiasm which blossomed as the job progressed that the townsfolk appropriated money and joined in to make the mosquito control project one fine example of community cooperation. Health instruction directed along lines such as these becomes a magnificent force not only for the personal health and welfare of the children and adults, but also for the promulgation of such worthy objectives as social efficiency and civic responsibility.

Question 4. What are the health problems and safety hazards in the state? Is the state in question any different from any other state? What do recent statistics, collected and made available by the county health department, reveal? Is it conceivable that Alabama might have problems different from Montana?

How does the state compare with the National Health Survey which indicates that pupil deaths from accidents lead the list, followed by cancers and leukemias, influenza and pneumonias, and congenital malformations? What about disabling difficulties? Usually respiratory disturbances rank first, followed by infections and parasitic disorders, and injuries. The accompanying figures are the result of a California health survey of the incidence of acute and chronic illness by sex for 1000 boys and girls, ages five to 14.

Incidence of Acute and Chronic Illness

Diagnosis	Male	Female
Common cold, sore throat, cough and nasopharyngitis	1,776	1,744
Accidents	1,010	848
Bronchitis and chest cold	254	175
Asthma and hay fever	223	133
Intestinal flu	209	270
Indigestion	205	213
Common childhood diseases	240	190
Allergies (other than asthma and hay fever)	169	118
Diseases of ear and mastoid, including deafness	120	100
Migraine and headache	98	128
Chronic tosillitis or sore throat	93	152

States, as communities of people, differ in many respects. Some are more agricultural; others are more industrialized. Some are reasonably warm all year round, while others are faced with an annual adjustment to cold and inclement weather. There are watery noses, sore throats, and cloudy skies in Cleveland, Ohio and Oswego, New York, while the sunshine blazes overhead in South Carolina. Farm safety is taught in the cornbelt states and industrial safety in Detroit. Water safety is of paramount interest in Minnesota, Wisconsin, and along the shores of the Great Lakes and seacoast states.

In Florida, hookworm is a major health problem of schoolchildren. Many individuals have contact with it some time or other. Children who go barefooted appear to be everywhere — and so are hookworm and other internal parasites. Vast numbers of elementary age children are treated by their county health unit through the schools. They stay free from the worms for only a short while following the cure, then they become infected again. And the chief reason for this is that they and their families will not put into practice certain beneficial health habits that have been brought to their attention by public health and school personnel. *The need, therefore, continues to exist for more effective health instruction. In fact, most of these children have more than enough knowledge on the subject to pass a written test with a high grade. What they lack is an intelligent understanding deep enough to create positive attitudes and changes in health behavior.*

One may focus attention on the state of Colorado and see how its needs affect health teaching as compared with certain northeastern states. The bone malformation disease of rickets, for example, has almost become a thing of the past in New England and most eastern states. It was a real problem 25 years ago when extreme poverty, ignorance, and low milk consumption were more common. Yet in southern Colorado the pigeon chests and bowed bones of rickets are seen in many towns and villages. The educational needs of many of the children of Mexican-American descent are greater than in other American communities. The same thing relative to needs could be said for the Puerto Rican-American area of New York City or the Italian–Chinese-American sections of Boston. In fact, health problems are more frequent among people of low economic standing in almost any part of the country.

Socio-economic backgrounds, climate and weather, prejudices and superstitions — even the terrain of the countryside — affect what is taught. In New Hampshire — a rugged state of forests, mountains, lakes, and streams, a state of less than half a million people — hunting and fishing are as much a part of one's education as any single subject in the public school curriculum. Every spring, on the first day of the trout season there is a school holiday throughout the state. Practically every boy and girl who can walk or hobble along goes fishing. During the year, and especially in the fall, great numbers of children and youth carry rifles and go hunting. This is not without educational implications. Firearms safety, initiated at the State Education Department level, has spread as a special health instruction topic to almost every city and rural school in the state. This is a concrete example of how a particular health and safety need can be met. It not only serves the immediate needs of the elementary age children, but also carries over to the older age groups. Proof of this exists in the unsolicited testimony of police department officials, game wardens, and sportsmen's club leaders.

Question 5. How does the local school environment furnish leads for health instruction? Are there poor physical facilities that may represent a safety hazard? Do children wonder why they are required to take physical education? What kinds of food do primary grade pupils choose in the school cafeteria? Do food selections differ for intermediate graders?

Opportunities to teach health topics in keeping with health needs and interests abound in the school environment. There are hardly two schools alike in facilities and equipment. Every laboratory, lunchroom, gymnasium and classroom suggest health items of interest and value to pupils. The cleanliness of corridors, walks, and rooms, the lighting, ventilation, temperature, playground equipment, and space all furnish leads to the observing teacher. And one should not forget the number and types of school accidents. Where do they occur and what can be done about them?

Question 6. What are the findings of medical examinations and screening tests? Do health histories and cumulative health record cards indicate any special findings which the instructional program may be able to remedy or improve? Do some children show a slow rate of growth?

Children with slight cases of malnutrition, postural defects, and similar deviations from normal need two kinds of attention. Primarily, they need to have remedial work started quickly, and secondly, they need information about themselves and their difficulty. There is no need to keep children in the dark about personal deviations, especially when their attitudes can be improved so much by a little understanding. Also, other elementary schoolchildren are generally very interested in the health problems of their classmates and how these may affect them. Furthermore, the child with a problem may become a real member of the group and feel quite at home in the class by being singled out as, for example, the teacher's helper for a lesson on posture and body mechanics. In one northern New York State elementary school the teachers have agreed among themselves to have children, returning to school after an absence due to illness, speak to their classmates and tell them about their experiences while ill. Very often the pupil who has been absent a few days with something like strep sore throat will stimulate a real show of interest in the broad area of upper respiratory diseases. Moreover, intermediate grade children want to know what they can do about it.

Question 7. Are there major student interests that relate to health education? Do pupils in the first three grades have specific interests that border on hazardous activity?

Young children are vigorous. Sometimes they are rough and adventuresome. Their play is serious, full of meaning—their way of life. Such children are too often unaware of the things they do that may influence their health and safety. Large muscle activities such as running, jumping, climbing, and wrestling are play activities that are at times hazardous. Climbing out on tree limbs, frolicking in the water in the summer, and testing the ice in the winter are potentially dangerous yet powerfully stimulating forms of recreation. Even interest in becoming Brownies or Cub Scouts presents leads for meaningful health instruction.

Student interests rise and fall according to school and local happenings. A major traffic tragedy, a local epidemic of Asian flu or scarlet fever, or a severe water shortage are current health events that may heighten pupil enthusiasm to the point where the alert teacher can take advantage of it and "make hay while the sun shines."

Current and immediate interests of children can be readily determined in a novel way by providing them with the opportunity of asking questions through a device such as the question box. This makes a bit of a game out of if. The teacher who is observant can determine children's health interests rather well by:

Taking note of what they do before and after school.
Talking with them.

Observing their actions in and about the classroom.
Listening as they talk together.
Watching their activities during leisure moments, unassigned periods, or at play.
Evaluating the stories and materials they bring from home.
Studying their paintings, drawings, crafts, stories, and letters.
Noticing their choices of books, clothing, and other materials.
Studying records of pupils of the same level, such as cumulative records, personal diaries, and class folders of the year's work.
Discussing them with parents and former teachers.

When young children are carefully observed one finds that they are interested in radio, television, movies, play activities, people of other lands, picture magazines, plants and animals, machines, the care of pets, their own body, and many other factual and creative items.

Health interests may also be checked through the use of a teacher-constructed questionnaire or pupil check list. Questions pertaining to medical and dental care, food habits, cleanliness, rest, and posture indicate a great deal in terms of pupil behavior and needs. A survey of individual health habits could be most revealing not only in terms of curriculum needs, but also in terms of health guidance. The Clarke Health-Habit Questionnaire has for a number of years proved to be a useful instrument in this area. It may be used for intermediate grade children and others to arrive at interests and additional health teaching needs.[10] Clarke asks questions dealing

---

[10] Printed copies of the questionnaire may be obtained directly from H. Harrison Clarke, University of Oregon, Eugene, Oregon. See also, Carl E. Willgoose. *Evaluation in Health Education and Physical Education.* New York: McGraw-Hill Book Company, 1961, p. 96.

with such things as living conditions, sleep habits, daytime naps, happiness and moods, hobbies, extracurricular activities, illnesses, meals, and dental visits. One of his final groups of questions is especially revealing to the teacher and the student who answers it:

Do you desire to be strong and physically fit? − − − − − − − − − − − −

Do you wish to be attractive? − − −

Are you satisfied with your present physical condition? − − − − − − − −

In the primary grades, direct questions which may be asked by the leader will indicate and stimulate interest in health. For example:

1. Do you wash your hands after going to the toilet?

2. What foods do you eat between meals?

3. Do you stay home when you have a cold?

4. When were you to the dentist last?

5. At what time do you usually go to bed at night?

6. How do you sit in your chair? Do you lean over or slide down in the seat?

Question 8. Have the pupils had experiences in other areas of learning which provide leads for needed health instruction? One might paraphrase Edgar Guest's expression that "it takes a heap of livin' in a house to make it a home," and say that it takes a heap of teaching in a place to change behavior. It takes many ideas from several study areas to educate for health. Experiences from one subject matter area carry over into another and enrich health instruction. The teacher plans for this in advance by correlating her materials with the content of other areas and the activities of other teachers.

Physical education games, dances, and stunts can be directly related to health instruction topics such as strength, vigor, nutrition, rest, and

social health. In fact, for children to have physical education activities and fail to learn why they are important to their health and welfare is indeed a shortsighted kind of education. Yet many opportunities are overlooked to explain why exercise, physical skills, and social contacts are necessary. The same may be said for the special areas of music and art. Do children know that healthy people, free from worry and organic drains, sing and paint better because they are happy?

Question 9. What is the relationship of the basic health needs of all persons to the health needs of children. This is the final question, and it is a broad one. A large part of Chapter 1 is devoted to the need for health education. This is brought out in terms of national and world health problems. Modern man, if he is to live the rich and full life today and survive in the centuries ahead, needs help in many ways. He needs to reduce drastically the incidence of degenerative diseases and accident rates; he needs to cancel out superstitions, gullibility, fads, quackery, misconceptions, and neuroticisms by increasing his application of scientific knowledge; and he needs to think more often in terms of future generations of mankind instead of aimlessly rushing along in the tense, materialistic, and turbulent stream of humanity.

Teaching for Understandings and Attitudes

When the questions on needs are all answered, it will be seen that there are a vast number of special needs which determine what to teach in any one particular locality and to any one particular class. There are also a number of other needs that elementary schoolchildren have in common. These needs are at the basis of the instructional program and designate the goals children must strive for and the kinds of experiences they must have. Helen Starr has made an excellent contribution to the health literature on this topic. Her list of understandings, attitudes and skills for schoolchildren adopted by many elementary school staffs, follows:[11]

Understanding:

To develop an understanding that health is a state of complete physical, mental, and social well-being.

To lay the foundation for an understanding for the physical, mental, emotional, and social nature of the human being.

To understand the importance of adequate rest and sleep.

To realize the importance of immunization as a protection against certain diseases.

To understand the importance of vigorous play and exercise to good body functioning and development of muscular strength and coordination.

[11] Starr, Helen. "What Emphasis in Health?" *Children in Focus.* Washington: American Association for Health, Physical Education, and Recreation, 1954, Chapter 9. (Used by special permission of the Association.)

To understand the effect of diet, exercise, rest, work, relaxation, and recreation upon growth.

To understand the responsibility of the individual for his own life and that of his fellow men in preventing accidents.

To develop healthful habits in one's own personal life.

Attitudes

To seek proper medical and dental advice.

To evaluate one's own health habits and make needed changes.

To appreciate the dignity and value of the individual and spiritual values in everyday living.

To use correct terminology and speak intelligently when discussing health matters.

To be an intelligent examinee at health examinations.

To organize time to provide for balanced living.

To be protected against communicable diseases.

To desire and appreciate the importance of mastering recreational skills.

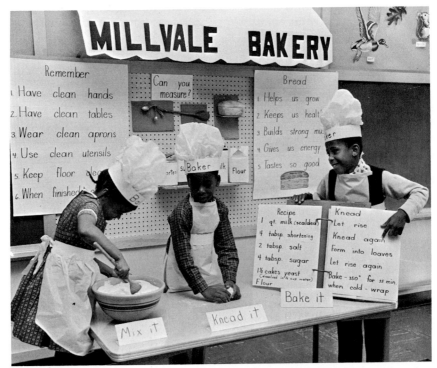

Figure 6–1   Permanent attitudes are formed through interesting activities. (Courtesy Cincinnati Public Schools.)

To secure and maintain good posture.

To use the body in efficient, graceful manner in sports and daily life activities.

To understand the basic daily foods essential to proper growth and health maintenance.

To be responsible for protection of oneself and others from accidents.

To take initial steps in administering first aid in an emergency.

To relate the importance of personal health to the health of a community and nation.

To respect health laws and regulations.

Learning Experiences:

To obtain accurate health information.

To share in planning for happiness and well-being of others.

To experience screening tests for vision and hearing once each year, dental screenings twice each year.

To be measured and weighed at least three times each year.

To care for oneself properly after exposure to the elements.

To bring to the classroom for study some of the health problems of the home and community.

To participate in well-rounded recreation and physical education programs.

To select and eat good meals.

To plan for emergency care in case of accident or sudden illness.

To plan for control of fire hazards.

To carry out essential practices of cleanliness and sanitation — the use of individual drinking cups, towels, soap, washcloths, toothbrushes, combs.

To examine the classroom, the school, and the community for health problems.

In view of the forementioned statements relative to understandings and attitudes, it cannot be overemphasized that it is a reasonably simple matter to teach facts, figures, and general knowledge about health.

For decades teachers have taught useful health information, yet the world is full of people who failed to apply what they apparently learned. Often the pupil who receives an "A" in the topic of dental health grows to adulthood harboring a mouth full of decaying teeth greatly in need of care.

The sixth grader who creates the finest project depicting the relationship of diet to overweight sometimes grows up to be a heavyweight with an attitude of complete indifference toward weight-gaining foods. And every social misfit in our country has been exposed to the influence of a number of reasonably good teachers. Rogers points out that "it has been estimated that during the future careers of any class of 40 children, 17 to 26 of them will ultimately be disturbed by conditions ranging from chronic unhappiness to criminal behavior or insanity."[12] Add to this the millions of cases of people involved in vocational failure, chronic unemployment, marital unhappiness, emotional instability, and other expressions of failure, and it becomes quite evident that teaching for understandings and attitudes is a most difficult task requiring the best in curriculum, methodology, and teaching.

Health Teaching

And you America,
Cast you the real reckoning for your
    present?
The lights and shadows of your future, good or evil?
To girlhood, boyhood look, the
    teacher and the school.
—WALT WHITMAN, in *Leaves of Grass*

Up to now, the discussion has been concerned with health instruction generally, with special attention being given to pupil characteristics, the kinds of pupil experiences in the program, and how they relate to group and individual needs. Very little has been said about the teacher as a person.

Instructional programs become effective in promoting pupil achievement when they have good teachers behind them. The finest fashioned

---

[12] Rogers, Dorothy. *Mental Hygiene in Elementary Education.* Boston: Houghton-Mifflin Co., 1957, p. 10.

course of study, carefully modified at the local level to consider immediate needs, is but words on a sheet of paper to the incompetent and unsympathetic teacher. Fortunately, however, most elementary schoolteachers like children and make an effort to understand and work with them.

Teaching has been defined in many ways, but in general it may be considered a procedure involving leadership. If education may be defined as a process of changing behavior toward certain preconceived goals, then teaching is the act of exercising leadership in this process. Good teaching can be so effective that children are taught numerous things without even being aware of it. "We are," wrote Lord Chesterfield, "more than half what we are by imitation. The great point is, to choose good models and to study them with care." This has a profound meaning for educators. Someone has said that "teaching is a process of making little images of the teacher in the minds of pupils." If such is so, and it appears to be, then teachers of impressionable youth and eager-to-learn children might well tremble at the thought of how much power they wield for good or evil. The thought of their responsibilities should shake them to the core and cause them to dedicate themselves more sincerely to the tasks ahead.

Teaching Health in a Democracy

Education is a function of the state primarily because a democracy can only grow and survive in terms of the skills, understanding, and general enlightenment of the citizenry. Literacy was the essential objective in the days of Thomas Jefferson, but something more is needed today. If democracy is to be preserved as a form of government, the teacher must "foster, pro-

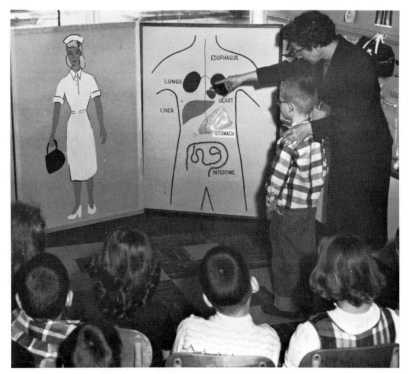

Figure 6–2 Each walk of life has its own elite.

mote, and develop it as a way of life." To go one step further is to state that teaching for health is necessary to make democracy succeed both as a form of government and a way of life.

There are two fundamental beliefs which may be referred to as principles of democratic leadership. One is the *principle of personal involvement.* This principle simply stated means that teachers and leaders must have a responsible personal connection with democratic action. They must not only preach democratic living; they must live it. A writer once asked Dr. Albert Schweitzer if he did not think that personally setting a good example was one of the best ways of influencing people. Dr. Schweitzer replied, "No! It's the *only way.*" The implication is clear that in order to really influence others in developing good health and democratic behavior, teachers must be fit themselves. The second principle of democratic leadership is the *principle of individual worth.* This is the principle that is sometimes referred to as "respect for the personality of the individual." Nothing should be rated above human personality. The teacher cannot be successful in a democratic society if she fails to equip young people with the necessary respect for the worth of the individual. When children have been treated as individuals in school, they will be better equipped to understand and practice the democratic way of life in the years ahead.

The future society depends not on how near its organization is to perfection, but on the degree of worthiness in its individual members. It is not hard to overlook the individual personality in our quest to secure collective opinion. Yet, as Albert Schweitzer points out, "Humanitarianism consists in never sacrificing a human being to a purpose." Furthermore, says Schweitzer, "The task immediately before us is to safeguard the integrity of the individual within the modern state.[13]

The Competent Teacher

"Each honest calling, each walk of life," says Conant, "has its own elite, its own aristocracy based on excellence of performance."[14]

There is little question that the teacher must be much more than an ordinary person. She must possess the characteristics, vision, and understanding of the clergy, the zeal and devotion of the medical worker, and the earthly human qualities of the missionary. She must be an idealist and aim higher than she can ever expect to go. Her enthusiasm for her teaching might well ring out the immortal words of Robert Browning: "Ah, but a man's reach should exceed his grasp, or what's a heaven for?" In short the *real* teacher has everything. This is demonstrated time and time again by the testimony of successful men and women who pay tribute to their teachers of earlier years.

Competency as a teacher is not something which automatically accompanies being hired to teach school. Almost anyone can get a job teaching. The question is, what constitutes a competent teacher? Certainly the example of competence is more than a teacher who approaches perfection.

It has been said that the competent teacher is neither a poem nor a paragon. In the words of Dean L. D. Haskew of the University of Texas, "A competent teacher—or a competent doctor, or a competent lawyer—is a person made up of assets and liabilities. His assets overcompensate for his liabilities, and his liabilities do not

---

[13] Schweitzer, Albert. *The Philosophy of Civilization.* New York: The Macmillan Co., 1949.

[14] Conant, James B. *The Education of American Teachers.* New York: McGraw-Hill Book Company, 1961, p. 183.

occur in crucial areas. He gets some desired results to a significant degree, and his undesired results are of minor significance. While he is not universally successful in accomplishing what teachers should accomplish, his successes decidedly outweigh his non-successes due chiefly to the fact that he knows his job and practices a profession of teaching."[15]

There are many excellent characteristics that might well describe the competent teacher. Certainly she should possess a number of superior traits—personally and professionally. Here are six earmarks or minimum essentials of the competent teacher:

1. *A Person with a Personality.* This is a live, warm person whose personality is such that she has a wholesome and constructive impact on young people. Everybody should have a nice personality; for the competent teacher it is part of her professional equipment. Moreover, for the teacher of health it is even more precious.

The all-inclusive personality—the perfect classroom teacher—is almost a figment of the imagination. At least it is probably a rare bird. In real life the desirable competencies are spread among several very fine teachers, none of whom is perfect.

Certainly the personality of a classroom teacher, who is aiming toward the successful teaching of health, must be one capable of registering a deep personal concern for the welfare of every pupil in the class. Children, influenced by the attitudes and practices of the teacher's warm, unflagging interest in them, receive an object lesson in what can be done by the teacher who really cares about the mental, physical, emotional, and social well-being of her students. Several years ago a Harvard University graduate

study indicated that this *feeling* of warmth and understanding (empathy) was the quality more instrumental in good teaching than anything else. Yet, one cannot legislate or command this quality by decree. Given a little help, it may be developed, especially among teachers who profess to like children.

Dr. James B. Conant, president emeritus of Harvard University, lists two top characteristics of first-class teachers: a contagious enthusiasm for the subject being taught; and a thorough enjoyment of the process of teaching.

Not all teachers have the personality that is desirable for school teaching. It has been stated that the chances are seven to one that in the course of 12 years of school a child will come under the thumb of at least two teachers with personality maladjustments. They may be unstable and neurotic or even seriously psychopathic. This is a most serious problem, not only for the health of teachers but also for the children they teach. The mental hygiene atmosphere of the classroom cannot transcend the mental health of the teacher. Inappropriate emotional response, faulty personality reactions, and devastating character maladjustments are invited and can be spread under bad classroom as well as bad home conditions. Teaching may indeed be a nerve-racking occupation. The person with the stable personality will find much to challenge it in education.

2. *A Person with a Significant Store of Useful Knowledge.* The competent individual must know his subject matter. A limited knowledge of the science of health cannot be offset by a broad understanding of educational philosophy and method. A balance of both is required.

Teachers of health need increasing knowledge. New medical discoveries and public health practices are occurring all the time. The well-informed teacher is one who has sought ex-

[15] From an address delivered before the Washington Conference, *Personnel Policies for Schools of the Future*, June 25, 1957. The National Commission on Teacher Education and Professional Standards.

tended instruction. In addition to this expanding knowledge of health, the competent teacher needs skill in mediating knowledge so that children may learn.

3. *A Person Who Has Considerable Success in Selecting Important and Strategic Things to be Learned.* The key word here is "select." Competent teachers, through study and training, know what they should select to teach, but because there is so much variety to choose from today, the selective function becomes an art. The fourth grade teacher, for example, knows that her students are interested and need some work in nutrition. With few exceptions, there is probably more written material available for classroom teachers in this area than for any other area in the field of health. It is conceivable that almost all materials are good. Some are better than others chiefly because they have been appraised and found to be more effective in the promotion of desired food habits and attitudes. Thus, the teacher's success in the selection of materials is somewhat related to her ability to evaluate them in terms of their contribution to preconceived pupil goals.

4. *A Person with Decided Skill in Arranging What Pupils Do in Order that Learning Will Take Place.* The key word here is "arranging." The ability to arrange the teaching situation so that children get the most out of it is high level skill. Today, with the many teaching instruments available — movies, field trips, libraries, and outside speakers — it takes a competent teacher to move from one to another so that all children receive maximum benefits. This holds true whether one teaches health or English.

5. *A Person Who Has Success in Establishing Constructive, Stimulating Relationships with Individual Pupils.* Although most personal contacts with children are made on a mass basis, the competent teacher knows how to go beyond the mass approach. She reaches individuals; she helps Sam with his problems, causes Sally to have a brighter outlook toward school work, or engineers a trip to the dental clinic for Mike. This characteristic in the competent teacher is the quality *par excellence,* for it gives meaning to teaching as an art. No matter how scientific teaching may become, it will forever remain an art.

6. *A Person with at Least One Well-Developed, Useful Specialty.* It is good for a teacher to be well-rounded, with many abilities useful in education. At the same time, however, excellence in some phase of educational endeavor seems to be a common characteristic of the competent teacher.

Faith in the Worth of Teaching. No discussion of the competencies of teachers of health would be complete without mention of the teacher's personal attitude toward teaching. This attitude may have more to do with successful health teaching than any other single factor. The teacher who likes the work and approaches the lesson with a pleasant and enthusiastic manner demonstrates a positive approach to the topic that sets the stage for optimum learning. The great New England pioneer in health teaching, Mabel Caroline Bragg, taught her teachers-to-be that the teaching of health — perhaps more than any other subject — calls for a teacher with dynamic vitality, an inspired interest in the welfare of children, and a faith in the worth of teaching. Miss Bragg herself was the magnificent example of this faith, for wherever she went, in college or grade school classrooms, she created an atmosphere of radiant, positive health. One must, therefore, possess a profound conviction of the worth of his work. There must be a sense of greatness in one's profession.

Finally, this faith in the worth of teaching is expressed through service. Through the basic concept of service the individual teacher establishes a place in the group. And through service the group takes on more significance. Unless man can be guided by a motive of service, selfishness and materialism eat at the roots of individuals and nations. Antoine de St. Exupéry attributes the fall of France to this lack of concept of service. In his *Flight to Arras* he says that if man insists upon giving only to himself he will receive nothing, for he is not a part of anything. Later when he is asked to die for something he will refuse to die, for his own interests will command him to live. There will be no deep love for something else strong enough to compensate for his death. Men do not die for tables and walls; they die for a home. They die for something bigger than themselves. Says St. Exupéry, "Men die only for that for which they live."

Health Guidance

It has been suggested several times throughout the text that the classroom teacher is in a unique position to influence pupil health. Through observation and simple screening practices, children with health abnormalities may be detected and referred to health services for remedial action. In addition to this there exist many fine opportunities to carry on individual health guidance.

Pupils with health problems have a much better chance to improve when the sympathetic and understanding teacher sits, like Mark Hopkins, on one end of the log with the pupil on the other. In the quiet of the teacher's office much can be accomplished. There is time to talk personally about cleanliness, foods, rest, pimples, or home life. This is health instruction at its finest. The teacher may listen, discuss, and make concrete suggestions. The pupil is relaxed, pleased beyond words that the teacher is interested in him, and is usually most willing to do as he suggests.

The number of schoolchildren who need this kind of assistance is increasing. There have always been a number of children with minor physical deviations needing attention, but in recent years more and more children have problems of adjustment on the mental-emotional plane. Although there are school psychologists, guidance counselors, and in some places school psychiatrists, there are nevertheless, far too few dedicated teachers who are both interested and capable of sitting down and talking at length with children in need of special consideration.

There are normal children and there are deviations from normal. Finding and working with the deviates is in itself a bona fide form of health instruction. The classroom teacher has the professional responsibility, therefore, to understand what is normal and to detect deviations from it.

Suggested Activities

1. In a recent article by Leo Kartman it is suggested that "the changing attitude of the patient helps to pave the way for an acceptance of the practice of clinical epidemiology." (See *Selected References.*) This would indicate that communicable disease can be traced and perhaps eradicated if patients will cooperate with physicians and public health workers. See what you can read on this topic. Follow this up with your comments relative to the probability of disease eradication if a health-educated citizenry is developed.

2. The pupil's learning process, the teaching method, and the health education course content are intricately related. Review the philosophy of Jerome Bruner relative to the "discovery method" in teaching. What do you think could be the influence of this method on health instruction?

3. Survey a class of primary grade pupils to find out their interests. Read what Paul Witty and Alfred North Whitehead have to say about interests. (See *Selected references.*) How may this information be used?

4. Study the list of nine *Imperatives in Education* set forth by the American Association of School Administrators. Discuss ways and means in which health education can contribute to the fulfillment of these points and help meet the needs of the times.

Questions for Discussion

1. What evidence is there that we are bridging the gap between health knowledge and health behavior? How can we better apply what the psychologists have learned about human motivations?

2. Have you noticed whether or not our health teaching is keeping pace with changing needs of individuals and society? Give a few examples from your experience.

3. To what extent do you believe parents receive health education through the health instruction program in schools?

4. From your experience, what seems to be the most effective way to tie up health instruction with physical education at the elementary school level?

5. What health instructional activities are suggested by the prepubescent growth spurt?

6. Carefully appraise a community in terms of local and state health needs. In general, what are your findings?

7. As civilization becomes more complex, is there a tendency for education to become somewhat divorced from life? Is this true for health education as contrasted with other subject matter areas?

Selected References

Bloom, S. W. *The Doctor and His Patient.* New York: Russell Sage Foundations, 1963, p. 157.

Brownell, William A., and Sims, Verner M. "The Nature of Understanding." *NSSE Forty-fifth Yearbook,* Part I. Chicago: National Society for Study of Education, 1946, Chapter 3.

Corliss, Leland M. "A Report of the Denver Research Project on Health Interests of Children." *Journal of School Health,* 32:355–359, November 1962.

Hodenfield, G. K., and Stinnett, T. M. *The Education of Teachers.* Englewood Cliffs, N.J.: Prentice-Hall, Inc., 1961.

Kartman, Leo. "Human Ecology and Public Health." *American Journal of Public Health,* 57:737–750, May 1967.

Whitehead, Alfred North. "In Deciding What to Teach." *Project on the Instructional Program of the Public Schools.* Washington, D.C.: National Education Association, 1963, pp. 27–28.

Willgoose, Carl E. "Health Education in Elementary Schools." *Education,* 82:131–133, November 1961.

Witty, Paul A. "Pupil Interests in the Elementary Grades." *Education,* 83:451–462, April 1963.

Planning the Health Curriculum

CHAPTER 7

Let us, since life can little more supply
Than just to look about us, and to die,
Expatiate free o'er all this scene of man;
A mighty maze! but not without a plan.

— ALEXANDER POPE

In the words of the philosopher-poet, there is order in the universe. But more than this there is behind it all a plan. In short, whether a project or undertaking is of great or small magnitude, its ultimate success and effect depend upon careful planning.

The curriculum in an elementary school is influenced chiefly by two prime factors: what a child needs and what society expects him to acquire. The curriculum, therefore, is a program used by the school as a means of accomplishing its purposes. Included in it are all of the experiences of children for which the school accepts responsibility. Obviously there are wide differences of opinion about the kinds of experiences children should have in school. This is good in a democratic society for it keeps education from becoming static. Just as the world today is far from being static, so also is the curriculum; it is always

subject to change, and in the face of criticism, attack, and counterattack, it has evolved to the pattern of the moment.

THE NATURE OF THE CURRICULUM

The present curriculum is one that has emerged from the time when the educational processes were conceived in terms of skills, memorized items, and a trained mind. In fact, the "disciplined mind" was something to aim for. Around 50 years ago there appeared a gradual emphasis on social usage as an important criterion in selecting curriculum content. The question of whether or not the child was learning anything conducive to living with other people in a society was raised. This led to the somewhat scientific selection of course content and grew into the scientific method. With greater emphasis through the

122

years on the science of education and a growing number of findings arising from the field of psychology, it was only a matter of time before the child-centered curriculum became known.

Types of Elementary School Curricula

Curricula are designated in a number of ways. The *separate-subjects curriculum* is regarded as the traditional curriculum. It is often called by such other names as the subject-matter curriculum and the scientific-subjects curriculum. Students study each subject that the school has to offer for a certain amount of time each day. Little attempt is made to relate one school subject to another. For example, physical education is taught without reference to health or social living. Health is taught as a subject by itself. Here, the tendency is for the student to learn isolated facts and pieces of information about health without seeing them as a part of the whole—as part of life in general. Interest is often low, and the teacher tends to concentrate on subject-matter achievement rather than on the adaptation of learning activities to the needs and capacities of the children.

Since 1925 the trend has been to employ the *broad-fields curriculum* in which closely related subject-matter areas are grouped together. Subject matter is organized, but the emphasis is on large fields or areas rather than on separate subjects. This type of curriculum may group such items as spelling, writing, reading, language-grammar-oral communication, and literature under the broad topic (field) of language arts. Health, safety, and physical education are often grouped together for they possess several things in common. Health may also be taught in the broad areas of science or social studies. This curriculum helps students to see relationships between several things learned in one general

area. For example, students learn from the broad field of health and social living that vitamins are more than something to be concerned about for personal health at the moment; they learn that they are related to historical accomplishments. The sailors who manned the ancient ships in the days of Columbus, Magellan, and Sir Francis Drake were somewhat limited in their capacities by vitamin deficiencies in the form of beriberi and pellagra.

When the number of subject-matter areas is reduced, the number of teaching periods is also reduced, and it is possible to lengthen the time of each period so that the teacher can work without interruption.

The third type of elementary school curriculum is the *activities-of-daily-living curriculum*. The learning activities are not organized into a definite pattern but are based on problems of everyday living which confront students. The emphasis is away from the mastery of subject matter and toward programs based on needs. Other curricula employing the same approach include the activity curriculum and the emerging curriculum. Of these types the emerging curriculum seems to call for the most understanding and creativity on the part of teachers and pupils.

The contemporary elementary school curriculum stresses the relationship of experiences to the learning process. The key word is *experiences*. The curriculum is organized for living and learning. These two words go together. No longer do we educate just for "later life." Education *is* life. It is concerned with the improvement of living—a better life for children and adults at the very moment—because of the *kind* of living that goes on in the school.

More and more curriculum theorists are calling for a curriculum which is organized into a planned series of encounters between the pupil, the teacher, and the wide community of persons and things. King and Brownell emphasize the necessity for the active involvement of children in the communities of discourse; they argue that this is the only way a vital curriculum can keep in close harmony with the changing conditions of the contemporary world of knowledge.[1] Goodlad makes a plea for action following understanding and commitment. In several of his publications he urges an abandonment of the ladder system in education, which requires each child to advance a grade a year, and proposes a non-graded system which will allow each child to advance at his own best rate.[2] In building his curriculum he stresses unifying principles rather than specific bits and pieces of knowledge.

Curriculum Development

Leadership in curriculum development has gone from the subject specialists and university and college professors to the "grass roots" of the community—to the teachers, supervisors, psychologists, specialists, and parents working together. The curriculum, in a sense, is part and parcel of the society, the local community, the classroom, and the pupils and teachers. All of these persons enter into the planning of the program so that the curriculum is viewed in the light of total influences. Materials and topics are carefully selected and developed cooperatively; supervisors and classroom teachers work together to rethink the curriculum periodically in terms of current problems which confront teachers in the school, the classroom, and the community. Where there is a need to make a change, a real effort is made to implement the findings rapidly.

Most of the larger schools have committees that are responsible for improving the program of studies, articulating it so that all elements of the school's offerings complement each other. This kind of planning guards against unnecessary duplication or gaps in the child's learning experiences. A good amount of long-range planning is necessary in both the broad subject areas and the special subject fields. Health topics, for example, need to be seen from the standpoint of their contribution to a broad area as well as from the single subject viewpoint. Planning, therefore, involves personalities and prepared courses of studies and available guides. Some of the many concrete elements that affect the teacher's planning in the health field are illustrated in this chapter.

The Curriculum Reform Movement. For a number of years curriculum specialists have been asking questions more insistently than ever. What priorities ought to be taught to children at any given stage of their development? How can the systematic testing of all new programs be carried out? What is the best way to encourage continuing experimentation with a variety of approaches to each field of study?[3]

So great has been the concern to restructure the curriculum and improve education in the United States that literally hundreds of separate projects have been initiated, completed, and put to use at state and local levels. Examples are numerous.

The widely used School Mathematics Study Group program (SMSG) was funded by the National Science Foundation for almost eight million dollars. The Biological Sciences Cur-

---

[1] King, Arthur R., and Brownell, John A. *The Curriculum and the Disciplines of Knowledge.* New York: John Wiley & Sons, 1967.

[2] Goodlad, John I. *School Curriculum and the Individual.* New York: Blaisdell Publishing Company, 1967.

[3] See especially the article by Robert M. McClure, "Trends in Curriculum Development," *Journal of Health, Physical Education, and Recreation,* 38:25–28, December 1967. See also John I. Goodlad, *The Changing School Curriculum.* New York: The Fund for the Advancement of Education, 1966, p. 15.

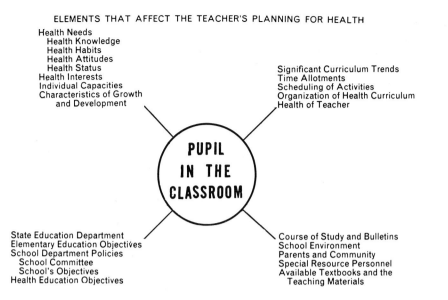

ELEMENTS THAT AFFECT THE TEACHER'S PLANNING FOR HEALTH

Health Needs
  Health Knowledge
  Health Habits
  Health Attitudes
  Health Status
  Health Interests
  Individual Capacities
  Characteristics of Growth
      and Development

Significant Curriculum Trends
Time Allotments
Scheduling of Activities
Organization of Health Curriculum
Health of Teacher

PUPIL IN THE CLASSROOM

State Education Department
Elementary Education Objectives
School Department Policies
  School Committee
  School's Objectives
Health Education Objectives

Course of Study and Bulletins
School Environment
Parents and Community
Special Resource Personnel
Available Textbooks and the
    Teaching Materials

riculum Study (BSCS) cost as much over the years 1959 to 1967. During this same period the high school physics program was overhauled by the Physical Science Study Committee (PSSC), and over 40 major curriculum projects were initiated in the social studies area in the last several years.

The School Health Education Study. The inadequacy of health education has been the concern of many groups and individuals for a number of years. In 1960 the NEA–AMA Joint Committee on Health Problems in Education recommended a survey of the nation's schoolchildren to determine the status of health education in the schools. Under a grant from the Samuel Bronfman Foundation in 1961, the School Health Education Study (SHES) was begun. Its purpose was to discover the status of health instruction and gain public support for reform measures.[4]

Large, medium, and small school systems were studied. Health behavior questionnaires were submitted to the students in the sixth, ninth, and twelfth grades in order to secure information which would reflect the accumulation

of health experience in the years prior to graduation.

The findings at all grade levels indicated serious misconceptions about health. Only one in five sixth graders brushed his teeth or rinsed his mouth regularly after eating. Sixth graders also scored poorly in safety education. This was not a strange finding, for it was discovered that health instruction practices were of poor quality throughout the country.

The School Health Education Study undertook a project to bring together health education specialists, supervisors, and classroom teachers to develop sample experimental curriculum materials based on a concept approach. These were carefully prepared and tested during the 1964–1965 school year in try-out centers in Alhambra, California; Evanston, Illinois; Great Neck–Garden City, New York; and Tacoma, Washington.

Beginning in 1966 SHES received support by the Minnesota Mining and Manufacturing Company (3M) to continue the development and publication of curriculum materials. In 1967, packets of materials pertaining to the first two concepts were available commercially, with the other eight concept areas scheduled to be available

---

[4] Sliepcevich, Elena M. *School Health Education Study: A Summary Report.* Washington, D.C.: SHES, 1964.

by 1971.[5] The ten curriculum concepts developed by the project are:

1. Growth and development influences and is influenced by the structure and functioning of the individual.

2. Growing and developing follows a predictable sequence, yet is unique for each individual.

3. Protection and promotion of health is an individual, community, and international responsibility.

4. The potential for hazards and accidents exists, whatever the environment.

5. There are reciprocal relationships involving man, disease, and environment.

6. The family serves to perpetuate man and to fulfill certain health needs.

7. Personal health practices are affected by a complexity of forces, often conflicting.

8. Utilization of health information, products, and services is guided by values and perceptions.

9. Use of substances that modify mood and behavior arises from a variety of motivations.

10. Food selection and eating patterns are determined by physical, social, mental, economic, and cultural factors.

The Health Concept Approach in Curriculum Development. It is appropriate at this stage of curriculum planning to consider outcomes of learning. In recent years, the two terms frequently employed to denote learning outcomes are *concepts* and *competencies*. Although they share a common ground, they are not the same. The concept is a point of view or idea held about something, whereas a competency is a solid ability or proficiency. Both are necessary in health education.

The concept approach offers the program planner a realistic pattern for the development of curriculum materials in health education. The topic has been well explored. (See especially the references to Bruner, Darrow, Phenix, and Woodruff at the end of this chapter.) Also, there have been several national curriculum studies that have used this approach quite successfully.[6]

A concept is a generalization about something. It is usually built from a number of related sensations, precepts, and images. Concepts range from ideas about very simple things to high-level abstractions. Woodruff has phrased a definition for curriculum planning which states:

> A concept is a relatively complete and meaningful idea in the mind of a person. It is an understanding of something. It is his own subjective product of his way of making meaning of things he has seen or otherwise perceived in his experience.[7]

To the individual pupil, a concept is a personal organization of a number of interpretations of things to which he has somehow been exposed. In this respect concepts cannot be taught as such. However, teaching is directed *toward* concepts. This means that the instructor is working with pupils in terms of whole ideas, even though pieces and bits of knowledges are being employed along the way. More specifically, the concept approach to learning is one in which all the facts, skills, and techniques are interdependent and interrelated. For too many

---

[5] Teaching-learning guides, together with the basic document (*Health Education: a Conceptual Approach to Curriculum Design, Grades K-12*) and printed originals for preparing overhead projection transparencies, are available from Visual Products, 3M Co., Box 1300, St. Paul, Minn., 55101.

[6] See Margaret Ammons and Robert A. Gilchrist, *Assessing and Using Curriculum Content.* Report of the Second National Conference on Curriculum Projects, Washington, D.C.: Association for Supervision and Curriculum Development, 1965.

[7] Woodruff, Asahel D. "The Use of Concepts in Teaching and Learning," *Journal of Teacher Education,* 20:81–99, March 1964.

years teachers of health have taught isolated vitamin facts in about the same fashion as history teachers have taught places and dates. The pupil learned his facts by rote memorization or repetition without seeing them as a part of a whole—a part of *his* life. They did not become a part of his value system. The dates, places, and vitamins were soon forgotten.

Therefore, the writers of the School Health Education Study materials realized that all health instruction activities must ultimately be related not only to the individual, but to the family and community at large. Health education attempts to unify man physically, mentally, and socially by developing health education behavior in the form of knowledges, attitudes, and practices with a dynamic focus on the individual, family, and community.

In a conceptual framework there are broad key concepts which represent the highest conceptual level of the health curriculum. In the School Health Education Study the three overriding concepts or processes affecting health behavior are:

> *Growing and Developing:* a dynamic life process in which the individual is in some ways like all other individuals, in some way like some other individuals, and in some ways like no other individuals.
> *Interacting:* an ongoing process in which the individual is affected by and in turn affects certain biological, social, psychological, economic, cultural, and physical forces in the environment.
> *Decision Making:* a process unique to man of consciously deciding to take an action, or of choosing one alternative rather than another.[8]

Practically all health education experiences can be fitted to the pattern of growing and developing, interact-

ing, and decision making. In the SHES project these key concepts were established as the three unifying threads of the health program from which the ten major curriculum concepts emerge. There are also subconcepts which were developed by elaborating on the basic ten concepts. These sub-concepts were set up in terms of physical, mental, and social dimensions. From this the long range goals were formulated in the *cognitive domain* (understanding, comprehending, realizing), *affective domain* (awareness, appreciation, consciousness), and *action domain* (developing, modifying, improving). Finally, the progression and sequence for the teaching-learning experience were developed.

Concepts have to be justified for each major health topic and each grade level. This was made clear by the members of the Curriculum Commission of the Health Education Division (AAHPER) when their report, *Health Concepts: Guides for Health Instruction*, was developed in 1967— after the crucial American health problems had been identified.[9]

A number of school systems have used concepts in the development of their local courses of study. *The Health and Safety Resource Guide, Kindergarten and Primary*, of the Waterloo (Iowa) Public Schools is especially well constructed with selected concepts for teaching and learning prepared for immediate teacher use. Of particular merit is the *Health Education Guide to Better Health*, grades K-six, for the state of Washington. Some 450 people helped prepare the guide in 1966. All units of study are set up in terms of one to six competencies, each supported by several well prepared concept statements. (A list of these competencies, together

---

[8] School Health Education Study. *Health Education: a Conceptual Approach to Curriculum Design.* St. Paul, Minnesota: 3M Education Press, 1967, p. 20.

[9] Health Education Division. *Health Concepts: Guide for Health Instruction.* Report of Curriculum Committee, Washington: American Association for Health, Physical Education, and Recreation, 1967.

with the respective concepts may be found in Appendix B.) This admirable design of concepts warrants a thorough study by the reader, for it is especially valuable for anyone about to begin the organization of a health instruction program.

Curriculum Scope and Sequence. Curriculum development deals specifically with the scope and sequence of the total program. When developing a program of health instruction for the primary and intermediate grades, one must also consider scope and sequence.

The word "scope" is used to define the breadth of the health curriculum. It tells *what* should be taught at all grade levels. The scope is wide or limited, according to the persistent and identifiable wants and desires of boys and girls. Sequence, on the other hand, refers to the *when* of the curriculum and determines the grade placement of the health learning experiences. It defines the curriculum vertically, whereas scope defines it horizontally.

DETERMINATION OF SCOPE. The basis for the scope of a health course is found in the necessities of life as revealed by close analysis, not by peremptory judgment. *The scope should present as great and as rich a selection of materials as possible. Teachers then do their own organizing. This is the modern elementary approach of stressing experience rather than subjects.* The better school systems are steadily moving in a direction beyond and above a static course of study and to a wealth of documentary materials based upon the needs of the group. Merely rewriting an old course of study in health does not necessarily improve the health curriculum, unless other documents are developed along with it to stimulate the classroom teacher to evolve her own organization and procedures — to develop a curriculum suited to a classroom of learners within a given community setting.

One who understands children will select, eliminate, and adapt experiences and materials to meet all the needs. The scope of the health curriculum, therefore, is made effective by greatly improving existing courses of study, by following guides to child development, and by using source units or course of study units. The last factor, the unit, is by far the most effective curriculum item. For example, in the health curriculum a very wide variety of learning and materials is organized into areas of experience, or in broad fields, or within single subjects, from which selections may be made. Health may be taught in the broad field of social studies or science, or it may be taught as a separate subject, or both. (It is most effective when taught as a separate subject.) Physical, mental, emotional, and social health embraces so much in the realm of human welfare and behavior that the scope of the health curriculum cannot easily be contained. There are limits, however, to the number and kind of topics that children should be introduced to at any one grade level. And there are obvious limits to the amount of emphasis or concentration afforded a particular topic at a certain grade level. All children, for example, are interested to some extent in foods, but the scope of the food topic in the second grade will be different from the sixth grade chiefly because of variations in interests, attention span, readiness, and maturity. The same could be said for sex education or any other elementary health topic.

In view of the vast scope of knowledge which has some relationship to present and future health needs of elementary schoolchildren, it has become more and more difficult for teachers and supervisors to select curriculum content in the health education area. It is necessary, therefore, that the scope be reviewed periodically in order to see what has been omitted that should be taught, to relegate to their proper places those health items that are only of minor importance, and to eliminate items that may be of a questionable nature. Moreover, scope must continually be related to needs, and carefully divorced as much as possible from human fallibilities, such as teaching a topic because it is easy or because it happens to be a personal preference.

DETERMINATION OF SEQUENCE. Sequence is defined in most elementary schools today, but it is not fixed with a rigid order of required topics for each school year. The trend is away from the fixed sequence to the more flexible one. The way to consider sequence is to have an overarching theme for each grade level and then suggest units. The teacher is perfectly free to plan with the pupils within the limits imposed by the theme. One should teach a unit when it is suited to the maturation of the pupils, when it provides for a coordination of learning experiences, when adequate materials are on hand, and when it is flexible enough to be of value in pupil-teacher planning.

It cannot be stressed too emphatically that the need for a planned course of instruction is essential for effective health teaching in the elementary school. The chief problem which faces most teachers is not what to teach in the major topical areas, but *how far one should go in the area at specific grade levels.* Solving this would help eliminate or minimize unnecessary repetition. Unfortunately, in many schools today health teaching is simply a "do-gooder" activity. The teacher, feeling sympathetic to the need for health instruction, decides to do "her bit" for the cause. She frequently teaches a little about the teeth, foods, and how to keep clean. This she does, all too often with no knowledge of what her pupils have already received in the way of knowledge from the year before or what they will be getting in the year ahead. Both scope and se-

quence are foreign terms in such a haphazard setup. A business run in this manner would go bankrupt in six months.

The only sound way to insure proper scope and sequence in health teaching is to set up the essential topical areas of instruction, under which are listed the knowledge and understanding that should be achieved at each grade level (in keeping with pupil characteristics, interests, capacities, and needs). Until this is done in every elementary school, health teaching will be at best only a "busy work" activity. (See latter part of this chapter and Appendix A, p. 407 for examples of health topics together with knowledges and understandings in sequence.)

Time Allotment and Scheduling. A health program can be definite enough to permit striving for preconceived objectives and flexible enough to provide for pupil needs. It may be taught quite informally, but it cannot be left to chance. It has to become a part of the total elementary school program by being scheduled; any program takes time to carry out. How much time should be spent on the health activities? Should a health curriculum, because of its wide scope, justify a rather large part of the school day? Is it conceivable that some teachers, extremely interested in a topic, might spend 30 to 40 per cent of a week's time on it? Who is to say whether this is right or wrong? Of course the classroom teacher must have a fair sense of value and use good judgment when allotting time to health instruction. Time ratios vary because of pupil factors relating to interests, experiences, and maturity; environmental factors involving facilities and materials; and the over-all curriculum plans of the particular school.

Many schools have a planned health curriculum which represents the results of long term study and research. This curriculum, coupled with state recommendations, may suggest a time allotment. For example, in New York

City 10 per cent of the time allotted to primary grades and 15 per cent in the intermediate grades is to be devoted to science and health teaching. In the state of California the law requires that "training for healthful living," "the nature of alcohol and narcotics," and "accident prevention and fire prevention" be taught, along with a number of other subjects, not in excess of 50 per cent of each school week. This permits flexibility, balance, and variety, and recognizes that unexpected events will appear, often as an interruption of school activities but of interest to all. In Kansas, for example, no specific time is even mentioned in the curriculum guides. It is simply stated that the day is no longer divided into short periods for recitation in each subject. Only a completely flexible program should be developed, with the weekly schedule existing chiefly for the teacher to determine whether she has made a fair and balanced distribution of her time.

Although primary graders have a short span of attention, they do not learn too effectively in very short periods day after day. Periods should be of sufficient length to have meaning, perhaps 15 minutes to half an hour. Several authorities prefer a set daily period for direct health teaching.

Daily classroom programs should also be planned so that different types of activity are scheduled for alternate periods; for example, active work following quiet work, such as project construction following reading, or physical education following arithmetic. There is little reason why classroom topics cannot be shifted around from week to week. Children like variety and innovations and respond very well to them. A health topic may be taught in the middle of the morning one day and just before lunch another day. If health is taught so that the class is interested in it, it might well be scheduled for a while during that period of time just before the noon hour when many children begin to slow down, show signs of fatigue, and have trouble concentrating on their arithmetic problems or some other subject.

Significant Health Curriculum Trends

If there is any one over-all trend in health curriculum planning it is to teach health understandings that yield proper practices and attitudes. This is being accomplished through a variety of experiences in a broad and flexible program. There are other trends:

1. The health curriculum is not limited to the activity and four walls of the classroom. It moves about the building. Primary grade children discuss playground accidents out where they might occur. Sixth graders visit the local sanitation department; they talk with restaurant owners about food handling and dishwashing practices. The health curriculum is alive and practical.

2. There is increasing emphasis on the manner in which principles and objectives influence the curriculum. Physical fitness is discussed in health classes at all grade levels. Exercise is cast in its proper role along with good nutrition, rest, and periodic medical check-ups. Classroom teachers are doing more testing for health behavior and physical fitness than ever before.

3. The health curriculum is being revised continually by classroom teachers working together with health services personnel, supervisors, and parents. Health needs change, and teachers are becoming more flexible in their teaching. They are more alert to the values of cooperative planning for health.

4. Health in the school is integrated with health in the community through the curriculum and teaching methods. Elementary teachers are learning more about their community health programs and agencies that can enrich their own health instruction.

5. Provision is being made in more

LARGE GROUP (80-250 pupils)	MEDIUM GROUP (30-36 pupils)	SMALL GROUP (10-15 pupils)	INDIVIDUAL TUTORIAL (individuals)	INDEPENDENT STUDY (individuals)

schools for formal, direct teaching of health in the elementary curriculum.

6. Health curriculum aids, such as bulletins, courses of study, and the state syllabus, are considered only as suggested guides for the teacher. The teacher must be sufficiently oriented to the modern elementary school purposes and instructional methods to be able to choose wisely those activities best adapted to the health learning situation in her classroom.

7. Because of the impact of advertising and quackery, a sharper evaluation is being made of health services and products.

8. The school nurse is more than ever an important member of the school health teaching team.

9. Sex and Family Living Education is being introduced in more elementary school health education programs.

10. There is slowly emerging a unified approach to health teaching in which all major health topics are properly considered instead of singling out one or two urgent topics (such as drugs and smoking) for special attention. There are fewer "one shot" assembly programs as token gestures of a health education program.

As indicated in a national committee report, elementary schools desperately need a school health coordinator, a designated, interested, and well-qualified faculty member who is responsible for the efficient operation of the health education program.[10] At present, the trend is slow along these lines.

Team Teaching. A number of new approaches to defining the functions of the elementary school teacher are being tried. One of these which has had an early success in Davidson County, Tennessee, and Lexington, Massachusetts, is *team teaching*. Here, an instructional team—free from the record-keeping clerical duties, teaches children in large or small groups or individually according to the nature of the subject matter. This arrangement, for example, makes it possible for all sections of an entire third grade to assemble for one type of lesson such as a superb film, a special lecture, or a speech by an outstanding resource person. More and more schools are experimenting with team teaching. Classroom teachers especially interested and talented in a phase of health may handle certain parts of the instructional program while others are free to develop new teaching materials or work with individual pupils.

The health curriculum lends itself to this kind of teaching. Although the large group will meet, often to introduce a unit of work, it is the medium group in which the bulk of the teaching is regularly done, so that teachers can have a continuing relationship with the same children over a period of time. The small group is especially valuable for carrying out vital discussions of health problems of interest to the age group. Also, there is ample room for individual tutoring within the school. Finally—and this is especially important—every pupil needs some time for a definite planned program of independent study. As the Trump Report suggests, this may be as much as 20 per cent of the instructional program.[11]

---

[10] See report of AAHPER Committee, "Needed Improvements in Elementary School Health Programs," *Journal of Health, Physical Education, and Recreation,* 38:28–31, February 1967.

[11] This report is especially well worth reading when considering the most effective organization for teaching. See J. Lloyd Trump, and Dorsey Baynham. *Guide to Better Schools.* Chicago: Rand McNally & Co., 1962.

In one large school in a suburb of Rochester, New York, all of the fourth grades studied a unit on digestion under team teachers. Working in small groups, each student posed questions that were placed on a large chart in the classroom and were subsequently answered. The team teachers found the approach challenging because children of various levels of ability could be reached. Moreover, the children enjoyed the format and greater flexibility that allowed for a more individualized instruction. The more able students acquired a sizable amount of information, as evidenced by their sophisticated reports and high test scores. However, as Polos suggests, there is no magic in team teaching, but in the light of many experiments it is effective in improving instruction.[12]

The Self-Contained Classroom. About three-fourths of all schools group students according to grade level in self-contained classrooms. The teacher gets to know the students well and has a chance to employ flexible grouping within the classroom. A well-prepared teacher can teach health effectively this way. In several places there is a health specialist, along with the music, art, and physical education specialists, who comes into the classroom to give a lesson.

Non-graded Classes. Approximately one large school system in three is currently using a non-graded sequence in at least some elementary schools. In this arrangement grade levels are removed from some or all classes, and the children who would normally be in these classes are placed in the non-graded sequence. This occurs mostly in the primary grades. Each pupil works according to his ability—beginning the new school year where he left off the year before.

Those who favor this organization point out that the pressure is off the

pupils, and material is better understood. However, non-grading requires close attention to record keeping in all subjects taught. Since boys and girls are no longer compared with each other, but only with themselves, the teachers need complete records on each pupil's progress.

Multi-graded Classes. Unlike the non-graded school, the multi-graded one retains grade levels. In a primary unit there would be an equal number of first, second, and third graders; and in an intermediate unit an equal number of fourth, fifth, and sixth grade pupils. About one-third of these pupils move on to the next unit each school year. This system of grouping permits students to advance at different speeds of learning. There is some evidence that it is more effective than the traditional organization of children. Superior teachers are required to teach within this framework.

UNIT TEACHING IN HEALTH

One of the most popular and often misused terms in education circles today is the "unit." Teachers loosely use the word, *unit*, to refer to a topic, an outline, a block of subject matter, a project, and even a chapter in a textbook. They divide and subdivide units at random and according to their own particular system of classification of instructional materials.

Most writers agree that a unit, whether for the teacher or the student, represents an organization of activities and information designed to develop useful understandings, attitudes, and appreciations which will contribute favorably to educational goals. Lee and Lee in their definition stress the implication that learning and socialization should be simultaneous. They say:

> A unit consists of purposeful related activities (to the learner) so developed as to give insight into, and increased control of some significant

---

[12] Polos, Nicholas C. *The Dynamics of Team Teaching.* Dubuque, Iowa: William C. Brown Co., 1965.

aspects of the environment; and to provide opportunities for the socialization of pupils.[13]

If a health unit stays within these definitions, one can hardly question its value. It begins with the health needs and interests of children who, with the help of the teacher, create and arrange an environment out of which will grow the purpose and enthusiasm for the work to be undertaken. Health units cut across subject-matter lines, thereby providing for integration. They furnish "grass-root" or first-hand experiences, and satisfy a number of innate drives to be active, to create, to dramatize, to communicate, and to construct. Lifelike opportunities in which the pupil may build something, experiment, read, share, interview, and express his ideas in various media are important parts of the units. The health unit centers in the present but stimulates an interest in future living. Early in its framework it encourages pupil discovery. Meaning is given to factual material when a unit requires problem-solving. Democratic group living is encouraged as desirable social habits are developed while children work on committees and in groups. Moreover, unit teaching stimulates critical thinking. It is rich in opportunities for children with varying degrees of ability and capacity to work along with others toward the success of the unit.

In addition to the numerous values of a unit, there are also certain rather well-defined characteristics which should be followed when constructing a health unit. Hanna, Potter, and Hagaman, in their extensive work on unit teaching in the elementary school, stress the following characteristics:

It possesses cohesion or wholeness.

It is based upon personal-social needs of children.

It cuts across subject lines.

It is based upon the modern concept of how learning takes place.

It requires a large block of time.

It is life-centered.

It utilizes the normal drives of children.

It takes into account the maturation level of the pupils.

It emphasizes problem-solving.

It provides opportunity for the social development of the child.

It is planned cooperatively by teachers and pupils.[14]

The Teacher's Resource Unit

A resource unit is simply a collection of suggested learning activities and materials organized around some central theme or given topic to be used by the teacher in preplanning. Often a resource unit in health is the product of a committee of teachers pooling their best ideas and then assigning to one teacher the responsibility of organizing the materials and to another the final writing. School nurses, dental hygienists, and even physicians may sit in and help with the unit. These units need not be complex or involved. They may be developed locally or at the state level. In either case they are not units of instruction but are chiefly collections of ideas and materials which may be helpful to an individual teacher in planning her work for the class.

It is worth repeating that the resource unit, no matter how complete, is not a teaching unit; it is strictly an aid to help the teacher and her students in planning a teaching unit. It usually is organized with a title and grade level designation, an introductory statement, a statement of proposed objectives, a content guide, suggested pupil activities, a list of

---

[13] Lee, J. M., and Lee, Dorris M. *The Child and His Curriculum*, 3rd ed. New York: Appleton-Century-Crofts, 1960.

[14] Hanna, Lavone A., Potter, Gladys L., and Hagaman, Neva. *Unit Teaching in the Elementary School*. New York: Rinehart & Co., 1955, p. 103.

teaching aids—books, pamphlets, music records, and films, and suggested evaluation procedures.[15] Ordinarily, the health resource unit is especially valuable for the classroom teacher, for it means that a considerable amount of research has been done to provide a number of useful ideas. As many or as few of these ideas may be used, depending upon the best interests of the particular class of learners at the time the teaching unit is being built.

Resource units in health may be built for a separate health course. Sometimes they are built to fit a broad-fields or core curriculum. They contribute to the core of a curriculum built around social living or science. This is sometimes thought of as a unit where there is a fusion of subject matter as part of the *integrating* experience which the unit provides. Certainly integration is desirable in health teaching. Children do not put knowledge in categories and classify it the way scholars do; life situations seldom fall within these artificial boundaries. The specialist in health education can be very helpful here in assisting core teachers. A number of classroom teachers will want to turn to the health educator for professional help in setting up units complete with problems to be studied, bibliographies for both pupils and teachers, and suggestions for school and community activities.

There follows below a brief example of the health aspects of a second grade resource unit. This was prepared for a core class studying the topic, "Living in Oswego, New York."[16]

---

[15] Klausmeier, Herbert J., and Dresden, Katherine. *Teaching in the Elementary School,* 2nd ed. New York: Harper & Brothers, 1962. Chapter 5.

[16] Because of the limitations of space, this is not the whole unit. It is a short edition of a resource unit, with a few examples of what might be found under each of the seven headings which relate especially to health teaching. One should keep in mind that the total resource unit would be sizable when it combines the subject-matter content from other fields.

I. Living in Oswego, New York
  1. Second Grade
II. Introductory Statement
  1. Second grade children like to talk about what goes on in their community. This is their world; it is rich, earnest, and full of meaning. It is alive with trucks, airplanes, bulldozers, mailmen, doctors, animals, children, and dozens of other things that move and fire the imagination.
  2. All towns and cities vary, yet all have things in common which most boys and girls gradually become familiar with and grow to understand.
III. Proposed Objectives
  1. These would include all of the understandings, values, skills, habits, and attitudes designed to favorably modify pupil behavior. For such a broad field as "Living in Oswego, New York" a rather lengthy list of objectives would be developed. Included in this list would be a number of references to personal and community health suitable for second grade pupils.
IV. Content Guide—Health Aspects Only—Problems to be solved
  1. How are trash and garbage collected?
  2. What kinds of homes are there?
    a. Do hotels, motor courts, and trailers all have heat, water, and clean toilets?
    b. Do some children live in homes where there are more accidents?
    c. Why do babies need so much care?
    d. How can we help our mother with the baby?
    e. Why are babies sometimes sick?
  3. How do people keep their surroundings clean?
    a. About the home?
    b. In the downtown restaurant?
    c. In the garage where the car is repaired?
    d. In the boys' and girls' room in school?
  4. Just how does one person's health habits affect the health of other people?

a. Why do people keep objects out of their mouths, cover sneezes, wash hands after toileting and before meals?

b. Is it a good idea to stay home when ill?

5. How does food keep fresh in the stores?

6. Where does our milk supply come from?

a. Why are paper milk containers better than milk bottles?

b. Why do the dairy farmers have to have a clean barn?

c. What kind of food do cows eat?

7. How does the policeman help the community?

a. What does the policeman in front of our school do?

b. Why is the policeman called "our friend"?

8. Where do we play in our community?

a. Why is play good for growing boys and girls?

b. What are the safety rules for swimming in Lake Ontario?

c. Do the fences around the playgrounds keep people in or out? Why is this?

d. How do beautiful parks in the city help to keep people happy?

9. How does our city take care of the sick?

a. How does the dentist help you?

b. How can the doctor tell when you are sick?

c. Why do people go to hospitals? How many reasons can you think of?

10. How do trucks and airplanes serve the city?

a. How many different kinds of trucks can you name? Airplanes?

b. Why is it colder up in the air than on the ground at the airport?

c. How is safety practiced by truck drivers?

V. Suggested Pupil Activities — Health Aspects Only

1. Arrange the room with pictures and other objects depicting community life in Oswego, New York.

a. *Pictures:* Of airplanes, the kind that land at the Syracuse airport as well as Air Defense Command jet planes and bombers; trucks that deliver milk, bread, laundry, oil; and trucks that collect garbage, repair telephone lines, haul logs; ambulances and patrol cars; department stores; public buildings such as City Hall, City Hospital, State grain elevator at the mouth of the Oswego river, Old Fort Ontario, Oswego harbor, water works, ships at dock in the harbor, the Niagara Mohawk Power plant with its four towering smoke stacks.

b. *Models and Exhibits:* Of food grown near by, such as small bag of onions, bunch of carrots, box of large Oswego berries (in season); children's model toys of earth moving equipment, milk trucks, bank trucks, fire engines; model of old time sailing ship; exhibits from Oswego County Historical Society; health models from Oswego County Health Association, clay model of breakwall in Oswego harbor, clay models of food, displays of home medical items including oral thermometer, box of Band-aids, open box of cleansing tissues, and cotton batting, boxes of hot and cold cereals found in the homes.

c. *Pamphlets and Books* of the milk, ice cream, and cheese making organizations in the community such as are represented by the National Dairy Council of Syracuse (especially adapted for second grade children); posters from local insurance company representatives illustrating optimum health; books for second graders:

d. PAMPHLETS (CHILDREN):

(1) *My Friend the Cow.* Grade

2. National Dairy Council.

(2) *A Visit to the Dentist.* Four-color booklet for second graders. American Dental Association.

(3) *Get Aboard the Good Ship Vitamin "C."* Colored pictures. Florida Citrus Commission.

(4) *Cuts of Meat in Your Grocery Store.* Pictures of various cuts of pork, beef, and lamb. National Livestock and Meat Board.

e. POSTERS:

(1) *School Safety.* National Safety Council.

(2) *Let's Be Safe Passengers.* Two-color drawing, relative to school bus boarding and leaving. National Commission on Safety Education.

(3) *Food Source Map.* Large U.S. map. Armour and Company.

(4) *The Rest Is Up to You.* Drawing of man in polka dot pajamas walking in sleep. Equitable Life Assurance Society.

(5) *Good Posture Pays Off.* Equitable Life Assurance Society.

(6) *It's Always Breakfast Time Somewhere.* Full-color chart. National Dairy Council.

(7) *We Help You Keep Fit.* Color chart on citrus foods. Florida Citrus Commission.

f. BOOKS (CHILDREN):

(1) Balet, Jan B. *Amos and the Moon.* New York: Oxford University Press, 1948. Story of boy searching for moon, in contact with butcher, fisherman, baker, and others.

(2) Barnum, Jay Hyde. *The New Fire Engine.* New York: William Morrow, 1950.

(3) Bianco, Margery. *Winterbound.* New York: Viking Press, 1948. Story of winter time in the community; what people do, and health concepts.

(4) Geismer, Barbara Peck, and Suter, A. B. *Very Young Verses.* Boston: Houghton Mifflin Co., 1945. Poems on cobbler, dentist, ice cream man, milkman, postman.

(5) Scott, William Rufus. *The Water that Jack Drank.* New York: William R. Scott, 1952.

(6) Steiner, Charlotte. *Wake Up! Wake Up!* New York: Grosset & Dunlap, 1952. Story stresses a good night's sleep for a vigorous, happy day ahead.

2. Have the boys and girls play with and handle the trucks, airplanes, the other models and exhibits relating to health.

3. Hike around the neighborhood observing community landmarks, not forgetting the grain elevator, the bakery, the fire station, and the hospital.

4. Talk about all the persons and things in the community that relate in some way to personal health. These are interest-arousing items.

V.A. Developmental Activities

1. Health activities used specifically to help acquire understandings, habits, and attitudes about health in the community. The following list of examples is incomplete. Many more would be necessary in a typical resource unit.

a. Read about life in the home. Discuss vacation time travels. Have children speak of the community's motor court and hotel accommodations.

b. Have children listen to stories about various health phases of community life. Creative children, with the help of the teacher, may want to dramatize a particularly interesting story or poem.

c. Discuss freely several elements of the community that definitely promote good health. Examples:

(1) How does the drug store help everyone in Oswego?

(2) Is it true that some sewage goes into the Oswego river?

(3) What do you think is being done about this?

(4) Where, along the lake shore, do most children swim? Do you think it is a safe place to swim?

(5) Many children go fishing from motor boats. How does one practice safety?

d. Employ appropriate films, film-strips, photographs, and phonograph records. Examples:

(1) *Play Safe.* National Safety Council.

(2) *Safety to and from School.* Young American Films.

(3) *The Fire Department.* Teach-O-Filmstrips, Popular Science Publication Co.

(4) *Common Cold.* Encyclopaedia Britannica Films, Inc.

(5) *A Smile Is to Keep.* American Dental Association.

(6) *Two to Make Friends.* Curriculum Films.

e. Use other community resources and materials. (Included here are field trips to dairies, and hospitals; material aids such as stick drawings, flash cards, displays, bulletin boards, graphs, special games, and puppet shows.)

f. Have children collect pictures from old newspapers (Oswego Palladium Times) representing health in the city of Oswego: pictures of city parks, recreation areas, drug stores, YMCA, swimming beaches, activities for crippled children, and scouting.

g. Display a very large sketch or picture of the common house fly and talk over how it carries dirt and germs between all the people in the city and county. Visit an open market and see the many ways foods are protected from flies.

h. Discuss individual cleanliness. Consider all the ways people in Oswego take baths (tub, wash tub, shower, and sponge).

i. Participate in school activities out-of-doors whenever practical. Ask the class the reason for this.

j. Visit a local restaurant, have morning milk and cookies. Have a small group represent the class and ask the restaurant owner questions about how he keeps the place clean.

k. Have the school or public health nurse show some of her equipment. Let the class ask questions. Have the nurse tell about her visits to sick people in and about Oswego.

l. Have a child bring his cat or mild-natured dog to class. Let the children see how friendly it is. Discuss having a pet show. Know that one must not tease pets around the community or play with strange animals.

m. Employ music to put across the concept that it is often the happy child who sings—and the happy child is normally the healthy child.

n. In art, encourage the painting of pictures depicting family life, crossing streets at the stop lights, turning the head to cough.

VI. Teaching Aids

1. Included here are as many materials and suggested resources for ideas as one can muster. These will include pertinent audiovisual aids, construction, experimentation, and demonstration materials, printed matter, posters, charts, exhibits, models, facilities useful outside the classroom, procedure for visits to the community, and procedure for bringing people from the community to the class.

VII. Evaluation Procedures
1. No matter how concentrated the resource unit is with materials, projects, activities, and ideas, only part of it will normally be employed in the classroom. A resource unit provides a source of readily available information for the teacher's use. Thus it is evaluated to some extent by the degree of usefulness it appears to have.
   a. Check sheets, developed in part by the class, are useful in observing habit and attitude changes toward community health problems and situations.
   b. At the beginning of the unit, "Living in Oswego, New York," a list of understandings of the moment might be prepared. It would be crude, but it could in part be compared to another such list prepared at the close of the unit. Children themselves, through self-evaluation, will offer many good suggestions to the question, "What have we learned about health in the City of Oswego?"
   c. Anecdotal records may be kept by the alert teacher. A number of check list methods are available for helping to organize behavior traits. If most of the class actively participates in a unit such as this one, each day there will be brought to the teacher's attention a number of pupil happenings worth recording. At the end of the unit when all records are combined, those concerning health habits and attitudes may be grouped for appraisal in terms of the original objectives.

The Health Teaching Unit

The essential difference between a teacher's resource unit and a teaching unit involves purposes. The purpose of a resource unit is to give the teacher a well fortified background in a particular area of study. In the teaching unit the organization is in terms of a given class. It is not nearly as broad and inclusive as the resource unit, it includes only those activities, materials, and evaluation techniques that will actually be used. Thus it is quite realistic and practical both in terms of time available and the nature of the learner. A teaching unit in the broad field of "Living in Oswego, New York" would differ from a resource unit of the same name, chiefly by being limited. Where a number of stories, films, and suggested activities appear in the resource unit, in the teaching unit the second grade teacher might read only one story, carry out two projects, and show one film.

Some planning of a teaching unit has to be done by the teacher in advance of meeting the class. Then the pupils are given a chance to select activities. They may examine or be given a choice of activities that appear in the resource unit. Those that seem to arouse enthusiasm may be selected for the teaching unit. This unit is then ready to implement. Needless to say, when pupils share in the planning of their own work in health they have greater retention of what they learn. Activities tend to be vital and are more apt to promote new health habits and appreciations. This is modern education at its best.

There is a difference in emphasis in health teaching between the primary and intermediate grades. It influences the building of the teaching unit. Health education in the primary grades is centered on helping children to live healthfully at home and at school. Much health is taught incidentally, indirectly, and informally in an effort to put across elementary health concepts and simple health practices. It would be very easy, therefore, for the teacher to "overorganize" the teaching unit in the kindergarten and first three grades. A few "tried and proven" ideas or activities may well make up the major part of the unit.

Obviously, during the planning stages of a unit, children come up with suggestions that are both excellent and impracticable (Figure 7–1). Through proper manipulation of the planning session the teacher guides the boys and girls into agreeing on the better suggestions. Evidence abounds in the primary grades to show that young, creative, and dramatic minds have imaginations that at times run wild. Gently curbing this wonderful quality, without at the same time reducing enthusiasm, is what makes teaching an art as well as a challenging profession.

Health teaching in the intermediate grades tends to be more specific, more formal, and generally planned in relation to broad areas of experience. Teaching units, therefore, are often constructed as subunits or integrated units of the broader field. Although they should not attempt to cover too much material in any one health area, nevertheless, it is difficult sometimes to strictly limit them. This is because health, in its fullest meaning, relates to physical, mental, emotional and social welfare. Practically everything that affects man may in some large or small way be connected to health teaching. Yet, it seems better to do a thorough piece of work on two or three projects or activities than attempt to rush through several. In the final analysis, limiting or extending the unit will depend on the nature of the pupils in the classroom.

Organization of Health Teaching Units. There are a number of ways to organize the teaching unit. Basically it needs some kind of introduction followed by objectives, a main body of activities, source materials, and finally some reference to evaluation.

Teaching units are generally organized along specific lines. This crystalizes the thinking of teachers and pupils. Klausmeier and Dresden use the same form that was employed in the resource unit. Various writers and educational groups have their differences and similarities in unit arrangements, but the similarities seem to outweigh the differences. Two examples of the organizations of teaching units follow:

KLAUSMEIER
  1. Title
  2. Introductory statement
  3. Objectives

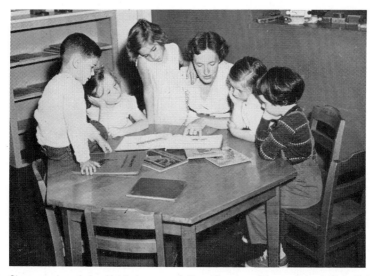

Figure 7–1 Class members help plan their own activities. (Courtesy Campus School, State University of New York, Oswego, N.Y.)

4. Content guide
5. Activities
6. Materials and resources
7. Evaluation

OBERTEUFFER AND BEYRER[17]

1. The title and statement of the problem
2. The objectives or outcomes sought in terms of behavior, knowledge, and attitudes
3. The content, problems, or subject matter of the unit
4. Student experiences or activities which will amplify content or throw light on the problems
5. The culminating or "wind-up" experience or summary
6. The resources available for developing the unit
7. Evaluating devices

Either of the above unit organizations can be used in health teaching. The pattern of the unit employed by Oberteuffer and Beyrer is concise and concentrated in seven topical headings. It is appropriate for this text.

Health Teaching in the Kindergarten

The health curriculum for kindergarten children may be quite informal. It is integrated with all other areas of instruction. Health topics are taught "as though you taught them not." The children are physically active, extremely individualistic, very imitative, dramatic, and imaginative. What they use in the way of material is largely manipulative and experimental. What they understand is generally developed through active participation and first-hand experience. Fantasy and reality appear to be the same to many children. The time-space concept is slow to develop.

Kindergarten boys and girls show interest in a number of items related to health. They are:

---

[17] Oberteuffer, Delbert, and Beyrer, Mary K. *School Health Education,* 4th ed. New York: Harper and Row, 1966.

Gaining confidence in themselves as persons.

Developing better motor coordination.

Speaking and acting spontaneously.

Assuming some responsibilities.

Learning to clean up and put things away.

Becoming observant of sights and sounds.

Becoming aware of the natural environment.

Gaining a number of specific health interests, such as:

Acting quickly and orderly in fire drills.

Practicing safe ways of going to and from school.

Visiting the school physician.

Carrying a clean handkerchief and covering the cough or sneeze.

Eating midmorning food and having a warm noon meal.

Resting between periods.

Having a relaxed atmosphere for classroom work and playground recreation.

Having proper toilet habits and practicing cleanliness.

Eating the right foods and caring for the teeth.

The observing kindergarten teacher will find numerous opportunities for health instructions every hour of the day. There will be times when it seems desirable to create situations which will appear to the pupils quite natural and unplanned. Daily health experiences in a healthful environment do much to build lasting impressions. Moreover, the kindergarten is a period of culturalization for children who have been neglected, "spoiled," or overprotected at home. It is a place for socialization, for getting to know people of one's age and what they are like.

The over-all kindergarten curriculum in health is much the same the country over. It is the emphasis that is different. In fact, there is considerable agreement between the various state courses of study and the curriculum specialists. Some of the kindergarten teaching areas common to most school situations today are covered rather well by an early bulletin of the New York State Department of Education:[18]

1. Health examinations and tests, including examination of teeth by dental hygiene teacher.
    a. Opportunity to make friends with the physician, nurse, and dental hygiene teachers and other members of the school health services staff.
    b. Opportunity to learn that everyone should have periodic health examinations by physician and dentist to help in keeping well.
2. Early morning checking time.
    a. Opportunity to inspect children, to recognize achievements and to care for health needs.
3. Weighing and measuring.
    a. Opportunity to arouse interest in growing and gaining and in doing things which will help children grow their best.
4. Mid-session lunch, noon lunch, real and play parties, preparation and tasting of real foods.
    a. Opportunity for practicing washing hands before touching food; sitting down to eat, relaxing, eating slowly and enjoying lunchtime, eating and liking certain foods; taking small bites, chewing food thoroughly and enjoying its flavor; touching only one's own food; washing and preparing food so that it is clean; discarding food which has

been dropped to the floor or ground; table manners.
5. Playground activities.
    a. Opportunity to arouse interest in activities in the sunshine and open air.
    b. Opportunity for fun, getting along happily with playmates, promoting physical development, increasing appetite and enjoyment of food, and maintaining or improving posture.
6. Rest periods.
    a. Opportunity to improve ability to relax and rest.
7. Cleanliness and health protection.
    a. Opportunity to learn desirable practices related to cleanliness of body and clothing, food and eating, use of handkerchief, protection of self and others when ill.
    b. Opportunity to learn to use toilet, handwashing, and drinking facilities properly.
8. Reading and other close eye work.
    a. Opportunity for learning proper position of books and other materials and adjustments of lights and shades.
9. Cooperation in keeping air in classroom fresh.
    a. Opportunity to help regulate air conditions by notifying custodian or by other appropriate means; to enjoy the feeling of a well-ventilated room; to become aware of the teacher's attention to the thermometer and air conditions.
10. Seating
    a. Opportunity to learn to select seats, desks, and tables so that the child may work and play in comfort and to change position to meet changing needs.
11. Clothing
    a. Opportunity to learn to put on and take off outdoor clothing and to care for it properly.

[18] Adapted from The University of the State of New York Bulletin, "A Guide to the Teaching of Health in the Elementary School," Bulletin No. 1328. Albany: The University of the State of New York Press, November 1, 1946, p. 89.

12. The total program
   a. Opportunity to enjoy and be reasonably successful in work and play, to get along happily with children and adults, to become increasingly self-reliant in caring for own needs and in helping others.
   b. Opportunity to participate fully in the daily program with decreasing need for adult guidance to the end that the child's own safety and the safety of others will be an important outcome of the program.

Research indicates that normal children of kindergarten age, though young in years, are quite receptive to ideas and are capable of learning many presumably difficult things. Because of the interest span and time factor, selecting what to teach is a necessary consideration. Many studies indicate that information on foods and safety is important. Research completed in the Los Angeles City Schools involving almost 1200 kindergarten pupils showed the need for emphasis in health instruction to be greatest in the following health areas:

Rest and sleep (correct bedtime and habit of taking a nap during the day)

Grooming (habit of hanging up clothes)

Growth and development (habit of sitting quietly and listening when others speak)

Prevention and control of disease (acceptance of immunization shots and habits of keeping hands out of mouth, and covering mouth and nose when coughing and sneezing)[19]

The new teacher, with the help of the children, will find it wise to build a series of teaching units covering the several areas of emphasis at the kindergarten level. These may be in skeleton form so that they can easily be amended during the period of use or kept flexible from year to year with appropriate modification.

Kindergarten Health Charts. One of the most effective health teaching items for the kindergarten age child is a series of 36 full-color charts (17 inches × 20 inches size).[20] Each chart presents a basic health concept in pictures — a method of learning most appealing and effective with youngsters of this age level. People, young and old, are portrayed in familiar situations stressing fundamental health and safety practices *with which children can identify.*

Teachers show these large charts (with spiral binding and easel-back for convenient viewing) to their class in order to provoke discussion relative to personal health practices. Figure 7–2 is a greatly reduced picture of chart No. 11 entitled *Warm and Dry?* In this particular illustration the teacher might begin the lesson by showing the chart and asking: "How do you know that it is a rainy, cold day? Do you think the children in the picture are wet or cold? Why not? Do you think the dog is cold? He certainly is wet. Why do you think this picture is called *Warm and Dry?*"

Health Teaching in the Primary Grades

The health curriculum for the first three grades is one in which the pupil is not held responsible for a great amount of specific health knowledge. Children may engage in a large number of experiences, but informality continues as it did in the kindergarten.

[19] Bobbitt, Blanche G., and Sellery, C. Morey. *Appraisal of Health Instruction in Selected Grades of Los Angeles City Elementary and Secondary Schools and Colleges.* Preliminary report to American School Health Association. San Francisco, Calif., October 30, 1960.

[20] Gallagher, J. Roswell, Spencer, Mary E., and Willgoose, Carl E. *Health Charts for Kindergarten (How About You?).* Boston: Ginn and Co., 1965. A *Teachers' Manual,* offering detailed suggestions for presenting the pictures, is included with the charts.

Purpose
To focus on the reason for staying warm and dry.

Related Outcomes
Developing understanding of use of clothing as protection for the body.
Showing importance of prompt removal of wet clothing.
Helping child understand need for proper care of wet clothing.

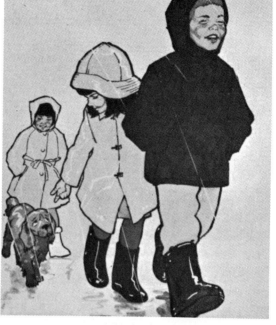

Figure 7-2 Kindergarten health chart. (With the permission of Ginn and Co., Boston, Mass. 02217.)

The approach is one of definite exploration of the important health practices. There will be opportunities for integration of the health instructional program with social studies, science, and physical education.

Since growth is a continuous process, there will be varying degrees of maturity, capacities, and interests among primary grade pupils. Where first graders are beginning to differentiate between fancy and reality, third graders will have pretty much established this differentiation. As children mature during the primary years they gain in ability to present their own ideas and problems orally and in writing. They gradually begin to appreciate cause and effect relationships, project their feelings more and more toward others, become less individualistic and possessive, and are more cognizant of adult opinion. Growth is slow and steady; they continue to tire less as they approach eight years of age, and show an increase in physical strength and dexterity.

Primary children show interest in a number of items related to health. They are:

Beginning to show some muscle growth

Advancing to a state of full visual fusion

Watching the first permanent teeth appear

Accepting greater responsibility for personal safety and appearance

Talking about nourishing food, going to bed early, playing out of doors and brushing teeth

Choosing lunch foods wisely

Practicing good sportsmanship

Aware of defective sight and hearing

Concerned with minor cuts and bruises

Curious about disease prevention

Beginning to develop some group responsibility, and are adjusting quite well to school.

The primary grade curriculum in health is designed to help children meet a number of health problems of the moment. This is presented not in great detail, but in the manner of an orientation so that a firm foundation

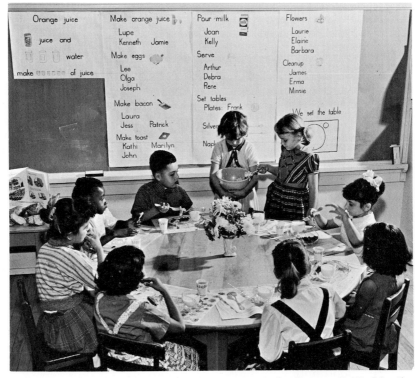

Figure 7-3 A carefully planned food tasting party arouses curiosity. (Courtesy *Health Education Journal,* Los Angeles City Schools.)

may be laid for the more advanced curriculum content in the intermediate grades. The big teaching task is to arouse curiosity, promote questions and lead pupils to give expression to their thinking.

The teaching areas common to most primary school situations may be seen by reviewing current courses of study. Opinions of health curriculum specialists are also valuable. Here are three examples:

KILANDER[21]

Personal health

Nutrition

Community health and sanitation

Consumer health

Mental health

Stimulants and depressants

Family living

Safety education

First aid

Home nursing

ANDERSON[22]

Physical Health

Personal and school cleanliness

Rest and sleep

Eating practices

Posture

Play practices

Dental health

Lighting

Common cold

Safety to and from school

Schoolroom safety

Playground safety

Home safety

Body growth

Mental Health

Sharing

[21] Kilander, H. Frederick. *School Health Education.* New York: The Macmillan Co., 1962, Chapter 16.

[22] Anderson, C. L. *School Health Practice,* 3rd ed. St. Louis: C. V. Mosby Co., 1966, p. 312.

Working together
Kindness
Being friendly
Orderliness
Depending on ourselves
Attaining goals

Community Health
  Home life
  Sources of water and milk
  Sunshine and health

TURNER, SELLERY, SMITH[23]
  Cleanliness
  Hands and nails
  Teeth
  Nose and mouth
  Hair
  Elimination
  Clothing
  Food habits
  Table manners
  Play and exercise
  Sleep
  Communicable disease control
  Sanitation
  Harmful substances
  Growth and health
  Mental and emotional health
  Safety

Health Teaching in the Intermediate Grades

The health curriculum for the fourth, fifth, and sixth grade pupils is one that builds on what has already been taught in the first three grades. The teacher approaches the health topics more objectively. There is greater depth in subject matter and a little more formality than in the primary grades. *The sole reason for this change is that the pupils are ready for more detail.* They know how and why to brush their teeth. Now their curiosity is aroused and they ask searching questions having more to do with the exception

---

[23] Turner, C. E., Sellery, C. Morley, and Smith, Sara Louise. *School Health and Health Education*, 5th ed. St. Louis: C. V. Mosby Co., 1966, pp. 299–301.

rather than the rule. They want to know, for example, why some man or woman of their acquaintance who never uses a toothbrush and eats haphazardly has such fine white teeth.

This is the age when the questions asked are often a real challenge to the teacher. It is a period in the growth of the nine, ten, and 11 year olds when there is a magnetic "awakening" to all that goes on around them. There is an adventurous spirit demonstrated by a willingness to try anything once, to look here and there, to explore eagerly. There is a heightened interest in science and machines—how bugs walk, what germs look like under the microscope, how the skeletal muscles hold up the body, and the effect a trip to the craters of the moon would have on man in a rocket. Here is a time when dreamers begin to look ahead and imaginative minds are literally "on fire." Health stories of adventure, mystery, travel, science, sports, animal life, and nature go over big.

In addition to placing greater emphasis on the fundamental topics of the primary grade curriculum, there is a need for special instruction in alcohol and narcotics. By the fifth and sixth grade period a number of pupils, boys in particular, have a desire to try a cigarette or taste alcoholic beverages. Both of these items are readily available in many homes today. This is the age when the "gang" develops, and boys and girls begin to conform to the wishes of the group. The ten or eleven year old shows an increase in self-direction and responsibility. The "wise guy" has a cocky walk and the rounded shoulders of the "man about town." He is seen all too often a block from school flicking the ashes from his cigarette as he heads for home. He is ready for a realistic picture of smoking directly from a classroom discussion.

Sex antagonisms grow and become acute by the sixth grade. Boys are interested in boys; girls in girls. Both profit from instruction pertaining to family relationships. Although sex education really begins at home, little is said about it in many cases. It should be integrated with the total health education program at all grade levels. It should not be singled out for separate or undue emphasis. In back of the 11 year old pupil's sex antagonism is a smoldering interest in the subject. It should be taught without apology by showing its nobility in terms of creative drive and family happiness.

When considering the areas for health instruction in grades four, five, and six, there is rather close agreement among curriculum committees and specialists. Here are the major health topics set forth in three different curriculum guides:

KANSAS STATE DEPARTMENT
OF PUBLIC INSTRUCTION[24]

Nutrition
Disease control
Dental health
Alcohol, tobacco, narcotic drugs
Personal hygiene
Family living
Safety
First aid
Mental health
Community health

DETROIT PUBLIC SCHOOLS[25]

Recreational safety
Nutrition
Conservation of vision and hearing
Disease prevention
Emotional health
(Sleep, rest, and dental health covered
in depth at K-3 level)

WATERLOO PUBLIC SCHOOLS[26]

Physical health
Necessary life functions

Eating
Play and exercise
Rest and sleep
Elimination
Care of the body
Cleanliness
Teeth
Sense organs
Clothing
Narcotics and stimulants
Social, mental and emotional health
Disease and its prevention
Communicable
Non-communicable
Life adjustment
Understanding ourselves
Understanding others
Safety
Precautionary procedure
Home
School
Community
Vacation
First aid
Sickness
Injuries
Civil defense
Signals
Practices
*Community resources and community
health*
Sanitation
Food, water
Waste
Health services
Professional care
Cooperative effort

These current lists, now being used as guides in thousands of elementary schools, should give some idea of the scope of the intermediate instructional program. The only trouble with these lists is that they are much too general. They cover the scope of all three intermediate grades instead of treating each grade separately.

At the present time the state guides teachers may find most helpful come from the states of Arkansas, California, Colorado, Florida, Kansas, Maine, Maryland, New York, North Carolina, Oregon, Vermont, Virginia, and Washington.

The Intermediate Grade Health Unit. Using the original resource unit as a guide for direction and ideas,

---

[24] Division of Instructional Services. *Health Education K-12, Guide for Curriculum Development.* Kansas State Department of Public Instruction, 1967, pp. 13–23.

[25] Division of Improvement of Instruction. *A Curriculum Guide for Health Instruction, K-6.* Detroit Public Schools, 1966, pp. 61–112.

[26] Board of Education. *Health and Safety Resource Guide.* Waterloo, Iowa: Waterloo Public Schools, 1964, pp. 99–142.

the teacher acts cooperatively with her class to plan a unit of work. At the intermediate grade level the unit or organization is the same, but the emphasis varies somewhat from that in the lower grades. Instead of embracing a multitude of activities suitable at the primary level and treating them somewhat superficially for orientation, the class generally agrees on a few carefully chosen activities or projects that have depth, sustain interest over a reasonable period of time, and stimulate research and discussion. It is probably better to have two or three top flight experiences in the unit than to lightly "browse" through a dozen less ponderable ones.

As previously indicated, the health unit at this level will need to be related to the other subject matter areas so that the health instruction will not only be practical in terms of the health area, but also meaningful in terms of the total curriculum at the moment. Opportunities for the integration and correlation of unit content and activities is also planned for.

The Graduated Program of Major Health Topics

In view of recent curriculum research, and especially the findings and recommendations of the President's Council on Physical Fitness and the School Health Education study relative to pupil interests, behavior and needs, it seems that the most appropriate health instruction curriculum for elementary school children is one that is spelled out in much more detail than the usual programs of the past. This means that teachers must get together and carefully plan for both scope and sequence in health teaching. Precisely, the major health topics or health areas for each grade level have to be established, along with a *graduated* list of knowledges and understandings (or concepts) to be achieved by pupils. This is not an easy task; it requires the combined

deliberations of several top teachers frequently under the leadership of the elementary curriculum specialist.

In order to insure a graduated program under each major health topic, *all of the desirable knowledges and understandings should be recorded for all six elementary grades.* This extensive list is then reviewed and arranged in such a manner as to place the easier-to-learn items first and the difficult-to-learn items last. It is then carefully divided into six divisions according to grade level with the more detailed knowledges and understandings falling at the fourth, fifth, and sixth grades. This kind of order prevents important topics from being omitted and other topics from being taught at an inappropriate time.

The *major health topics* for the elementary school are as follows: (P-Primary Grades; I-Intermediate Grades)

1. Personal cleanliness and appearance (P, I)
2. Physical activity, sleep, rest, and relaxation (P, I)
3. Nutrition and growth (P, I)
4. Dental health (P, I)
5. Body structure and operation (P, I)
6. Prevention and control of disease (P, I)
7. Safety and first aid (P, I)
8. Mental health (P, I)
9. Sex and family living education (P, I)
10. Community health (P, I)
11. Tobacco, alcohol, and drugs (I)
12. Consumer health (I)

Notice that the topics of Tobacco, alcohol, and drugs (No. 11) and Consumer health (No. 12) are introduced at the intermediate level.

By way of example, the following graduated material is outlined for the dental health topic for each of the six grades. It is a brief selection of knowledges to which other related knowledges may be added. Note that there is some overlapping, yet there is progression toward more difficult material:

DENTAL HEALTH

KNOWLEDGES AND UNDERSTANDINGS

Grade One

When and how to brush teeth
Loss of first teeth and appearance of first
   6-year molar

Grade Two

Care and brushing of first teeth
Using toothpaste or powder
Care of the toothbrush
Raw foods that help keep teeth clean
How sweets affect teeth
Value of regular dental care

Grade Three

How teeth may be cleaned without brush-
   ing
Foods that build strong teeth
What the dentist does for us
The appearance of clean teeth
The cause of toothache

Grade Four

Structure of the tooth
Harmful effects of decayed teeth
Practices that injure teeth
Importance of good teeth for talking and
   digestion
Some schools employ dental hygienists to
   help children about the care of their
   teeth

Grade Five

Relation of structure to the function of
   teeth
The significance of malocclusion
The meaning of good dental health
Personal tooth care and regular visits to
   the dentist
Importance of orthodontia

Grade Six

Progress of sixth graders toward the development of a full set of teeth
Equipment and the special skills used by
   dentists for many purposes
Appraising dentifrice advertisements

Turn to Appendix A (p. 407) for a graduated list of suggested knowledges and
understandings for *each* of the major health
topics, grades one to six. This may be employed as a guide in building a course of
study.

It should be pointed out that planning for the first six grades must be
done in terms of future junior and
senior high school programming. In
the above dental health example it is
obvious that more technical knowledge and understanding is not called
for here, but with this foundation the
student is prepared for more detailed
study in grades seven or eight. Moreover, a detailed structuring of knowledges, understandings, or concepts
should be included in the finished
curriculum guide or course of study.
If, for instance, this structuring were
applied to Grade Four above the more
specific knowledges to be attained
might be elaborated as follows:

Grade Four

Dental Health. Teeth that are
clean and growing properly are an asset to an individual in at least three
ways: talking, appearance, and
digestion.

The tearing and grinding function of
teeth aids the process of digestion.

The four kinds of permanent teeth
—incisors, cuspids, bicuspids, and
molars are each helpful in a special
way.

The tooth structure consists of the
crown, neck, root, enamel, cementum,
nerves, and blood vessels.

Decayed teeth may cause illness and
a disturbance in other bodily processes.

There are a number of practices injurious to the teeth.

The school dental program exists
for the benefit of all schoolchildren.
The dental hygienist is employed to
help teach children how to care for
their teeth.

Organizing Major Health Topics

How does one organize the major health topics in the instructional program from grades one to six? Is each topic referred to each year? Is there a danger of too much repetition on a yearly basis? Is there merit in a cycle plan in which certain topics are omitted or simply reviewed every other year?

Certainly it has been the custom to have a considerable spread of information through the grades rather than a concentration at certain grade levels. Each major health topic has been taught at each grade level rather than being omitted at any grade level. Sometimes this insures healthy repetition and frequently acquaints the pupil with something that may have been missed the year before, especially in schools that do not follow a planned health instruction curriculum.

It is common knowledge that it is extremely difficult to keep from repeating too often what is said in the second grade to the children in the third grade. Health teaching may be more effective when there is a concentration of instruction on certain health topics on an every-other-year basis instead of spreading a limited amount through each of six or eight grades. Where the *total* elementary school health instruction program has been carefully planned there may be real value in such a cycle plan.

The cycle chosen may vary slightly for each major health topic. Almost all topics should be introduced in the first grade. It may be wise to introduce "nutrition and growth" to first and second grades, skip the third and continue in four and six. The same thing may be true in "safety." Obviously, there is much safety teaching to accomplish right away in the first three grades. Here, one might skip the fifth grade and proceed to the sixth. There is so

Summary of Topics by Grades

	1	2	3	4	5	6
Nutrition and growth	x	x	R*	x	R	x
Personal cleanliness and appearance	x	R	x	R	x	R
Dental health	x	x	R	x	R	x
Accidents and safety	x	x	x	x	R	x
Mental health	x	R	x	R	x	R
Sex and family living education	x	R	x	R	x	R
Body structure and function	x	x	x	x	x	x
Disease control	x	R	x	R	x	R
Community health	x	x	R	x	R	x
Physical activity, sleep, rest, relaxation	x	x	x	x	R	x
Tobacco, alcohol, and drugs					x	x
Consumer health			x	R	x	R

*R = Review year (brief treatment of topic).

much to cover in "body structure and function" that the topic might be spread through all six grades. In the planning stage, a chart would be constructed to reflect the organization.

This cycle plan seeks to get away from needless repetition—repetition that all too often is deadly, because it smothers curiosity and kills the interest of normally intelligent boys and girls. Frequently children are bored with lessons on such subjects as brushing the teeth, or standing tall, or something similar; they see nothing new, fresh, and stimulating. Much of this may be prevented when the major health topics are thoroughly covered on the "on" year and very simply reviewed on the "off" year.

Critical Areas for Attention. There are at least two major health topics today which require special attention when the health curriculum for the elementary school child is being planned. These are safety education and sex and family living education. Each of these topics is big enough to stand by itself in the elementary curriculum. There are, in fact, school systems where these two topics are considered separately from the health curriculum.

In singling these areas out for special emphasis one runs the risk of giving the impression that other health topics are less significant. Obviously, all major health topics are important. Moreover, this is an era when health educators are striving for a unified approach in health teaching and when *all topics* command a proper amount of attention in a balanced and sequential program. (See Chapter 8 for ways and means of implementing these major health topics.)

Both safety education and sex and family living education have been selected as critical areas for attention because of the widespread interest associated with them.

SAFETY EDUCATION

The Emphasis on Safety

Today, in the face of mounting accident rates, the elementary grade programs stress education for safe living. Teachers are in duty bound to put forth their finest efforts in this area.

It is worthwhile to spend a little time discussing the significance of this major health topic, for safety education is more than just an offspring of health education; it is practically a full-fledged area by itself. There are signs that safety education may well turn out to be what Malfetti calls a "block off the old chip." Accidents are epidemic in the United States. They kill more persons under 46 than any other "disease"; more between ages 15 and 24 than all other causes combined. They cause serious injury to millions of people annually. Moreover, at ages five to 14, accidents cause half the deaths among boys and a third among girls—a toll that has been rising in recent years. (See Fig. 7–4.) Recognizing the enormity of this, the U.S. Public Health Service recently expanded its accident prevention program. This officially makes accident prevention equal with the study of mental illness and of cancer, heart disease, and other leading killers.

Although accident statistics do little to convince children that they should exercise safe conduct, they do serve to point up the seriousness of the situation, and especially the need for group action.

Children and Accidents

As already indicated in Chapter 1, all accident statistics are frightening indeed. Moreover, in every accident category the number of deaths and injuries related to children alone is suf-

MORTALITY FROM LEADING TYPES OF ACCIDENTS AT AGES 5–14
United States, 1963-64

Type of Accident	At Ages		
	5–14	5–9	10–14
Average Annual Death Rate per 100,000			
Boys			
Accidents—All Types	25.5	24.1	27.0
Motor vehicle	11.0	11.7	10.2
Traffic	10.7	11.3	10.0
Pedestrian	4.9	7.0	2.6
Nontraffic	0.3	0.4	0.2
Drowning*	5.3	4.6	6.1
Firearms	1.9	1.0	2.8
Fires and explosions	1.7	2.2	1.2
Falls	0.8	0.7	0.8
All other	4.8	3.9	5.9
Home Accidents†	4.2	4.5	4.0
Girls			
Accidents—All Types	11.4	13.2	9.5
Motor vehicle	5.7	6.3	4.9
Traffic	5.6	6.2	4.8
Pedestrian	2.5	3.6	1.2
Nontraffic	0.1	0.1	0.1
Fires and explosions	2.1	3.1	1.1
Drowning*	1.3	1.3	1.3
Firearms	0.4	0.4	0.3
Falls	0.3	0.3	0.3
All other	1.6	1.8	1.6
Home Accidents†	3.0	4.1	1.7
Accidental deaths as a percent of all deaths			
Boys	49%	47%	52%
Girls	33	35	30
Motor vehicle accident deaths as a percent of all accidental deaths			
Boys	43	48	38
Girls	50	48	52

*Exclusive of deaths in water transportation.   †Also included in other accident categories.
Source of basic data: Reports of the Division of Vital Statistics, National Center for Health Statistics.

Figure 7–4 Accidents among school age children. (Courtesy Metropolitan Life Insurance Co., *Statistical Bulletin*, September, 1967.)

ficient to cause parents and teachers to think in terms of prevention.

Children are everywhere. They play with fire and get burned. They discharge misplaced firearms, fall out of high places, and drown while swimming, boating, and fishing. Large numbers of non-swimmers and poor swimmers have neither the skills nor the knowledge so closely associated with water activities. Like many of the adults who have boating accidents, they are careless and negligent around the water.

Children are injured and die in automobile accidents because they and their parents are willing to pay the enormous price for our "rubber-tired

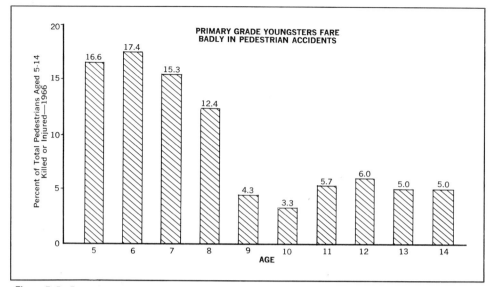

Figure 7-5   Percentage of school children killed or injured in pedestrian accidents—1966. (Courtesy American Automobile Association.)

existence." Yet, it is possible through safety education classes to demonstrate how the seat belt and the shoulder strap work to save lives. Children who understand this frequently prod adults into using seat belts instead of sitting on them when they drive. Seat belts will not prevent accidents, but, like insurance, they soften the blow if the worst happens.

Pedestrian accidents are high among younger children. Over 50,000 children are injured each year, many permanently. In an American Automobile Association study the schoolchildren in the first three grades fared poorly in pedestrian accidents as compared with older groups. (See Figure 7–5.) These figures are not surprising since primary graders are prone to cross streets at the wrong time, pass between parked cars, and dart into the street during their informal play activities.

It has been researched and demonstrated that a school site can be safe for pedestrians through careful building engineering and traffic control, and through responsible education of the young pedestrian.[27] In a number of places in which buses are not used children are being guided relative to the "safe route to school." In the same manner, older children have received guidance relative to bicycle routes to school in an effort to reduce a sizable number of bicycle injuries.

The National Fire Protection Association indicates that there were 7100 school fires in 1965. Fortunately, such fires have been held to a minimum because of changes in the physical makeup of the school itself, the addition of protective devices, and the pupil-teacher fire drill training. Actually, the need is great for fire safety precautions in the home, in which 200 children die a year.

Young Children and Accidental Poisoning

An estimated 1,000,000 poisonings occur each year, most of them among

[27] See especially *Guide to a School Pedestrian Safety Program*. Washington, D.C.: Automotive Safety Foundation, 1965. See also Sam Yaksich, Jr., "Afoot Among Wheels," *Safety Education*, September–October 1967, p. 13.

children; over 500 children die from the effects. Public health officials blame at least part of the deaths on widespread misconceptions about what constitutes a poison. About a quarter million products designed for use in the home contain toxins, and many of these seem to be attractive to youngsters for chewing, drinking, and eating. Products such as cleaning and polishing agents, detergents, shoe polish, cosmetics, paint, plant and food sprays, and a variety of medicines have all been involved in accidental poisonings. Efforts to decrease the number of home poisonings led to the passage in 1960 of the Hazardous Substance Labeling Act. It requires the labels of household aids and medicines to list poisons, antidotes, and recommendations for use. An important innovation in poisoning treatment procedures is the poison control center, organized by physicians and coordinated by the Department of Health, Education, and Welfare. There are almost 500 such centers in hospitals throughout the nation. Here the poison contents of thousands of trade-name products are crossindexed. These are primarily information centers. However, neither the law concerning hazardous substances, nor the poison control centers can help to decrease the number of poisonings, if parents do not do their share.

Teachers have a real role to play. Once a year they should be instrumental in getting the message to all parents of primary grade children that poison hazards can be reduced by:

1. Placing drug cabinets high on the wall and locked, or securely fastened.

2. Keeping carbon tetrachloride, contained in dry-cleaning fluids and polishes, out of the way of children.

3. Keeping aspirin out of the reach of the young.

4. Checking the labels on children's toys to be sure that the paint used for the often bright and cheery colors is not deadly.

5. Determining whether or not unused medicine should be saved. Unusable medicine should be thrown away to avoid the hazard of medicine which has become toxic with time.

Man's Friend the Dog

The dog-bite rate is about 400 per 100,000 population or 800,000 cases a year. The figure is probably low, as many bites are unreported. In most cases the dog doing the biting is labeled as "friendly" by both owner and victim. Female dogs and young dogs are more likely to bite. Incidence of bites generally doubles when the warm weather comes and dogs and children are out of doors more. Man has not learned how to live with dogs; he treats the dog as a completely domesticated animal when, in reality, the animal is partially wild. To enjoy the companionship of these pets with safety young people should be taught:

Do not hold your face close to the dog

Do not permit your dog to stray. In one city a leash law resulted in a 50 per cent drop in dog bites

Do not pet a strange dog

Do not tease a dog, pull its tail, or take away food, a bone, or a toy with which he is playing

Why Accidents Happen

With the poet-philosopher we can say "to err is human," but in the next breath we must admit that "to err" is relative. It is relative to the thinking ability of man. This is where the problem really lies, for only about 15 per cent of accidents are due to hazardous conditions in the environment; it is man's behavior that counts.

Involved in the human factor at the elementary age level are essentially four elements:

Lack of knowledge and experience regarding the laws of cause and effect—the underlying reasons behind accidents and accident topics, i.e., fire, electricity, and water safety

Lack of skill in such activities as swimming, using playground apparatus, shop equipment, and crossing busy highways

Improper attitudes and personal traits—a "daredevil" or foolhardy manner that makes it easy to "take a chance"

Inadequate emotional health, coupled with unrestrained emotions and yielding an "accident-prone" state

The last factor is especially interesting. A close study of accident causes shows too often that injuries are not accidental as they first appear. A small number of people have a higher percentage of accidents. Even when they move to new locations they keep on getting hurt. These individuals are termed "accident-prone." They have an accident habit or pattern which usually develops early in childhood. Accidents have become their way of solving problems and frustrations. Thus the careless child who has frequent injuries and many minor accidents becomes the concern of medicine, psychology, and safety education. More specifically, this child has more emotional outbursts, lacks self-control to a greater degree, is apt to be more impulsive, and acts more hastily than other children.

The Prevention of Accidents

What is suggested here should be quite clear; that is, avoiding accidents is not a simple matter. Overcautious teachers, for example, may fill a child's world with "don't"—"don't swim alone," "don't run down the stairs," implying that if he sits in the corner he will be safe. In reality his safety requires skill, judgment, and common sense to meet daily problems with successes. The relationship between feelings, emotions, and actions is fundamental. Thus accident prevention involves the promotion of good mental

health as well as day-by-day opportunities for children to practice safe behavior.

From the viewpoint of education, the topic of safety must be taken seriously. This was pointed out as long ago as the 1960 White House Conference on Children and Youth:

> . . . safety education [should] be in the school curriculum as early as possible (Rec. 46) . . . community programs of accident prevention and public education [should] be intensified . . . (Rec. 48).

These recommendations suggest a school-community wide program of safety-education. This involves the planning efforts of many people. It means that in the elementary school administrators, supervisors, health service personnel, physical education and industrial arts instructors, custodians, together with classroom teachers must plan and implement the safety education program. This is probably the only way to prevent the soul-shaking accident statistics. The campaign must begin in the early grades.

The School Safety Program

The school safety effort calls for a number of things. It calls for the provision of a safe school environment, one that is supervised and surveyed periodically. Across the land there are 800,000 accidental injuries to school pupils while under school jurisdiction.[28] There should also be an accurate accident-reporting system. First aid, medical procedures, and fire drills must be set up on "standing orders." Community personnel must cooperate with the schools. And finally, the classroom instruction program must be carefully structured so

---

[28] *Estimated Pupil Accidental Injuries in U.S. Elementary and Secondary Schools.* Chicago: National Safety Council, 1967.

that pupils completing a unit of work on safety will be quite aware of hazardous situations in the school and community and how to adjust to them satisfactorily.

The content of the safety instruction program might easily dominate the whole health education offering. Care, therefore, has to be exercised in limiting teaching to the essentials at each grade level.

At the primary and intermediate levels the accentuation is as follows:

Primary Level

1. Safety in the home
2. Safety to and from school
3. Classroom safety
4. Playground safety
5. School building safety

Intermediate Level

1. Safety patrols
2. Bicycle safety
3. Traffic safety
4. Fire prevention and drills

5. Home and farm safety
6. First aid procedures
7. Harmful substances

A more specific kind of safety curriculum planning will result in a program with a proper sequence of topics. The following knowledges and understandings are presented in brief form. Subtopics should be developed under each item:

SAFETY EDUCATION

Grade One

How to proceed to and from school safely
General safety practices in the classroom
Safety during and after school hours
Particulars concerning personal identity when lost
Where to seek help for injuries or illness

Grade Two

How policemen and firemen protect children
How to use playground equipment

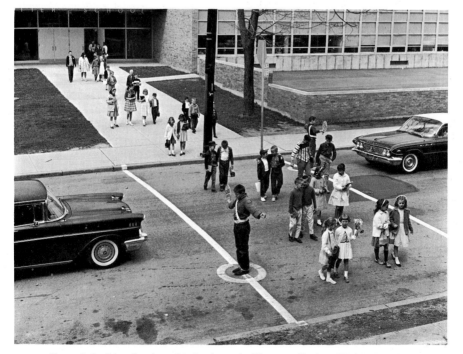

Figure 7–6 Education for safety begins early. (Courtesy Cincinnati Public Schools.)

Treatment of strange animals and strange
   people
How to report accidents and illnesses
Safety on the water

Grade Three

Safe play in all seasons of the year
Bicycle safety: rules, skills, maintenance
Eyes, ears, and face protection
Fire prevention and fire safety
Personal responsibilities

Grade Four

Purification of drinking water
Elementary first aid practices
Safety out of doors (insect bites, sunburn,
   and poison ivy)
Accidents in the community
How to assist younger children in acci-
   dent prevention

Grade Five

Fire prevention at home and in the community
Water safety methods including artificial
   respiration
Leadership in safety patrols and school
   safety councils
How to prevent eye and ear accidents

Grade Six

First aid practices for minor injuries (cuts
   and burns)
Details of personal safety at home (medi-
   cines, automobiles, rugs, stairways, and
   electrical outlets)
Safety in recreational pursuits
Food products safe to eat
Survival in the nuclear age

By the sixth grade more attention
is directed toward firearms safety
and other significant aspects of safety
within the community. Certainly, in
a town or city where there are a number of lakes and streams, some specific
instruction is called for in the area
of water safety. A growing number of
the newer elementary schools have excellent swimming pools. In such cases
instruction pertaining to personal
safety is taught directly to pupils of

all ages. This is done through the
development of skills in swimming
and the handling of boats and canoes.
These experiences in physical skills
are followed by classroom discussions.
This kind of "skill-knowledge" experience is extremely effective. Carryover value, in terms of habits and
attitudes, is long lasting. Here is a
kind of educational instruction which
gives considerable support to those
who advocate experiences in the elementary school program.

The reader is referred to Chapter 8
for complete details relative to teaching the topic of safety. Comments pertaining to first aid for teachers can be
found in Chapter 3. A full treatment
of safety practices in the school environment can be found in Chapter 4.

SEX AND FAMILY LIVING EDUCATION

If our aim is adults who will use their
sexuality in mature and responsible
ways, we cannot begin sex education
later than earliest childhood.
        —Mary S. Calderone, M.D.

It has been wisely stated that sex is
not something we do—it is something
we are. Therefore, sex will never be
thoroughly understood until it is related to the total adjustment of the individual in his family and his society.
Ultimately, everyone must define his
sexual role and establish a value system. The combined efforts of the home,
church, and school are required in
order to bring about a full understanding and acceptance of human sexuality
at all age levels.

From Silence to Publicity

Because there is such an abundance
of evidence to show that most boys and
girls are not receiving adequate sex
education at home or elsewhere, the
schools by the hundreds throughout
the land are awakening to their respon-

sibility. The pendulum has swung from silence to publicity. Progress has been so fast that it has created problems, including a shortage of qualified teachers and considerable uncertainty about what form instruction should take.

It is agreed that there is an immediate need for an educational program to offset the half-truths and general misinformation that children are constantly exposed to through the commercial exploitation of sex and erotica by modern mass media. Children have grown up to become adults who believe that sex is simply a plaything, or at best a biological phenomenon—a reproductive item. They have not understood it as an integral part of total personality. Quite the contrary, they see it as genital-centered—the exact opposite of what should be the goal.

It is difficult to develop responsible sexual morality in personal and family situations when the "anything goes" philosophy of life permeates the minds of primary graders and adults alike. As the old taboos die and the permissive society takes shape, only a calculated sex and family living education can hope to be an effective counteracting agent. This is not easy. It is a difficult undertaking in an era of endless seductions, raw and obscene language, increasing nudity, suggestive posters and films, homosexual frankness, and an almost constant celebration of the erotic life.

Confusing genital-centered sex with true sexuality is recognized by the major faiths and parent groups as an unfortunate contemporary fact. Its relationship to sexual experimentation, venereal disease, promiscuity, pregnant teenagers, and unwed mothers is clear. The statistics are frequently overwhelming. (Review the evidence in Chapter 1.) Moreover, the numerous expressions of sex are as important to the health of the marital relationship and to the solid foundation of the family in twentieth century society as are its procreative aspects. Both home and church, therefore, are working closely with the schools to define purposes and establish programs.

The Role of the School

It is the function of the school to cooperate with community leaders in the early exploration and planning of a curriculum in sex and family living education, from the kindergarten through high school. Failure to do so has almost always resulted in misunderstandings and less than adequate programs. Local groups of citizens should realize that they do indeed have a say in what the school does. Also, they have a responsibility to back the school in its efforts.

From the start it should be made clear that the objective is to eliminate anxieties and misunderstandings pertaining to sex through the development of an adequate knowledge of the physical, mental, social, emotional, and spiritual processes involved. The primary purpose is "to establish man's sexuality as a health entity."[29]

Sex education is to be distinguished from sex information. It implies that man's sexuality is integrated into his total life development as a health entity and a source of creative energy.

In Anaheim, California, where the program is considered one of the best in the country, it is noted that:

Family life and sex education is a continuous process in which the development of attitudes and conduct are most important so that the individual's sexual nature will contribute to his self-development and happiness, and at the same time conserve and advance the welfare of society.

[29] This is the chief purpose of the Sex Information and Education Council of the U.S. (SIECUS), an organization devoted to the dissemination of knowledge relative to human sexuality. The SIECUS Newsletter is especially valuable (1790 Broadway, New York, N.Y., 10019).

Such a statement as this helps to overcome the difficulty all known societies have had in dealing with sex — the tendency to take a partial view of it, to see it in terms of only one of its dimensions.

Historically, the learned organizations and their prophets have been urging the schools to get started. In 1941 the American Association of School Administrators recommended that sex education be included in the school curriculum. It was recommended again in 1960 at the White House Conference on Children, and by the middle 1960's a number of state and national groups called for action. Several states have developed excellent policy statements regarding sex and family living education. One of the finest, put forth in a 24-page booklet and complete with 26 admirable objectives, is the one from Illinois.[30] Another policy statement, short and clear, was prepared by the New Jersey State Board of Education and given wide distribution throughout the state and beyond. The full statement follows:

A POLICY STATEMENT ON SEX EDUCATION

(ADOPTED BY THE STATE BOARD OF EDUCATION ON JANUARY 4, 1967)

Sex education is a responsibility which should be shared by the home, church, and school. The State Board of Education and the State Department of Education support the philosophy that each community and educational institution must determine its role in this area. Therefore, the State Board of Education recommends that each Local Board of Education make provisions in its curriculum for sex education programs.

---

[30] Illinois Sex Education Advisory Board. *Policy Statement on Family Life and Sex Education.* Springfield, Illinois: Office of the Superintendent of Public Instruction, 1967.

Sex is a major aspect of personality. It is intimately related to emotional and social development and adjustment. Being boy or girl, man or woman, conditions one's sense of identity, ways of thinking and behaving, social and occupational activities, choice of associates, and mode of dress. Sex cannot be understood simply by focusing on physiological processes or classifying modes of sexual behavior. Human sexuality — the assumption of the individual's sex role — can best be understood by relating it to the total adjustment of the individual in his family and society.

The primary purpose of sex education is to promote more wholesome family and interpersonal relationships and, therefore, more complete lives. It is not a subject that lends itself readily to "lecturing" or "telling." An approach which encourages open discussion and solicits the concerns of the individual is needed to help young people develop appropriate attitudes and understandings regarding their sex roles. This approach is possible if parents, clergy, teachers, health personnel, and others responsible for the education of children are informed and secure in their own feelings about sex.

Sex education is a continuing process throughout life and therefore must be planned for during the entire school experience of the child. Schools are important agencies in the development of healthy habits of living and moral values. Therefore, the Department of Education recommends that appropriate programs in sex education be developed by educational institutions cognizant of what is desirable, what is possible, and what is wise.

Sex Education as Health Education

In the field of health education school boards and administrators are urged, at one time or other, to provide special time in the curriculum for as many as 30 categorical topics, including smoking, drug abuse, alcohol education, venereal disease, accident prevention, tuberculosis, and cancer, in addition to sex and family living education.

Aware of the present emphasis on sex and family living education, the Joint Committee of the National School Boards Association and the American Association of School Administrators published a statement in which they set forth the firm belief that the only way in which the school can fulfill its responsibility for meeting the health needs of youth is through a comprehensive program of health education from the kindergarten through the twelfth grade. Such a program establishes the organizational framework for meeting the health needs, interests, and problems of the school-age group. Reports the Committee:

> Including sex and family life education with the other categorical health topics in one sound, interrelated, and sequential program not only saves time in an already-crowded curriculum, but assures that all topics will be part of a long-range program and will receive more complete and detailed consideration at the appropriate level of the student's development. . . .
>
> The Committee wishes to emphasize that it must be recognized that the school curriculum is already overloaded. Literally, if something new goes in, something must come out. There is neither time nor justification for separate courses in any of the categorical areas advocated by specialized interest groups.
>
> Health is a unified concept. It must be approached with consideration of the total human being and the complexity of forces that affect health behavior. It is concerned with the health attitudes and behavior of the individual, his family, and the community. It is concerned with knowledge, attitudes, and practices—that is, health behavior in its totality.

This cannot be achieved with a piecemeal approach.[31]

Teach Sex Education Early

An early start in the sex and family living area builds a firm foundation of understandings and attitudes before complex and emotional problems confront boys and girls in their teens. Thus, Glen Cove, New York kindergarten children discuss the coming of a new baby into the family group. Moreover, the baby was not "got" at the hospital, but grew inside the mother until the doctor helped bring it out.

In numerous elementary schools programs have been carefully planned to meet local needs. These needs are much the same everywhere. Whether it is Washington, Illinois, or Oregon, the teacher is the key to a good program. No teacher should be forced to teach in an area in which she feels uncomfortable. Fortunately, many elementary school teachers are usually "at home" discussing the world of persons and families, both formally and informally in their classrooms.

The following selected references are especially useful in building a rationale for teaching sex and family living education early in the grades, and for appreciating the need for a sequence of experiences which will contribute to the development of appropriate concepts of sexuality in the later years:

Adams, John B., and Sestak, Michael. "Sex Education—a Sensible Approach." *Journal of School Health,* 37:222–224, May 1967.

Benell, Florence B. "Eliminating Barriers to Sex Education in the Schools." *Journal of School Health,* 38:68–71, February 1968.

Bracher, Marjory. "The Martinson Report: Im-

---

[31] Statement by the Joint Committee of the National School Boards Association and the American Association of School Administrators. *Health Education and Sex/Family Life Education.* Washington, D.C.: National Education Association, 1968.

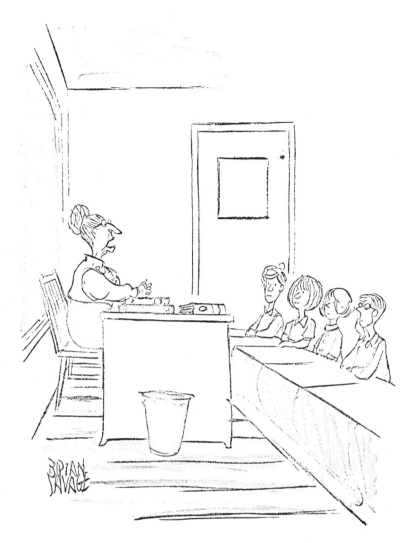

"The Board of Education requires me to give you some basic information on sex, reproduction and other disgusting filth."

plications for Sex Education." *Journal of School Health,* 37:491–498, December 1967.

Broderick, Carlfred B. "Sexual Behavior Among Pre-Adolescents." *Journal of Social Issues,* 22:6–21, April 1966.

Calderone, Mary A. "Goodbye to the Birds and Bees." *American Education,* November 1966.

Calderone, Mary A. "Planning for Sex Education: a Community-wide Responsibility." *NEA Journal,* January 1967.

Foster, Greg R. "Sex Information vs. Sex Educa-

tion: Implications for School Health." *Journal of School Health,* 37:248–250, May 1967.

Guidance Associates. *Sex Education U.S.A.: A Community Approach.* New York: Harcourt, Brace & World, 1968.

Kirkendall, Lester A. *Sex Education.* SIECUS Discussion Guide No. 1, October 1965 (1790 Broadway, New York, N.Y., 10023).

Kirkendall, Lester A., and Cox, Helen M. "Starting a Sex Education Program." *Children,* August 1967, p. 136.

Levine, Milton I. "Sex Education in the Public Elementary and High School Curriculum." *Journal of School Health*, 37:30–38, January 1967.

Manley, Helen. "Sex Education: Where, When and How It Should Be Taught." *Journal of Health, Physical Education, and Recreation*, 36:17–20, March 1965.

Simon, William, and Gagnon, John H. "The Pedagogy of Sex." *Saturday Review*, November 18, 1967, p. 79.

Teachers Publishing Corporation. "Sex Education: How It Is Being Taught in Elementary Classrooms." *Grade Teacher*, May-June 1967.

Time Essay. "On Teaching Children about Sex." *Time*, June 9, 1967.

Sex and Family Living Curriculum

There is a reasonably good amount of experience to draw upon when it comes to structuring a program. The list of communities with effective elementary programs is rather extensive. Among the better known examples, in which sex and family living programs have operated successfully for some time, are the following communities:

University City, Missouri
Glen Cove, New York
Evanston, Illinois
Denver, Colorado
Anaheim, California
Washington, D.C.
Cleveland, Ohio
Longview, Washington
Kansas City, Missouri
Great Neck, New York
Oxnard, California
El Dorado County, California
San Diego, California
Bedford, Massachusetts
Detroit, Michigan
Los Angeles, California
San Francisco, California
Eugene, Oregon
Hinsdale, Illinois

A number of these communities have extensive curriculum guides available for a modest cost. Here are a few of the better ones:

Human Growth Outline. Lincolnwood School District No. 74, E. Prairie, Lincolnwood, Illinois.

A Curriculum Guide in Sex Education by Helen Manley. Social Health Association of Greater St. Louis, State Publishing Co., St. Louis, Mo., 63136.

Workbook for Planning Elementary Curriculum. El Dorado County Schools, P.O. Box 710, Diamond Springs, California.

Human Growth and Development. Oxnard School District, Department of Educational Services, 255 Palm Drive, Oxnard, California.

Family Living Guide, Kindergarten Through Grade Four. Evanston Public Schools, District No. 65, Cook County, Evanston, Illinois, 60201.

Sex Education and Family Life: Growth Patterns and Reproduction, K-12. A curriculum guide for school personnel, reproduced in *Journal of School Health*, May 1967.

Personal and Family Living for the Elementary School. Curriculum Resource Bulletin, Public Schools, District of Columbia, Administration Annex No. 7, North Street, N.W., Washington, D.C., 20007.

A Pioneer Program in Health Guidance in Sex Education. Glen Cove Public Schools, Glen Cove, N.Y., 11542.

Sex Education in the Schools. Educational Research Council of Greater Cleveland, Rockefeller Building, Cleveland, Ohio.

Guide to Social Health Education, by grades, San Diego City Schools, San Diego, California.

Although the emphasis differs, there is a fair amount of agreement as to primary and intermediate grade content in sex and family living education. This is particularly true when one compares the courses of study that have been periodically revised in the several communities where established programs have been in operation for some time.

Some idea of the scope of the program, kindergarten through sixth grade, can be appreciated by looking over the Sex and Family Living Education outline as it appears in Appendix A (page 407). A further example from an on-going program in Glen Cove, New York appears below:

GLEN COVE PUBLIC SCHOOLS, N.Y.

Kindergarten

1. Know sex differences between girls and boys.
2. Give direction toward male or female role in adult life.
3. Learn correct names for body parts and terms concerned with elimination.
4. Understand that human baby develops inside body of mother.
5. Understand baby gets milk from mother's breast by nursing.
6. Appreciate that there are good body feelings.
7. Learn to recognize signs of love and devotion within family.
8. Develop idea of continuity of living things — incubate eggs.

First Year

1. Understand egg cell is basic to new life.
2. Learn that some animals hatch from eggs and others develop inside body of mother until birth.
3. Appreciate wonder of human body.
4. Develop sense of responsibility for own body.
5. Appreciate efforts of mother and father for family members.
6. Recognize influence of emotions on body health.

Second Year

1. Learn that different animals need different amounts of time to get ready to be born.
2. Understand that the egg cell does not develop into a baby by itself — role of father.
3. Learn that some animals are born live through a special opening in the mother's body.
4. Recognize that growing up brings responsibility.
5. Appreciate importance of mutual love and consideration in family.
6. Understand composition of family does not necessarily determine happiness of family.

Third Year

1. Understand that each person's unique heredity is determined at moment of fertilization.
2. Observe influence of heredity in your family.
3. Know that growing up means more than just getting bigger.
4. Develop increasing sense of responsibility to self and family.
5. Understand relationship between a healthy body and mind.
6. Study life cycles of various animals, including humans.

Fourth Year

1. Learn that certain glands control body growth and development.
2. Recognize importance of protecting vital body parts from injury, i.e. during sports.
3. Appreciate miracle of reproduction and maternal care among various forms of animal life.
4. Appreciate superiority of brain of man over instinct reaction of animals.
5. Learn meaning of responsible behavior in peer and family groups.
6. Study circulatory and digestive systems and realize their functional potential is influenced by habits being developed.

Fifth Year

1. Learn role of sex glands at puberty and emotional changes they bring.
2. Understand menstruation occurs as a natural part of a girl's growing up.
3. Understand seminal emissions occur as a natural part of a boy's growing up.
4. Learn that although nature readies our bodies for reproduction at puberty, several years more are needed to prepare for marriage and responsibility of parenthood.
5. Discuss importance of wholesome life attitudes and values as manifested in responsible behavior.
6. Discuss acceptable and unacceptable ways of showing emotions.

One of the most thorough reports to appear in recent years was prepared by the Committee on Health Guidance in Sex Education of the American School

Health Association.[32] An outstanding feature of this extensive publication is that specific concepts and attitudes are set forth for each grade level in a manner readily understood by the teacher.

AMERICAN SCHOOL HEALTH ASSOCIATION

Kindergarten and Grade One

A. **Concepts.** As a product of their experiences in the study of this unit, it would be hoped that some such concepts as these would be formulated by children in kindergarten and the first grade:

1. All living things reproduce. Life comes from life.
2. The creation of new life is one of nature's greatest miracles.
3. Every child has a mother and a father in the beginning.
4. Every person needs to have a feeling of belonging.
5. Each member of a family is an important member. Children and parents working and playing together help to make a home a happy place to live. There are many ways in which children can help to make their homes happy ones.
6. Each member of a family is interested in the well-being of every other member.
7. Using good manners lets other people know that we like and respect them. Thoughtful boys and girls are courteous to each other, to their mothers and fathers, their brothers and sisters, and to everyone else.
8. Every person desires privacy at some times. Each person has a right to privacy, and each should respect the privacy of others.
9. Each part of the body is an important part of the whole person,

and there is nothing shameful about any part of the body.
10. We should be cautious in dealing with strangers. Although some strangers who offer rides or candy to children are trying to be kind, others are not. We should always refuse such offers and should tell our parents and teachers about them.

B. **Attitudes.** As an outcome of this unit, it is to be hoped that the student will form some such favorable attitudes as these toward himself, others, family living, and reproduction:

1. An appreciation for the role of each family member.
2. An appreciation for his own importance as a member of his family and a desire to contribute to his family's well-being.
3. A respect for the rights of others.
4. A sense of wonder in regard to reproduction.
5. A wholesome respect for all parts of the body and a desire to learn and to use correct terminology in referring to them.

Grades Two and Three

A. **Concepts.** As a product of their experiences in the study of this unit, it would be hoped that some such concepts as these would be formulated by children in the second and third grades:

1. All living things grow and reproduce.
2. Every child has a mother and a father in the beginning.
3. Parents or guardians take care of their children in many ways until children grow up and are able to take care of themselves.
4. Human babies and children live with their parents or guardians for many years because it takes a long time for them to grow up and to learn how to do for themselves all the things that parents do for them while they are young.
5. Human beings grow in many ways—physically, intellectually, emotionally, socially, spiritually.
6. All living things have basic needs which must be fulfilled for optimal growth.

[32] "Growth Patterns and Sex Education: a Suggested Program K-12," *Journal of School Health*, May 1967. This total in-depth issue of 136 pages is available for a small cost from American School Health Association, 515 E. Main St., Kent, Ohio, 44240.

7. We need many different kinds of food to help us grow.
8. The food we eat is changed and used by our bodies to help us grow.
9. Optimal growth depends in part upon how well we utilize the food we eat.
10. Babies need special foods for optimal growth.
11. Everything we do helps us to learn more about ourselves, other people and the world we live in.
12. We can do our best work and have the most fun when we are happy.
13. Being neat and clean helps to make us feel good about ourselves.
14. Boys and girls enjoy playing and working with other boys and girls who are neat and clean.
15. There are many ways that mothers and fathers and children can show that they love each other.
16. Using good manners is one way we can let members of our families, other grown-ups, and other boys and girls know that we like them.
17. Fathers do many kinds of work in the community, and all of them can help to make the community a better place in which to live.
18. Mothers help the community in many ways — by making the home a healthy and happy place to live, by working at jobs outside the home, or by participating in community activities which they enjoy.

B. **Attitudes.** As an outcome of this unit, it is to be hoped that the student will form favorable attitudes toward himself, others, family living, and reproduction:

1. An appreciation for the roles of each member of the family as an individual and as a contributing member of the family unit.
2. A desire for optimal nutrition.
3. A desire to develop or to continue personal practices which lead to cleanliness and good grooming.
4. An appreciation for clothing that is clean and functional, regardless of its "fashionableness."

5. A respect for other persons as individuals and a desire to show respect for others by treating them courteously.
6. A growing regard for masculine and feminine roles in our society.
7. An appreciation for the ways in which adult men and women contribute to the community and the desire to become future contributing adult members of the community.
8. A sense of wonder concerning the complex nature of the human personality and its development.
9. An appreciation for the effect that a pleasant manner has upon one's relationship with others.

Grade Four

A. **Concepts.** As a product of their experiences in the study of this unit, it would be hoped that some such concepts as these would be formulated by children in the fourth grade:

1. We are made of many cells which have important tasks to do in making it possible for us to live and grow.
2. Blood carries food to the cells and waste products away from the cells to places where they can be collected and excreted.
3. A person's heredity refers to those personal characteristics that have been passed down to him from his parents through genes and chromosomes.
4. Each person receives half of his inherited characteristics from his mother and the other half from his father.
5. Each person's inherited characteristics are determined at the moment of conception when his father's sperm fertilizes his mother's ovum.
6. A person's heredity influences the way he grows, what he will look like, and how tall he can grow to be.
7. What a person becomes is determined by his heredity, his environment and, to some extent, what he wants to be.
8. Each member of a family contri-

butes to the well-being of the whole family and each of its other members.

9. The health of each family member affects the well-being of all family members.

10. There are many activities that all members of a family can participate in and enjoy together. Playing together and working together helps mothers and fathers and children know each other better and strengthens the family as a unit.

11. Having a hobby is one way a person can use his leisure time constructively. Hobbies add enjoyment to living. Sometimes the members of a family enjoy sharing the same hobby.

12. A friend is someone who likes you and whom you like. A person can have many different kinds of friends among people of all ages.

13. One of the best ways to make new friends is to be friendly to other people. Being friendly lets others know that we would like to have them as our friends.

B. **Attitudes.** As an outcome of this unit, it is to be hoped that the student will form favorable attitudes toward himself, others, family living, and reproduction:

1. An appreciation for one's family heritage, both hereditary and environmental.

2. An appreciation for the influences that heredity and environment have upon growth and development.

3. An appreciation for the ability one has to control the direction of his own development and a desire to exercise this control to the greatest extent possible.

4. A regard for the effect that the health of each family member has upon that of all other family members and upon the family as a unit.

5. A desire to have one's own health status and practices contribute to rather than detract from family well-being.

6. A willingness to understand and adjust to the health problems of all members of the family.

7. An appreciation for the contribution that children this age can make to the leisure-time activities and fellowship of the family and a desire to help plan and participate in such activities with other members of the family.

8. An appreciation for the values and enjoyment that can be gained from constructive solitary activities.

9. A desire to select and pursue some activities that one can do on his own.

10. A respect for the desire others have to engage in solitary activities and a regard for their right to do so.

11. An appreciation for the different kinds of friendships one can develop with many different persons of various ages.

12. A desire to be a friend to others.

Grade Five

A. **Concepts.** As a product of their experiences in the study of this unit, it would be hoped that some such concepts as these would be formulated by children in the fifth grade:

1. Although the general pattern of growth and development is the same for everyone, each person follows this pattern at his own individual rate.

2. At some times in their lives, girls are taller than boys, but boys catch up later and usually become taller than girls.

3. A person's growth and development are determined by hereditary potential for growth and development and by the influence of the many kinds of experiences he has in his environment.

4. Hormones are responsible for the changes in appearance that occur as boys develop into men and girls develop into women.

5. Hormones influence not only a person's growth and physical development, but also the way he feels and behaves.

6. As boys and girls become men and women, their feelings and

actions toward themselves and others change.

7. As people grow older they are able to assume more responsibility for their own care and for the well-being of others.

8. Although most habits are helpful to us, some of the habits people form can interfere with their well-being and ability to get along with others.

9. Seminal emissions are nature's way of releasing stored-up sperm.

10. Menstruation is a normal, healthful function which indicates that a girl is becoming a woman who will be able to conceive and have children.

11. The creation of a new life is one of the most wonderful acts of Nature.

12. Parenthood is a privilege and a responsibility.

13. Each new life begins with the union of a single sperm from the father and a single ovum from the mother.

14. The fertilized ovum divides into many cells which have different structures in order to assume different tasks. Cell division and differentiation begins at the time of conception and continues in order to form a fully developed human being.

15. As a baby lives and grows and develops inside the mother, the placenta and umbilical cord bring it food and oxygen from the mother and carry its waste products to the mother for elimination.

16. The blood of a developing baby is formed in its own body. Its circulatory system is separate from the mother's. Food and oxygen and waste products are exchanged between mother and baby through the process of osmosis.

17. The amniotic sac and fluid create an environment which protects the fetus until it is ready to be born.

18. The best way to assure that one's body will continue to function efficiently and well is to give it the normal care and attention it requires.

19. As a person grows and develops from a child into an adult, his changing body requires additional kinds of care in order to keep functioning at its best.

20. Although some children do not grow as rapidly as others, this is not an indication of any abnormality.

B. **Attitudes.** As an outcome of this unit, it is to be hoped that the student will form favorable attitudes toward himself, others, family living, and reproduction:

1. An appreciation for normal individual differences in rates of growth and development and an acceptance of one's own rate.

2. A desire to seek information pertaining to sex and sexuality from reliable sources as replacement for unscientific information and hearsay.

3. A persistent regard for medical services and health consultation from scientific sources.

4. An appreciation for the uniqueness of each individual and for the ways in which all individuals are similar.

5. An appreciation for the contributions that families make to the total development of each person.

6. A desire to contribute to wholesome family living by participating in family activities.

7. An appreciation for the constructive expression of one's sexuality through the reproductive processes and within the framework of the family unit.

8. A desire to respond to increased privilege by displaying a growing sense of responsibility for self and others.

9. A desire to form habits which will contribute to one's well-being and to eliminate or avoid developing habits that may be destructive to optimal growth and development.

10. An appreciation of one's sexuality as a healthful expression of his personality.

11. A wholesome acceptance of one-

self as a sexual being and of those physiological processes (e.g. menstruation and seminal emissions) related to this aspect of one's being.

12. A regard for both the privileges and responsibilities attendant upon parenthood.

13. An increasing appreciation for the complexity of the human personality.

14. A persistent regard for the nature of the phenomena involved in the creation of a new life.

15. A respect for one's body as a tool for creative self-expression and the desire to give it the care it requires and deserves as such.

Grade Six

A. **Concepts.** As a product of their experiences in the study of this unit, it would be hoped that some such concepts as these would be formulated by children in the sixth grade:

1. Cells have different kinds of structures which enable each kind to perform its specialized function.

2. A person's emotions affect the way his body functions.

3. The hormones secreted by the endocrine glands regulate many physiological functions. They prepare the body for action during periods of emotional stress.

4. Emotions are natural human feelings existing in all persons. They are aroused in response to other people and to situations in one's environment.

5. Emotions need to be expressed in some way. There are constructive and destructive ways of expressing emotions.

6. Emotions can be expressed in the most constructive way when their expression is controlled by the use of one's ability to reason.

7. One of the tasks involved in becoming a mature person is that of learning to control the emotions in such a way that their expression helps, rather than hurts, both oneself and other people.

8. Maleness and femaleness refer to biological characteristics unique for each individual.

9. Although boys are mostly male and girls are mostly female, no person is all male or all female. There is some degree of femaleness in all boys and some degree of maleness in all girls.

10. Masculinity and femininity refer to patterns of behavior that are characteristic of males or of females in a particular culture. These patterns of behavior are not present at birth, but are learned through the experiences one has in his family, his school, and his community. As boys and girls grow up, they learn how to be masculine or feminine by observing and behaving like the men or women they know and admire.

11. The process of growing and developing from children into adults is very complex and involves many physical, emotional and social changes and adjustments.

12. The growth and development of a baby from one fertilized cell into a complex human being is one of nature's greatest and most miraculous achievements.

13. An appreciation of "maleness" and "femaleness" is an important aspect of becoming an adult.

14. There are such normal variations in physiological activity in each individual that it is important to recognize, understand and accept the many characteristics which may be common to both sexes.

B. **Attitudes.** As an outcome of this unit, it is to be hoped that the student will form favorable attitudes toward himself, others, family living, and reproduction:

1. An appreciation for the integrated nature of man.

2. An acceptance and appreciation of the emotional dimension of being and of the human quality that emotional expression gives to personality.

3. A desire to express one's emotions in constructive ways.

4. A willingness to explore a variety of alternatives in the attempt to

learn how to channel one's emotions into constructive outlets.

5. A growing acceptance of and appreciation for the sexuality of oneself and others.

6. A desire to adopt the behaviors natural to and characteristic of one's assigned sex role in our culture.

7. A sensitivity to, acceptance of, and appreciation for behavioral characteristics which may be exhibited by members of both sexes, which are natural to both sexes, but which may be culturally expected of one sex rather than of the other.

8. An acceptance of and appreciation for the complex physical, emotional, and social changes that one undergoes in the process of growing and developing into an adult.

When it comes to implementing the sex and family living education program there are a number of comments that can be made and effective student activities which can be recommended. This discussion is included as a part of Chapter 8 (p. 247). Further details relative to useful stories for boys and girls, posters, records, and appropriate films and filmstrips for the primary and intermediate grades are listed in Chapter 11 (p. 379). There is today an excellent selection of these materials. The films are especially good.

OTHER ASPECTS OF
THE HEALTH CURRICULUM

The Emphasis on Physical Activity

The role of exercise in the health of the individual pupil has long been recognized. In recent years it has become a very popular school activity due primarily to the age of automation, the era of the overfed, overprotected and underactive child. Thus teachers of health should seek to cooperate with physical education instructors so that the vigorous physical activity in the gymnasium or on the playground may be related to such items as weight, diet, fatigue, personal cleanliness, and general well-being as taught in the classroom.

Where there are no special physical education teachers it will be necessary for classroom teachers to teach the games, dances, stunts, and exercises themselves. Carefully planned activities are effective in raising individual pupil physical fitness. This has been ably demonstrated by the President's Council on Physical Fitness. Where ongoing programs exist failures on tests of physical fitness are around 25 per cent or less, but where there has been no previous program of physical education the test failure rate runs around 45 to 55 per cent. Professional leadership in physical education, therefore, is conducive to a far better health program in the elementary school.

The School Lunch Program

In many schools today a special, and somewhat formal effort is made to improve the nutritional status of children, while at the same time increasing their knowledge and appreciation of foods, through the school lunch program.

In 1946 Congress enacted the National School Lunch Program as a "measure for national security, to safeguard the health and well being of the nation's children, and to encourage the domestic consumption of nutritious agricultural commodities and other foods." This program is carried on today on a non-profit basis without physical segregation or other discriminations by the school against any child because of his inability to pay the full cost or any part of the cost of the meals.

A school plan with such worthy objectives as these certainly cannot go unnoticed as a means of further implementing the health instruction program. One cannot dismiss the educational implications of an activity that serves over two billion lunches to millions of children. Surveys, however, indicate that school personnel are not capitalizing on the opportunities inherent in the school lunch situation and little is said about the school lunch as a learning laboratory.

The school lunch offers a place to teach diet and food habits in their natural setting, making the lunch program an educational operation rather than a business function. Here, boys and girls may learn to be self-sufficient, to make decisions, and to spend their money wisely. There are meals to plan and serve, sanitation to be considered, and numerous chances to promote climates favorable to appetite, to growth, and to mental-emotional health. There are few total school activities so conducive to a practical, down-to-earth kind of teaching as that afforded by the school lunch operation. This is a real-life situation where the teacher can find in a single lunchroom an assortment of eating patterns — from the plate lunch to the à la carte lunch; from the home lunch supplemented with school lunch items to the all too typical box lunch with the weak combination of a jelly sandwich and a piece of cake.

Beginning in the primary grade classroom with the study of foods, the teacher encourages her class to share their thoughts relative to school lunch menu planning. The planning, especially in the third grade and above, may begin with a school survey of current dietary practices or a study of the components of a well-balanced lunch as a part of the total daily diet. Other ideas include the following:[33]

Discussions may be directed toward overcoming food dislikes. Foods left on the trays may provide a basis for such a study.

New foods may be accompanied by a class discussion on the values of the foods and ways of acquiring a taste for them.

Assisting with the serving of lunches gives pupils a first-hand opportunity to learn about proper sanitary practices.

Help in the preparation of food and cleaning up the lunchroom after the meal may be arranged. Where this is done, pupils should be rotated so that all have an equal chance.

Survey the school lunch facilities and consider ways of implementing their findings.

Observe the social graces. Take turns as hosts and hostesses. This is a social hour for pupils and teachers. It is pleasant and enjoyable — a tonic to learning.

Where proper studies have been conducted, the school lunch has proved to be an effective medium for developing good eating habits — a fact that has been sustained throughout the school year.[34]

Perhaps the biggest difficulty in the school lunch program has been with the children who bring lunches from home. Many schools and homes have cooperated to improve the home-packed lunch. In Petaluma, California, for example, the school health council and local PTA got together, established the nature of the problem through a city-wide survey, cooperatively prepared a *Guide to Home-Packed School Lunches,* and took steps to revise the health curriculum to integrate this nutrition work into the classroom situation.[35]

[33] Some of these are adapted from the booklet, *Health Aspects of the School Lunch Program: Report* of the Joint Committees on Health Problems in Education of the National Education Association and the American Medical Association. Washington: National Education Association, 1962.

[34] Martin, Ethel Austin. *Roberts' Nutrition Work with Children.* Chicago: University of Chicago Press, 1955, p. 457.

[35] Manning, W. R., and Olsen, L. R. "Home and School Cooperate to Enrich the Home-Packed School Lunch," *Journal of School Health,* 32:87-89, 1962.

	something hearty	something crisp or juicy	something toothsome	something drinkable	something to surprise
M	Corned beef sandwich *Rye bread* *Corned beef*	Dill pickle	Skewered pineapple chunks and orange segments	Milk	Coffee cake or sweet roll
T	Egg salad sandwich *Enriched bread* *Chopped egg,* *piccalilli, mustard* *(Add lettuce* *before eating.)*	Carrot and cucumber sticks	Cluster of grapes	Cocoa (in vacuum bottle)	Popcorn balls
W	Chicken leg *Whole wheat bread* *and butter sandwich*	Small whole tomato	Wedge of apple pie	Cream of mushroom soup (in vacuum bottle)	Crossword puzzle
T	Dried beef-cream cheese sandwich *Enriched bread* *Chopped dried beef,* *cream cheese*	Green onions or scallions	Small orange	Milk	Cinnamon bread and butter sandwich
F	Tuna sandwich *Enriched bread* *Flaked tuna,* *crushed pineapple,* *green pepper*	Shiny red apple	Chocolate cupcake	Milk	Deviled egg

	something hearty	something crisp or juicy	something toothsome	something drinkable	something to surprise
M	Peanut butter-orange sandwich *Enriched bread* *Peanut butter,* *orange rind and juice* *(Add lettuce* *before eating.)*	Celery hearts	Bing cherries	Milk	Waffle wafers
T	Hamburger sandwich *Enriched bun* *Hamburger pattie*	Waldorf salad *(Add dressing* *before eating.)*	Wedge of blueberry pie	Milk	Prize riddle
W	Baked bean sandwich *Enriched bread* *Baked beans,* *chili sauce*	Peach halves	Cookies	Milk	Stuffed celery with Bleu cheese or cheddar cheese
T	Ham-Swiss cheese sandwich *French bread* *Sliced ham,* *sliced Swiss cheese*	Dill pickle	Banana	Lemonade	Cream of potato soup (in vacuum bottle)
F	Salmon salad sandwich *Whole wheat bread* *Flaked salmon,* *chopped celery,* *apple sauce*	Cucumber and green pepper strips	Whole apricots	Cocoa (in vacuum bottle)	Doughnut sandwich

Figure 7–7   Some suggestions for a school lunch. (Courtesy American Institute of Baking.)

In Long Beach, New York, a very complete booklet entitled *For Your Children at Lunchtime* was developed by the PTA for parents. The school health council and classroom teachers assisted.

Questions for Discussion

1. Select one of the following topics and prepare a resource unit for use in a primary grade of your choice:
   a. Safety
   b. Dental health
   c. Sleep, rest, and relaxation
   d. Communicable disease control

2. What is the relationship between health knowledge and health attitudes? How does this relationship affect the planning of unit activities? Give an example to illustrate this.

3. What seem to be the major health interests of pupils in the primary grades? In the intermediate grades?

4. What health and safety problems are most frequently discussed in news items, health columns, and complete articles in daily newspapers and popular magazines?

5. From what you have been able to observe, what are some of the needed improvements in elementary school health programs?

6. List several ways of achieving both scope and sequence in planning a health education curriculum. Also list the references on curriculum development that you consulted.

7. Visit the college library and look over a number of curriculum guides in health education. List some of the ways they differ and some of the ways in which they are similar.

Suggested Activities

1. In his book, *The Changing School Curriculum* (The Fund for the Advancement of Education, 1966) John Goodlad points out that "health has never been a clearly defined study in our schools." Ask two or three elementary classroom teachers how they feel about this statement. Is it generally true or generally false?

2. In the past decade curriculum changes have been more widespread and intensive than at any time in the history of American schools. One should ask if the curriculum changes are really significant. Do children learn better in the new programs than they did in the old? Suggest several means of finding out how valuable certain curriculum changes are in a school. See also the article by Jack R. Frymier on "Curriculum Assessment— Problems and Possibilities" in *Educational Leadership,* November 1966, pp. 124–128.

3. Look into the School Health Education Study (SHES). Examine some of the instructional materials. Try out some of the overhead projection transparencies. What are your comments relative to these new health education materials?

4. Read some of the material that has been written about the advantages of team teaching. From the point of view of health instruction does it seem to be more or less practical to teach by the team method or the method frequently employed in the self-contained classroom unit? Support your answer.

5. Formulate your own list of concepts suitable for a grade of your choice which pertains to the area of sex and family living education. Examine several curriculum guides and the May 1967 edition of the *Journal of School Health* before putting your list in final form.

Selected References

Bair, Medill, and Woodward, Richard G. *Team Teaching in Action*. New York: Harcourt, Brace & World, 1966.

Bruner, Jerome. *Toward a Theory of Instruction*. Cambridge, Mass.: Belknap Press of Harvard University, 1966.

Combs, Arthur W. "Fostering Self-Direction." *Educational Leadership*. February 1966, pp. 373–376.

Darrow, Helen F. "Conceptual Learning." *Childhood Education*, 287–288, February 1965.

Goodlad, John I. *School Curriculum and the Individual*. New York: Blaisdell Publishing Company, 1967.

Goodlad, John I. *The Changing School Curriculum*. New York: The Fund for the Advancement of Education, 1966.

Kilander, H. Frederick. *School Health Education*, 2nd ed. New York: The Macmillan Company, 1968, Chapters 12 and 16.

King, Arthur R. J., and Brownell, John A. *The Curriculum and the Disciplines of Knowledge*. New York: John Wiley & Sons, 1967.

Klausmeir, Herbert J., and Dresden, Katherine. *Teaching in the Elementary School*, 2nd ed. New York: Harper and Brothers, 1962, Chapters 4 and 5.

Kuopman, G. Robert. "School Lunch—A Concept in Learning." *The Nations's Schools*, 30:37–38, February 1957.

Lehman, Edna S., Schumacher, Corrine, and Vitek, Mildred. "The Conceptual Approach to Health Education." *Journal of Health, Physical Education, and Recreation*, 38:32–35, February 1967.

Means, Richard K. "The School Health Education Study: a Pattern in Curriculum Development." *Journal of School Health*, 36:1–11, January 1966.

Oberteuffer, Delbert, and Beyrer, Mary K. *School Health Education*, 4th ed. New York: Harper and Row, 1966, Chapters 4 and 5.

Phenix, Phillip H. *Realms of Meaning*. New York: McGraw-Hill Book Company, 1964.

Plesent, Emanuel. "Kindergarten Through Twelfth Grade Curriculum in Three Weeks." *Journal of School Health*, 38:113–115, February 1968.

Sliepcevich, Elena M. "School Health Education Study: Appraisal of a Conceptual Approach to Curriculum Development." *Journal of School Health*, 36:145–153, April 1966.

Woodruff, Asahel D. "The Use of Concepts in Teaching and Learning." *Journal of Teacher Education*, 20:81–99, March 1964.

Implementing the Health Curriculum

Much has already been said about health instruction, the nature of the learner, the capabilities of the teacher, and the organization of the health curriculum in the modern elementary school. A large part of this has dealt with numerous items which might be categorized as "forerunners" or prerequisite considerations for putting the health program in action. Implementation of the health curriculum actually begins when the class enthusiastically settles down to work on the unit. This is the time when the planned activities either measure up or fall short in meeting the needs of the pupils. Moreover, this is the time when all the favorable educational influences are manipulated in such a way that the purposes of health education may ultimately be attained.

PHILOSOPHY OF THE BROAD AND VARIED PROGRAM

The heart of the health curriculum is what the boys and girls actually do; it is the activity itself that provides the learning experience. An awareness of the fact that children differ widely immediately suggests that the program of health instruction must be a broad and varied one. This is true not only because of needs, but also because of personal interests. Even children of the same chronological age, the same level of maturation, and with a similar degree of aptitude for learning will vary widely in their interests. Few children are alike; "what is one man's meat is another man's poison." It is important, therefore, that the activities selected for any one area of study have some variety. In this way sooner or later every child will find something that he likes very much. That which he likes is more apt to be a successful undertaking, and his success tends to breed more success.

Where it is not easy to have variety in content, there should at least be variety in the teaching techniques or aids employed. For example, the teacher of an intermediate grade topic on safety may want the class to concentrate on two or three rather weighty activities. It is altogether possible that

173

some students will require more moti-vation in order to become really inter-ested. Varying the approach from what has been done in previous health units may prove beneficial in stimulating interest.

It has been said that "there are sev-eral ways of skinning a cat," any one of which may get the job done. The phi-losophy of the broad and varied activ-ity program is simply one in which the teacher is urged to let her imagination loose and guide the class in a number of different experiences so that every pupil will have a truly stimulating les-son on a number of occasions during the school year.

THE HEALTH CURRICULUM — AN IMPLEMENTATION PROBLEM

Probably one of the biggest prob-lems facing teachers and supervisors in the realm of health instruction to-day is tied up with implementing the various health topics. This is a con-tinuing problem. It involves more than pupil interests, needs, methods, and materials; it is related to the personal likes and dislikes of the teacher and the ease or difficulty with which cer-tain items may be taught in the school. It is somewhat evident that the present curriculum emphasis on health educa-tion is not a matter of deciding when to teach a topic such as safety or nutrition, but rather of deciding what aspect of the safety or nutrition topic a particular group of pupils needs. Obviously all grade levels do not need the same de-gree of emphasis in any one area of health instruction.

The overlapping of subject matter materials may be good, because it is true that the ceaseless whisper of cer-tain verities has in time a positive ef-fect. On the other hand, overlapping as such is not economical in terms of time available to teach. There is too much to cover. The selection of topics and the content under each of these topics

needs to be done carefully. Merely in-sisting, for example, that primary and intermediate graders should be ex-posed to the sleep, rest and activity area is not enough. The activities se-lected to implement a topic need care-ful scrutiny. The Harvard Report admirably points this out:

> Selection is the essence of teach-ing. Even the most compendious sur-vey is only the rudest culling from reality. Since the problem of choice can under no circumstances be avoided, the problem becomes what, rather than how much, to teach; or better, what principles and methods to illustrate by the use of informa-tion.[1]

Although a number of research stud-ies have been carried on relative to pupil interests, major health problems, the nature of the elementary school health curriculum, the major topics for elementary school study, and the particular knowledges and under-standings for each grade, very little has been done regarding specific *teaching activities* in the major topi-cal area of instruction. This has re-sulted in a conglomeration of activities and experiences under a particular topic, with or without reference to properly stated outcomes. Needless to say, every activity employed to teach a health topic, whether it be an experi-ment, a story play, a poster drawing, or a field trip, should contribute to the predetermined objectives.

SUGGESTED ACTIVITIES FOR MAJOR HEALTH TOPICS

A number of special health topics for elementary schoolchildren follow below. These topics are the ones that make up the health curriculum and were set forth in some detail in Chap-ter 7. In order to do justice to current

[1] Report of Harvard Committee. *General Education in a Free Society.* Cambridge, Mass.: Harvard University Press, 1948, p. 63.

courses of study and at the same time be complete, a total of 12 categories or topics are covered. They are (1) Personal Cleanliness and Appearance; (2) Physical Activity, Sleep, Rest, and Relaxation; (3) Nutrition and Growth; (4) Dental Health; (5) Body Structure and Operation; (6) Prevention and Control of Disease; (7) Safety and First Aid; (8) Mental Health; (9) Sex and Family Living Education; (10) Community Health; (11) Tobacco, Alcohol, and Drugs; and (12) Consumer Health. These topics have been set up separately, together with a number of suitable activities for the primary and intermediate grades. The teacher should find this arrangement useful when considering how far to go with any one particular grade. Although primary grade children are quite different from intermediate graders as a group, there will be times when there is considerable overlapping of interest between children of different grades. More specifically, a precocious third grade child may be ready for a suggested experience or project suitable for the typical fifth grade class.

Another reason for presenting a wide range of activities under each topic is that in many parts of the United States there are schools administratively set up in such a way that one teacher may teach one or more grades in one classroom. It is not uncommon in some remote areas to find combined grades, such as second and third or fourth and fifth. In one state there are a number of junior-primary units where the teacher has a class made up of the first three grades. In such a situation a great amount of attention is given to individual pupil differences, and boys and girls make progress in their subjects more or less at their own rate of development and often without the pressure to complete a specified quantity of work in any one year.

The activities suggested for the primary and intermediate grades are not all-inclusive nor are they offered as ideals or "musts" in any way. They are simply a collection of appropriate experiences for a particular category of health instruction. No teacher will carry out all of the suggestions, but she may use those most applicable to her particular grade. Practically all of the activities have been tried in one school or another and found to be worthwhile in promoting a greater understanding of health. Many of them are suitable for initiating a unit of study. When employed with appropriate questions, they contribute to the discovery method of instruction. Obviously, depending on local circumstances or local teachers, some of the activities are better than others in their tendency to change behavior and promote acceptable health practices and attitudes.

In using this suggested material, keep these points in mind: (1) the effectiveness of the activities will be increased after a review of the chapters on methods and materials; (2) evaluation techniques (Chapter 12) will help measure the worth of the activities selected; and (3) sources of materials to accompany these activities (films, filmstrips, charts, posters, pamphlets, and stories for children) should be used. These are listed in detail in Chapter 11.

SUGGESTED ELEMENTARY SCHOOL ACTIVITIES AND EXPERIENCES

1. Personal Cleanliness and Appearance

Desirable Outcomes (Primary Level)

To understand why cleanliness and grooming are important to personal health and appearance.

To be able to wash the hands when necessary, use toilet facilities properly, brush teeth, keep bodies clean, use the handkerchief, care for the clothing, comb the hair.

To understand and develop habits in the care and protection of the eyes, ears, and nose.

Desirable Outcomes (Intermediate Level)

To know why clothing needs to be changed frequently, and in keeping with weather conditions.

To develop habits of cleanliness related to food and eating practices.

To understand something about the structure and function of the skin and the elimination of wastes through the skin.

To appreciate the relationship between appearance and daily living, social success, and self-respect.

Comments

The child entering school is faced with the somewhat new idea of being responsible, more than ever before, for his personal cleanliness and appearance. As he progresses through the grades he grows in understanding the reason why cleanliness and grooming are important to personal health and appearance. He becomes aware of how cleanliness helps to prevent the spread of disease and how it makes him more acceptable to his classmates.

Although standards of cleanliness vary, most homes are equipped with the basic facilities for helping children keep clean. When children, through no fault of their own, fail to meet accepted standards of cleanliness or appearance, care should be taken not to humiliate them unintentionally.

In the intermediate grades the type of cleanliness may be related to the prevention and control of disease. After learning the characteristics of bacteria and their relationship to disease, the habit of keeping clean becomes more closely related to a real desire to make a good appearance and to preserve health. Cleanliness then becomes a social asset.

With the active aid of the students, cleanliness and neatness in the class-room can be achieved. With a little encouragement children take pride in the condition of their books, desks, and materials. The alert teacher recognizes that it is only a step from such individual accomplishments to the development of pride in the group. Such things as work tables, floors, blackboards, bulletin boards, the coat room, the toilet room, and lockers can become objects of group concern and of group action in keeping them clean and presentable. The NEA-AMA Joint Committee on School Health Problems clearly points out that "when a child feels that a desk is *his* desk and when children feel the classroom and everything in it is *their* classroom, they will act and react differently from times of stubbornness when they feel they must do certain things simply because they are told. Class lessons in cleanliness become important because of their personal application."[2]

Suggested Activities[3]

PRIMARY LEVEL

1. Conduct informal talks every morning. Talk about the need for bathing, cleaning the teeth, combing the hair, wearing neat clothes.

2. Take turns dusting the room, books, bookcases, and arranging shelves and clothing racks.

3. Draw pictures illustrating taking a bath, washing clothes, ironing shirts, and cleaning fingernails. A first grade child can draw a meaningful picture of himself washing his face in the bathroom at home without much difficulty. Have several children illustrate their own story of cleanliness by holding their pictures up for all to see.

4. Discuss the different ways people take baths (full tub, wash tub,

[2] National Education Association—American Medical Association. *Health Education*, 5th ed. Washington, D.C.: National Education Association, 1961.

[3] For a list of teaching aids and sources to be used with these and the following major health topic activities, see Chapter 11.

shower, sponge, or steam baths). Read the poem *After a Bath* by Aileen Fisher.

6. Visit the school nurse for a personal inspection. This may be quite rewarding, especially if done with a little advance planning.

7. Have the students demonstrate to the class the proper method of:
    a. Washing and drying hands
    b. Combing the hair and cleaning the hairbrush
    c. Covering coughs and sneezes
    d. Blowing the nose properly
    e. Drinking from a drinking fountain

8. Have a child bring his pet cat or dog to school and show the class how he brushes it and keeps it neat.

9. Appoint all class members as "Health Detectives." Before the weekend begins ask everyone to keep his eyes open on Saturday and Sunday and note what he can see involving the cleanliness and appearance of people, animals, buildings, roads, walks, lawns, and gardens. On Monday permit everyone to tell what he saw. This may be made more interesting by having the group make little cardboard badges which may be worn right away on Friday afternoon:

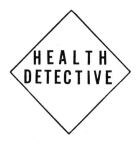

10. Talk about the care of clothing. Secure a mirror for use in the room to check personal appearance each morning. First and second graders generally love this activity.

11. Give each child a coat hanger for his clothes. Give each child a large number cut from a calendar. Play a game with the numbers until each child can tell his own. Then he can paste it over the hook where he hangs his clothes.

12. Dramatize the proper clothing for each season of the year. Organize this in the form of a fashion show. The 41-frame filmstrips, *You and Your Clothes* (Young American Films), may help to vitalize this dramatization further (applicable for second grade).

13. Appoint a committee to prepare an exhibit of different types of clothes for different occasions. Work clothes, rubbers, raincoats, riding clothes, snowsuits, bathing suits are all designed for special purposes. Appoint another committee to collect various types of hats which express native customs, i.e., felt hat, cap, turban, straw hat, fez, fur hat, hood (applicable for third grade).

14. Create a classroom store and engage in buying and selling experiences which will help to provide a better understanding of the kinds of clothing best suited to health needs and appearance.

15. Talk about the protective covering of animals, fish, birds: the fur of the bear, fox, squirrel, raccoon; the feathers of the wild duck; the shells of clams and oysters; the bark of the trees.

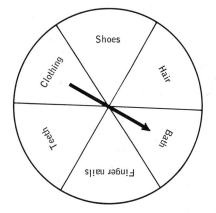

16. Invite the school custodian to class to talk about how the school is kept safe and clean.

17. Construct a Health Check

Wheel. Use a wheel 20 inches in diameter. Use a brad to fasten an arrow to the middle of the wheel. Use pictures of health practices made by pupils or illustrations from magazines. Ask a pupil to spin the arrow to select a health practice to be checked for the day.

INTERMEDIATE LEVEL

1. Look in the class dictionary for words pertaining to cleanliness.

2. Discuss ways and means of making the classroom more attractive.

3. Formulate a list of characteristics admired by a fourth, fifth, or sixth grader (as the case may be) that has to do with cleanliness and neatness. Have a self-check against the list and make plans for improvement. This self evaluation may be accomplished informally by each child at his desk.

4. Discuss what respect means. What does it mean to have self respect? What does it mean to have others respect you? What does it mean to be popular? How does keeping yourself clean and neat help to increase your self respect and popularity (applicable for fourth grade)?

5. Examine the skin on the back of the hand with a magnifying glass. See the creases and folds when the hand is relaxed. See also the dirt which will disappear after washing (good for a fifth or sixth grade class). Have the class note the pores and tiny hairs. Discuss perspiration and body odors. Note oil and hair glands and tell what they do for the skin and one's appearance.

6. Have the class bring in pictures from magazines depicting how the skin works. Pictures, such as a man shivering from the cold or sweating from the noonday sun, or of a little boy burning his finger over the hot stove, are good examples. Magazine advertisements for beauty aids may also be discussed. Do the aids do everything the ads claim they do?

7. Discuss injuries to the skin which may affect health and personal appearance. Talk about cuts, bruises, blisters, burns, and splinters. Show the class or have the nurse demonstrate how to treat a blister and remove a splinter of wood from a finger.

8. Prepare an article for the school paper on some topic of cleanliness.

9. Experiment with the wearing of wet clothes by taking a piece of dry cloth and a piece of wet cloth and placing both on the skin. Ask the class which feels cooler? Which takes more heat from the body? What conclusion should be drawn? Proceed from there to study types of seasonal clothing. Refer also to clothing used in tribal areas and other sections of the globe.

10. Discuss germs and how they cause disease when the hands, tableware, and family utensils are not clean. Use the microscope to see the germs. Point out that germs are both helpful and harmful, that washing with water may remove a few, but only careful washing with soap and hot water will remove enough of the germs to protect our health.

11. Show how "hidden dirt" stays on the skin, even when a pupil thinks he is clean, by rubbing the back of the hand with a small piece of cloth dipped in alcohol. Let the class see the cloth before and after rubbing the skin.

12. Study clothing in terms of color combinations, wise selections, care, and wear. Put a color chart up in front of the classroom. Dress a model or dummy.

13. Find out how Jenner, Pasteur, Koch, Reed, and others have benefited humanity.

14. Visit the school cafeteria to inspect and observe the methods used to maintain sanitary conditions. The same approach may be made at a park, picnic area, or public beach to note hygienic conditions.

15. Show the relationship of posture to personal appearance.

16. Plan, find out, report on, make,

draw, collect, write, discuss, and sing about cleanliness and neatness. Notice that the words above suggest activity—*doing something* with the topic.

17. Collect pictures of a variety of hair styles.

2. Activity, Sleep, Rest, and Relaxation

Desirable Outcomes (Primary Level)

To understand how a proper balance of exercise, work, sleep, rest, and relaxation will provide for optimum achievement in physical and mental well-being.

To appreciate the need for play and large muscle activity, sunshine, daily relaxation periods, and a wide variety of leisure time activities.

To recognize why sound sleep in quiet surroundings is healthful, and why quiet activities before bedtime or mealtime are beneficial.

Desirable Outcomes (Intermediate Level)

To understand how exercise builds and maintains health and the importance of outdoor play and recreational activities.

To know the real value of sleep and rest, and how to rest and relax.

To observe regular hours of retiring and rising together with other personal requirements for sleep and rest.

To employ hygienic practices when engaging in physical activity at school and in the community.

Comments

Boys and girls at all age levels should reach the end of the day free from fatigue and irritability. They should rest a while before eating and engage in pleasant and quiet activities before going to bed. They should arise in the morning rested and ready for schoolwork or play. What could be more simple? Yet, getting this knowledge across to all elementary school pupils and having them modify their living habits accordingly is indeed a difficult task.

Health teaching on this topic relates to a number of significant variables. Children themselves vary in their sleep requirements. Those from four to eight years of age need a total of 12 or 13 hours of sleep. For 11 year olds, 11 hours is generally sufficient. By age 12 or 13, ten hours is usually enough. But the quantity of sleep is not nearly as important as the quality. The quality is affected by numerous home and community stimuli. In every neighborhood there are items such as street noises, factory noises, industrial odors, barking dogs, older children at play, and other factors which have a negative effect on the quality of the night's sleep.

Parents must have an understanding of sleep and rest needs, of wholesome physical activities, of signs of fatigue, and many more conditions conducive to adequate growth. When parents fail to guide their children properly at home, the efforts of the classroom teacher may seem quite meager. Late evening programs, movies, television shows, radio, and after dinner visits tend to cut into the optimum sleep requirements for growing children. Over a period of time pupil behavior is affected. Children in such instances become more fatigued, lose their keen appetites, drop in scholarship, and frequently demonstrate a less social behavior.

Although children are more discriminating than they used to be in what they choose to watch on television, there are still many who spend hours per week sitting and watching. There are, of course, many excellent offerings on television, but numerous children stay up too late watching.

There is an excellent opportunity for the teacher to work with the home, to see that all pupils receive their due share of vigorous growth-stimulating physical exercise, relaxation, and sleep each day. Probably more bacterial and virus diseases get a foothold in the human organism because of chronic fatigue than from any other hygienic shortcoming. Children need school activities which will point up the fact that satisfying school work, outdoor play, rest, sunshine, proper food, and happy associations at school and in the home neighborhood help them to secure a restful night's sleep.

Today, more than ever in the past, considerable attention must be given by the teacher to the role of physical exercise in the maintenance of organic health.

Physical fitness is the prerequisite to everything else. It is the wherewithal that permits movement; it is in a very real sense the capacity for activity—any and all activity. Tyler says that the muscles are the "organs of the will." Since the muscular fitness items of strength and endurance (which relate to organic health and mental-social health as well) cannot be stored, it is necessary that daily attention be directed to vigorous physical exercise. Although most students appear quite active, a knowledge of the benefits of exercise needs to be stressed aca-

demically in the classroom, as well as directly on the playgrounds and gymnasiums. There are numerous boys and girls today who are under their normal strength and well below a minimum level of muscular fitness. Their physical efficiency is too low for them to live fully and function as they should. The quiet, chore-free activities of a somewhat sedentary adult population have reached the schoolchildren. Even those pupils a few blocks from school ride the bus; others sit and watch much of the time; still others are tense and emotionally on edge due in part to the rapid pace of modern civilization. With overeating and underactivity it becomes clear that education for health is more important than ever. Suitable activities which are carried on in a pleasant atmosphere, free from the pressure and rapid pace of modern society, can be most profitable.

The role of the classroom teacher is to demonstrate clearly to her particular grade that exercise, nutrition, and rest build a quality of physical fitness that is a forerunner for all other activities. This means that the classroom teacher is a physical education teacher and as

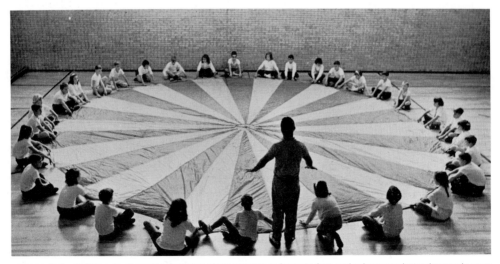

Figure 8–1 Children in physical education class prepare to jump to feet and raise parachute vigorously overhead. (Courtesy Baldwinsville Schools, Baldwinsville, N.Y.)

such is a teacher of health. The value of physical skills cannot be over-emphasized, for fitness in later life is related to skills acquired during the early years. Emerson, in his *Essay on Education*, refers to "educated eyes in uneducated bodies." In so doing he makes a strong point in favor of phys-ical efficiency and skills.[4] Thus each instructor of youth, particularly at the elementary level, teaches the mi-metics and story plays, the games, the rhythms and dances, and the recrea-tional skills that contribute to growth and understanding at the moment.

A large percentage of classroom teachers carry on their own programs of physical education. It is the minor-ity that have the services of the trained specialist to teach activities. It is im-portant, therefore, that each teacher be well acquainted not only with the behavior characteristics of the age group, but also with the appropriate activities for each grade level, season, and facility. The program must be a broad and varied one so that all child-ren have a number of experiences and find something that they are interested in. It is the concomitant learnings asso-ciated with these games and dances that foster social efficiency, cultural appreciations, and moral ethical values. This becomes emphasized when one considers that "activity — play, games, stunts, rhythms, and dance — is to the child as work is to the man. It is serious, special, and full of meaning — the child's way of life. Through it he learns about himself, the people and the things around him."[5]

----

[4] "... let us have men whose manhood is only the continuation of their boyhood, natural characters still; such are able for fertile and heroic action; and not that sad spectacle with which we are too often familiar, educated eyes in uneducated bodies."

[5] The National Conference on Physical Edu-cation in the Elementary School. *Physical Edu-cation in the Elementary School.* Washington, D.C.: The Athletic Institute, 1951.

Suggested Activities

PRIMARY LEVEL

1. Discuss the relationship of physical activity to "feeling good." Show how overactivity relates to fatigue, sleep, and relaxation.

2. Have the class tell about the games and dances they enjoy playing most. Play one or two favorite games in the classroom as an illustration of something "we like" to do, or do the same thing on the school playground.

3. Put the following poem on the blackboard in big letters:[6]

WE ARE PLANNING OUR DAY

WE PLAN OUR WORK
WE PLAN OUR PLAY
TO MAKE A HAPPY
BUSY DAY.

Have the class plan the work, play, and rest periods for the day. Point out the balance between these three items. Ask the class to tell why they think this kind of planning may make them happy.

4. Teach some exercise which will strengthen abdominal and back mus-cles and contribute to good posture and body mechanics. Play games to release tensions built up in concen-trated activities. Engage in funda-mental rhythms such as walking, marching, skipping, hopping, sliding, twirling, and jumping to music (ap-plicable to kindergarten and first grade).

5. Have fun acting out mimetics such as story plays that are full of ac-tions. Dramatize such things as going to a fire, swimming along the shore, rowing a boat on a fishing party, tree branches bending before the force of the wind.

6. Ask the class to tell some of the

----

[6] Reprinted through the courtesy of the Metro-politan Life Insurance Company.

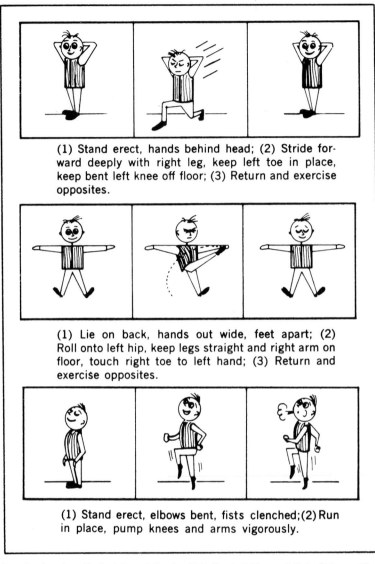

(1) Stand erect, hands behind head; (2) Stride forward deeply with right leg, keep left toe in place, keep bent left knee off floor; (3) Return and exercise opposites.

(1) Lie on back, hands out wide, feet apart; (2) Roll onto left hip, keep legs straight and right arm on floor, touch right toe to left hand; (3) Return and exercise opposites.

(1) Stand erect, elbows bent, fists clenched;(2) Run in place, pump knees and arms vigorously.

(Adapted from the American Medical Association booklet, *Physical Fitness*, A.M.A., Chicago, Illinois, 1966.)

humorous things that happen in their work and play. Point out that these little happenings make us happy.

7. Bring a kitten to class. After the class has been under way awhile, tell everyone to look at the kitty. See how many children have pets. Have them tell how their animal friends rest or sleep. Ask where birds go to sleep.

8. Make a clock out of cardboard. Place the pointer at a reasonable bed-time. For first graders set it at 7 P.M. Inquire as to when the various children go to bed.

9. Bring a globe of the world to class. Explain daytime and nighttime by pulling the shades to darken the room and holding a flashlight over the globe to represent the sunshine. Notice in what countries people are sleeping when it is daytime in America.

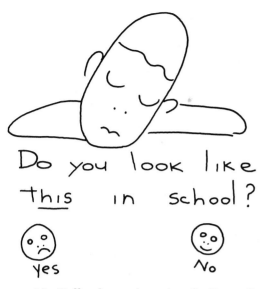

Do you look like this in school?

yes   No

10. Talk about the nice feeling of going to bed. Let the pupils suggest how nice the sheets feel and the softness of the bed (first grade).

11. Check on the number of children having baby brothers or sisters. Have the children answer questions on how long the babies sleep, what awakens them, and why they need

more sleep than older children (first grade).

12. Ask the question: "What do we do after dinner at night?" Put the answers on the board. After a representative list of activities has been written down, have the class pick out the activities that appear best in terms of pleasantness and relaxation. Guide the group toward the selection of items such as happy, quiet play, listening to stories, reading, and well-selected home duties.

13. Take the opportunity to capitalize on the daily rest period in school. Listen to soft music before the rest period (kindergarten to second grade). Examples: *Lullabies For Sleepy Heads*, Dorothy Olsen (RCA Victor), *The Swan* from *Carnival of the Animals* by Saint-Saens.

14. Construct a model bedroom on a large table. Use doll furniture and doll people. Show a comfortable room with clean bedclothing, opened window, and other optimum physical factors. Put a clock on the wall set for bedtime.

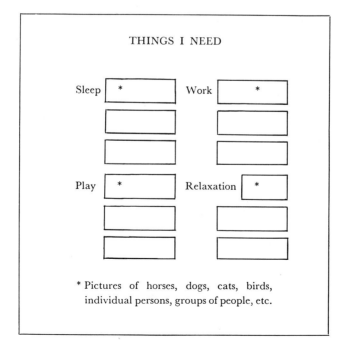

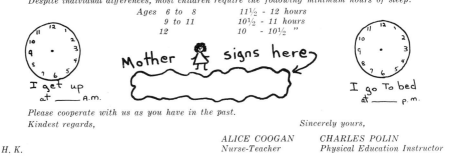

EAST SCHOOL

Dear Parents,   *Long Beach, N. Y.*

Are you willing to give your children a longer sleeping hour?

For many years we, at East School, have been interested in your child's good health. We know you, too, are concerned. With this in mind, we feel it is necessary that you help us with a serious problem that has come to our attention. We have observed the students and find that a great many of them are tired and sleepy. After further investigation, we learned that too many children go to sleep at a rather late hour. This, combined with a late wake-up time, results in fatigue, as well as neglected toilet habits and insufficient time for a nutritious breakfast. The children are, therefore, poorly prepared for a day's work and play, and are at a low level of efficiency.

We can overcome this undesirable situation by insisting that the children retire at a reasonable hour, receive the proper number of hours of sleep, and awake at 7 a.m. They are then prepared for school, and have a nourishing breakfast and are ready for a full day's work.

Despite individual differences, most children require the following minimum hours of sleep:

Ages	6 to 8	11½ - 12 hours
	9 to 11	10½ - 11 hours
	12	10 - 10½ "

Mother signs here

I get up at ____ A.M.

I go To bed at ____ P.M.

Please cooperate with us as you have in the past.

Kindest regards,   *Sincerely yours,*

ALICE COOGAN   CHARLES POLIN
Nurse-Teacher   Physical Education Instructor

H. K.

15. Learn quiet games to play before bedtime.

16. Make pictures or posters suggesting activities conducive to play, sleep, or relaxation.

17. Prepare a wall board with pictures brought to class depicting sleep, work, play, and relaxation (second and third grade).

18. Plan a program of action with children and parents. In one community a letter sent home was quite effective.

INTERMEDIATE LEVEL

1. Formulate a well-balanced daily schedule that makes ample provision for each of the functions of exercise, relaxation, and sleep which affect the growth and development of the human body.

2. Discuss the values of muscular work as a health measure. Point out that a muscle in good tone is firm and ready to act; muscle tone is the foundation for further development of strength and skill; sufficient strength and endurance reduce fatigue and permit a child or adult to keep going longer; agility, flexibility, speed, and precision are improved; increased heart action results in a more efficient heart with more blood being pumped together with fewer beats per minute; oxygen is better distributed to tissues; all organic functions in the body are improved; and general health is advanced (fifth or sixth grade).

3. Use a wall chart to show how the muscular system works and how its use puts demands on the other body systems; the demands in turn tend to keep the other systems organically and functionally healthy.

4. List on the board a number of physical activities that may be engaged in around the home. Number these activities according to the degree of vigor required. Do the same for occupations in the community and for sports and games in the school physical education program.

5. Display pictures of prominent athletes or pictures of athletes in action. Magazines such as *Life, Look,* and *Sports Illustrated* abound in ex-

cellent pictures of swimmers, golfers, tennis players, baseball batters, football carriers, and ice skating champions.

6. Plan a hiking, camping, or bicycling trip. Make the trip if possible.

7. Practice relaxing. Have the class stand by their desks with both arms extended above the head. On command, relax only the hand by allowing the wrist to "break." Then relax to the elbow joint, and then the rest of the arm. Repeat by relaxing the whole arm on command. Point out how difficult this seems at first (fifth and sixth grades).

8. Discuss the meaning of recreation. Ask the children what their parents do for recreation. Suggest and list on the board several reasons that play is not a waste of time.

9. Prepare a hobby exhibit. Show pictures of the hobbies of prominent people. Suggest to the class that they illustrate some of the hobbies of their older brothers and sisters and their parents.

10. Encourage informal discussions of why we tire, how rest affects posture, work, and play, and why anxiety, fear, anger, and eating before bedtime may affect sleep.

11. Keep individual records of the number of hours sleep each night for one whole week with notations on "How I felt in the morning." Dis-

cuss the records at the end of the week. Bring into the discussion the advantages of sleeping alone, the kinds of mattresses slept on, restlessness in sleep, and sleep habits (sixth grade).

12. Count pulse rates before and after a period of exercise. Note also the respiratory rate, its increase and return to normal. This may be made quite interesting. Have the children stand by their desks and count their own pulse beats for 30 seconds. Multiply by two and record on a piece of paper such as the example below. Then run quietly in place for one minute and quickly take the pulse rate again for 30 seconds. Record in the proper place on the paper. Sit down and rest. Take the pulse two minutes later and record.

Find out who had the greatest rise in pulse rate. How many came close to returning to their original pulse rate? Discuss what has happened in the body, with particular reference to physical condition and fatigue.

13. Interview the school nurse regarding the relationship of excessive fatigue, inadequate sleep, and activity to the common cold.

14. Make a pie graph that will show how to budget a 24 hour day for school, work, play, and rest.

15. Invite the physical education teacher into class to talk about ath-

---

MY SLEEP RECORD

Day	Hours Slept	How I felt in the morning
Monday		
Tuesday		
Wednesday		
Thursday		
Friday		
Saturday		
Sunday		

```
┌─────────────────────────────────────────────────────┐
│                                                       │
│                    PULSE RATE                         │
│                                                       │
│     Before exercise  ───────────────                 │
│                                                       │
│     Immediately after exercise───────────────────     │
│                                                       │
│     Two minutes later  ── ───────────                 │
│                                                       │
└─────────────────────────────────────────────────────┘
```

letes he has known. Encourage questions from the class relative to the eating, sleeping, and resting practices of athletes.

16. Appoint a committee of three to find out about the Harvard Step Test of Physical Fitness for elementary age pupils. Give the test and check individual student scores.[7]

3. Nutrition and Growth

Desirable Outcomes (Primary Level)

To understand that well-balanced, daily nutrition includes food from each of the four basic food groups and why such a variety of food is needed by the body for growth.

To acquaint children with a variety of nutritious foods, good eating habits, customary social behavior at mealtime, and the planning of balanced meals.

To understand that energy is necessary for work and play, that some foods provide more energy than others, and that appetite can be improved by careful planning of work, play, and rest.

To be aware of the fact that being tired, sick, and unhappy is often related to poor nutrition.

Desirable Outcomes (Intermediate Level)

To understand how a well-balanced diet helps to achieve success in work and play, and how it relates to one's emotional outlook.

To know that foods contain various

nutrients, minerals, and vitamins which have something to do with disease, personal vigor, and enthusiasm.

To understand how food is used in the body and that the body is composed of cells which need wholesome food for proper growth and development.

To know something about the foods used in other parts of the world and how food is handled, preserved, and stored.

To desire and be able to personally choose suitable meals when the child must select his own, and to be familiar with some common food fads, misconceptions, and superstitions.

To understand that coffee and tea do not contribute to the growth of young boys and girls.

Comments

One might begin thinking about foods and nutrition by wondering whether there is a definite need for this kind of work with children. There is both evidence of progress and evidence of need. In the first place there has been a great reduction in the number of nutritional deficiency diseases such as rickets and scurvy. Children are taller and heavier than they were generations ago, and, despite continual parental ignorance and poverty, the diet of the schoolchild has also improved during the last half century. In addition, more is known about the factors which affect foods and food habits of adults and children, and school and public service agencies have done much to promote proper food consumption.

On the other hand, there are several

---

[7] Adequate instructions may be found in Carl E. Willgoose, *Evaluation in Health Education and Physical Education.* New York: McGraw-Hill Book Company, 1961, pp. 117–118.

studies, such as the one by the School of Medicine of the University of Washington, which show that a large number of boys and girls are significantly overweight. The studies indicate that girls frequently lead a soft existence — underactive, overeating, passive, and very dependent on parents. Also, Mayer's studies at Harvard University of obese girls indicates that they are far less active than girls of normal weight.

Moderately severe and prolonged undernutrition in children can produce alterations in brain activity which may never be corrected.[8] Through improvement in diet, the child may catch up to his peers in physical size, but limitation of nutrient

---

[8] Coursin, D. B., "Effects of Undernutrition on Central Nervous System Function," *Nutrition Review*, March 1965. See also Philip L. White, "Nutrition and Genetic Potential," *Journal of School Health*, 36:341–345, September 1966.

intake during the early years occurs during the period that normally produces some 90 per cent of normal brain structure. In addition, recent research indicates that malnutrition delays puberty and slows the development of mental ability. This is frequently expressed through a lack of mental vigor and reduced ability to concentrate.

It is not easy to tell when a child is malnourished. It may help, however, to check the characteristic deviations in appearance and behavior listed in Chapter 5. A familiarity with these signs will not only be beneficial in terms of individual cases of malnutrition, but will also suggest items for study in the food instruction program.

Improving nutrition rightfully begins in the home. Much is also being done in the community. Significant food improvements are continuing and are often noticeable. Some of these include the enrichment of bread, flour, corn meal, grits, and rice, the

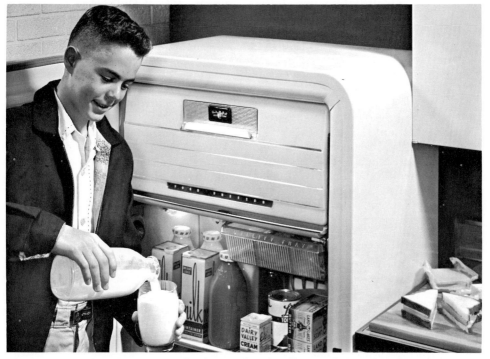

Figure 8–2   Post a picture of a classmate in action. (Courtesy National Dairy Council.)

iodization of salt, the fortification of margarine and milk, the development of selected varieties of foods, and the fluoridation of drinking water. Moreover, group feeding practices, some of which offer considerable instructional value, are becoming more common. Some of these which should be of special interest to elementary school-teachers are group day care centers, the school lunch, homes for children, social adjustment schools, and summer camps.

There are certain essentials one must bear in mind for effective nutrition teaching. This should never become a fixed or stereotyped area of instruction. The teacher needs a knowledge of nutrition coupled with an appreciation of home-school-community relationships. To check herself on her own methods she may ask such questions as these:[9]

Do I relate classroom experiences and other activities to the daily food practices of children?

Do I make clear to the children the habits that are desirable for them to establish?

Do I provide parents with information and solicit their suggestions so that I may expect full cooperation from them in habit formation?

Am I guided by the needs of children and the community in selecting learning situations?

Most nutrition educators point out that nutrition teaching to be most successful should begin early in the grades. This is the time when the school supplements the home, and here, perhaps more than ever again, there is mutual interest of parent and teacher.

In the primary grades there is a breadth of teaching possibilities built around growing big and strong, farm

[9] Martin, Ethel A. *Roberts' Nutrition Work with Children*. Chicago: University of Chicago Press, 1955, p. 412.

and market visits, growing vegetables in the classroom or school garden, preparing foods, tasting foods, enjoying foods, and the sociability of the occasion. The list of possible teaching units in nutrition is lengthy indeed. One can fire the imagination of the enthusiastic child with such headings as, "Getting Ready for Our Picnic," "The Animal Way," "Off to the Farm," "To Market with Mother," or "Making Butter the Hard Way." Moreover, the list of available top-rate films on nutrition is extensive; many are excellent. For example, *The King Who Came to Breakfast* (17 minutes, color, Association Films) depicts Bil Baird's marionettes who tell the story of wheat from 15,000 years ago to the present, showing how wheat developed in the deltas of Africa, spread north and west with various civilizations, and has come to play a key role in our way of life. A most helpful elementary teacher's guide is *Better Breakfast Activities*, distributed free by the Cereal Institute, Inc. It consists of 15 pages of top ideas, experiments, and activities that have been tried and found successful with children.

One more excellent example of how to make the topic of food interesting comes from the National Dairy Council. (See current address of national office in Chapter 11.) This organization produces *Animals that Give People Milk*, a two-page world map showing animals that give people milk and the habitats of the animals. Each animal is numbered. The numbers in the larger circles show the animals that are the largest source of milk in the continent or area in which the circle appears. This map provokes discussion almost immediately.

In the intermediate grades the good food and living habits which were started in the primary grades continue to grow, but with more answers and meaningful experiences provided. Children now learn more specifically what foods will do for them with a

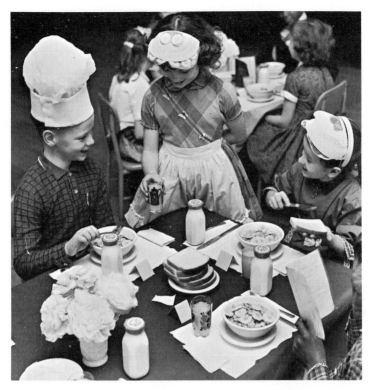

Figure 8-3 Try a breakfast party at school. (Courtesy Cincinnati Public Schools.)

minimum of emphasis placed on technical names.

Simple, outstanding functions should be selected for emphasis. Such an example might be growth and energy. Too many functions confuse pupils and sometimes make them feel that each food does all things for them. Social studies sequences involving the kinds of lands and peoples must be taken into account. In addition there should be a chance to exercise group planning and judgment involving real nutrition problems — problems such as arranging for field trips, carrying through a school garden project, thoroughly investigating the effect of stimulants such as tea, coffee, and Coca-Cola, or making a tape recording of advertisements for food heard over the radio. Otherwise the topic of foods may come and go without measurably moving the class toward the desirable outcomes.

Suggested Activities
PRIMARY LEVEL

1. Explain the *Guide to Good Eating* and stress the need for food each day from the four basic groups. The *Guide to Good Eating* (in color) is made available by the National Dairy Council (third grade).

2. Keep a record of height and weight. Interest in growth, especially through the individual pupil's readily visible characteristics, is generally high. Particularly useful charts may be obtained free from the Horlick Malted Milk Corporation, Racine, Wis. (second and third grades). Attach personal pictures if available.

3. Establish the EE and FF club. Copy the daily lunch menu on the board. Children read this and compare the food items with a food chart also on the board. Everyone goes to the cafeteria knowing what they are eating and *why*. On return, the pupils

My Name --------------- Age -----		
Month	Weight	Height
Sept		
Oct.		
Nov.		
Dec.		
Jan.		

report themselves as EE (eat everything) or FF (fussy feeder). Then they discuss why they think they acted the way they did (first and second grades).

4. Plan a balanced menu for lunch. Consider the possibilities for both winter and summer. Plan with attractiveness in mind, and call attention to the fact that it *is* attractive. A number of excellent food projects may be obtained free from the Cereal Institute.

5. Visit the local milk bottling plant or bakery to see how foods are preserved through sanitary and other processes. Arrange for samples of the product ahead of time. Be certain, also, that the class knows what to look for.

6. Study color in foods. Begin by asking the class to bring in colored pictures of foods. In the fall of the year a blue hubbard squash cut down the middle is brilliant. So is a pumpkin, a sweet potato, a box of freshly picked cranberries, a handful of sweet apples.

7. Ask the class where their food came from. Some foods come from seeds, others from fruits, leaves, stems, roots, and animals. The class may bring in special foods to illustrate this point.

8. Display several animal bones and human teeth. The children may have samples of first teeth at home and are usually happy to bring them to school. Then discuss the makeup of bones. Calcium and phosphorus are obtained from a number of items which the teacher may take, one at a time, from a large basket on a table at the front of the class: milk, celery, hard cheese, eggs, almond nuts, dried beans, turnip tops, and broccoli, peanut butter, and a piece of lean meat (liver, kidney, heart). See also the excellent wall chart, "For the Calcium You Need," Evaporated Milk Corporation (free).

9. Make clay and cardboard food models which can be used in building combinations for meals. Models already made in appetizing colors may be obtained free from the National Dairy Council. Make place mats and place cards for the table. Discuss and arrange flowers for the table (first grade). The Dixie Cup Co., Easton, Pennsylvania, will be happy to send the teacher a sample place setting which is complete. This is attractive, durable, and may be used very well over a period of time.

10. Make paper cups by folding clean sheets of paper. Enjoy drinking water from them.

11. Visit a farmer in the chicken yard or in the fields raising grain. See turkeys at Thanksgiving time. Have one brought to class in a cage if the class cannot visit a farm. Notice how foods like milk, butter, cheese, and bread are kept safe from dirt and flies.

12. Play grocery store; pool the knowledge of the class for an efficient operation. Use real canned goods and

OUR CHILDREN suggest

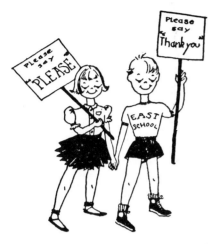

solid vegetables such as potatoes, onions, and carrots.

13. Dramatize good behavior at mealtime. Use host and hostess at midmorning snack or at lunch. Express gratitude for food by saying grace.

14. Prepare and taste fruit and milk drinks. Milk may be flavored with honey, chocolate syrup, peanut butter, or bananas.

15. Look over various food advertisements brought to class. Post the better ones so that they may be seen. Discuss accuracy. Talk about food values, truths, and half truths (third grade).

16. Prepare a cookbook made chiefly of pictures instead of words. Each pupil will collect all kinds of colored pictures of foods. Past issues of popular magazines may be cut up at home or in class. These pictures are then pasted on sheets of paper in groups, and the sheets may be combined into one small booklet.

17. Conduct an experiment in which two tomato plants are used—both plants to be given sunlight, air, and water, but one to be planted in poor soil and the other in good soil.

18. Use the clock when talking about regular meal habits, sleeping, work, and play.

19. Make large posters showing the body engine in action, such as hopping, running, dancing, skating, swimming, playing games.

20. Find out how many ways milk is used in the home.

21. Make butter in class; then spread it on crackers to eat as a midmorning snack. (Obtain instruction leaflets for all class members from the National Dairy Council.)

22. On different days prepare and serve raw vegetables: cauliflower, carrots, turnips, lettuce, celery, spinach, broccoli, cabbage, tomatoes. Serve a small bit of the vegetable which is broken and washed by the children.

23. In discussing breakfast foods, make a display or "store front" of empty cereal boxes brought from homes of the children.

24. Using a large map of the United States, find and mark the places from which meat comes. Locate the sources of the different kinds of fish.

25. Keep a weekly record of the basic four groups eaten every day. (Use chart distributed by Maltex Company, Burlington, Vt.)

26. Hold a mothers' breakfast at school.

27. Prepare menu booklet. Suggest that some menus be tried at home.

28. Have a "Crazy Milk Day" in the classroom. Help the children make butter to eat on crackers, buttermilk, cottage cheese, yogurt, and cream cheese. Call attention to cheese with some "Did You Know?" posters:

DID YOU KNOW?

... that in Switzerland, when a baby is born, a wheel of Saanen cheese is marked with his name? On all the holiest occasions of his mortality his private cheese is served. When he dies the mourners consume the last of this ceremonial Wheel of Life.

... that the holes in Swiss cheese form themselves naturally through the chemical changes that take place during aging?

A Guide To Good Eating
USE DAILY...

Most people are motivated to follow a food guide more closely when they understand why certain foods are em- phasized. On the next pages you will find ideas that may help you explain the importance of each food group.

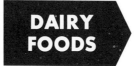

DAIRY FOODS

3 TO 4 GLASSES—CHILDREN
4 OR MORE GLASSES—TEEN-AGERS
2 OR MORE GLASSES—ADULTS

CHEESE, ICE CREAM AND OTHER MILK-MADE FOODS CAN SUPPLY PART OF THE MILK

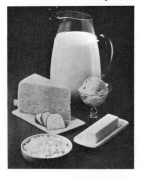

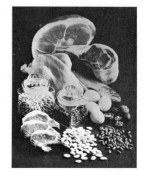

2 OR MORE SERVINGS

MEATS, FISH, POULTRY, EGGS, OR CHEESE—WITH DRY BEANS, PEAS, NUTS AS ALTERNATES

MEAT GROUP

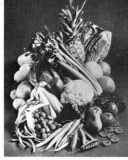

VEGETABLES AND FRUITS

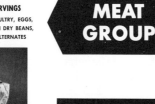

4 OR MORE SERVINGS

INCLUDE DARK GREEN OR YELLOW VEGETABLES; CITRUS FRUIT OR TOMATOES

4 OR MORE SERVINGS

ENRICHED OR WHOLE GRAIN ADDED MILK IMPROVES NUTRITIONAL VALUES

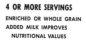

BREADS AND CEREALS

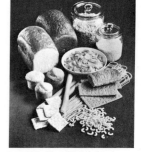

This is the foundation for a good diet. Use more of these and other foods as needed for growth, for activity, and for desirable weight.

The nutritional statements made in this guide have been reviewed by the Council on Foods and Nutrition of the American Medical Association and found consistent with current authoritative medical opinion.

Figure 8-4   A daily reminder. (Courtesy National Dairy Council.)

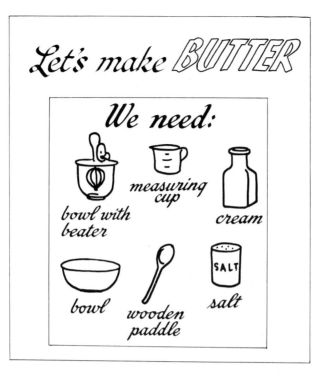

INTERMEDIATE LEVEL

1. Discuss the statement, "It's smart to eat a good breakfast." How much breakfast should one eat, and what kind? The Iowa breakfast studies and a number of others show that 25 to 30 per cent of the day's nourishment should be provided by breakfast. The bacon and eggs type of breakfast can be equaled by one consisting of milk, cereal, toast, and butter. Present-day cereals have a far greater food value than most people realize. A single serving of Cream of Wheat, for example, contains as much iron as a serving of liver. And many cereals are rich in high vitamin wheat germ.

2. Prepare several breakfast menus. Divide the class into "Try Out" committees. Each committee will try out two or three menus, considering such things as ease of preparation, taste, cost, food values, and personal preferences (sixth grade). Further discussion might center around the factors involved in establishing personal preferences.

3. Study food dishes from other lands. Consider the nationalities represented by pupils in the classroom. Possibly an Italian dinner, Greek lunch, or Brazilian breakfast could actually be served in the school with or without parental assistance. In the dairy areas of. Brazil, for instance, a breakfast would consist of a hard roll (*pãozinho*), butter (*manteiga*), mineiro cheese (*queijo mineiro*), and warm milk flavored with coffee. A Chinese meal complete with chopsticks, plate, and spoon affords quite an experience. See *It's Always Breakfast Time Somewhere* (National Dairy Council) for suggestions and facts of particular interest to middle grade children.

4. Arrange a food tasting party. Several kinds of vegetables, fruits, and breads may be brought to class and arranged on paper plates in an appetizing manner by student committees. Experiences may be gained through this activity which in time may raise the "food likes" above "food dislikes." In one school the class elected

a monitor for the cafeteria to see if each pupil at least tasted their food. The monitors became so interested that they began spoon feeding those who had not tasted the food. This resulted in a number of pupils returning to their classrooms and saying such things as, "I didn't know I liked stewed tomatoes, but they are pretty good."

5. Request the local or county agent to visit the class to explain some of the problems of local agriculture and animal husbandry. Before he arrives, have the class prepare a list of questions that they would like to have him answer (fifth and sixth grades).

6. Request the state agricultural college or county agent to send some samples of various types of soil for actual use in the classroom. Fertilizing additives may be used to stimulate plant growth and to demonstrate why the farmer must employ crop rotation to insure the return of certain elements to the soil after a crop has been harvested. One New England school has for years demonstrated the necessity for proper fertilizers by having an experimental garden in the classroom. Seed quality may also be demonstrated this way.

7. Correlate such factors as rainfall, temperature, altitude, and frost dates with the food belts for corn, wheat, cotton, or dairy products.

8. Look over a simple diagram of the digestive and elimination tract. Answer questions on digestion, appetite, hunger, assimilation, and the elimination of waste. Most children enjoy talking about appetite — good and bad.

9. Investigate the "romance" of food. Milk in Holland is churned into butter. Lobsters in Maine are a state export item of considerable significance. Chile con carne from Mexico can be discussed first and tasted afterwards; Heinz, Libby, Campbell, and others pack it in cans. Massachusetts is the "land of the cod." Why? (A help-

ful booklet on the story of fresh fruits and vegetables may be obtained free from United Fresh Fruit and Vegetable Association.)

10. Secure several recordings of music and experiment with each while the class eats. How do marches compare with soft string music as a background for eating?

11. What is meant by a pleasant, cheerful atmosphere at meal time? Post the following poem just before lunch period.

When supper's almost ready
We rest a little while
And think of something funny
That will make the family smile.

12. Introduce the class to cranberries and cranberry juice — an excellent hot weather drink. Try it out in class and compare its vitamins and minerals with other fruits and vegetables. Information leaflets may be obtained from Ocean Spray Cranberries, Inc., Hanson, Mass. (fourth grade).

13. Conduct an animal feeding experiment with white rats, hamsters, or baby chicks.[10] This is especially good for a fourth grade class. Two 65-gram rats, weighed each Monday over an eight week period, may yield startling results. In an Indiana classroom one rat was fed the regular school luncheon diet and grew to 180 grams. The other rat was fed only hard candy, vanilla wafers, unenriched bread, jelly, and soft drinks; he wasted away to 55 grams. (For more on this see Chapter 9.)

14. Investigate food fads, dieting, and calories. Build calorie charts for

---

[10] Local National Dairy Council offices are generally able to meet requests for these experimental animals (free). See also *White Rat of Hawkins Halls*, a story of a white rat experiment, Evaporated Milk Association.

MY CALORIE RECORD

Day of Week_____

Calories Consumed

Breakfast
(list foods here)_____

Lunch
(list foods here)_____

Dinner
(list foods here)_____

Total calories for day_____

typical quantities of common foods. List foods consumed during previous day and calculate calorie intake. Excellent calorie lists which may be obtained in quantity free of charge are contained in the following booklets:

> *Breakfast Source Book.* Cereal Institute, Inc.
> *Nutrient Content of Various Food Products.* National Dairy Products Corporation, 605 Third Ave., New York, N.Y., 10016.

Compare differences within the class. Compare daily activities of the various pupils at home and at school, and relate to food intake.

15. Keep a record of the "Foods I Eat" at lunch over a period of one week. Study these in terms of the four basic food requirements. Especially useful are records already prepared for classroom use by the National Livestock and Meat Board. Also, the colorful *Good Health Record,* which can be kept for four weeks, is especially useful and is published (free) by the Kellogg Company.

16. Collect food superstitions and discuss these in terms of scientific knowledge.

17. Examine a grain of wheat—the wheat berry (see page 195).

18. Discuss the varieties of cheese. Make cottage cheese in class. Add a touch of onion or chives and serve in class on crackers. For excellent content information obtain *An ABC of Cheese* and *The World of Cheese* from

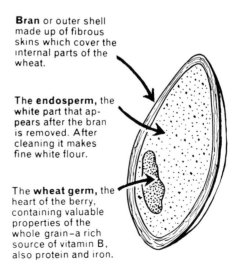

Bran or outer shell made up of fibrous skins which cover the internal parts of the wheat.

The endosperm, the white part that appears after the bran is removed. After cleaning it makes fine white flour.

The wheat germ, the heart of the berry, containing valuable properties of the whole grain—a rich source of vitamin B, also protein and iron.

Kraft Foods. Most children will be amused to discover that the ancient Greeks trained on cheese and dried fruits and that the Romans developed cheese-making into an art.

19. Calculate the cost per quart of dried, fresh, whole, and evaporated milk. To make this really worth while, taste each kind of milk. Taste buttermilk too.

20. Arrange a centerpiece of vegetables for a school party.

21. Cook dried fruit. Make a fruit salad. Make chopped vegetable sandwiches using dark bread. Serve in class following a discussion of the food values involved.

22. Take husks from oats and have the children roll them with a rolling pin to make rolled oats. Discuss how oats are rolled in the factory.

23. Conduct an experiment using chickens to show the need for green, leafy, or yellow vegetables. Give one chicken feed without vitamin A. Give the other the same diet, but add one of the many sources of vitamin A.

24. Construct and post on the bulletin board a diet for some special people: the Olympic athlete, the Arctic explorer, the astronaut.

25. Volunteer to stage a special school assembly program: "Food and Energy Around the World" with special costumes, props, music, dances, and narration.

26. Interview officials of the local health department regarding food protection practices.

27. Read and report about some of the harmful effects of overweight and underweight (sixth grade, independent study).

28. Under committee leadership, conduct an "experimental kitchen"; prepare and try out nutritious snacks, sandwich spreads, and drinks. Examples:

Hot Spiced Cider
Heat apple cider with lemon slices and lemon peel. Spice with cinnamon sticks, cloves, and allspice.

Party Treats
Wrap dates with bacon and broil. Drizzle heated yellow cheese over popcorn and stir until kernels are coated. Make balls of cream cheese and roll them in shredded coconut.

29. Ask the school nurse to explain red cell blood count. Have pupils study foods which provide iron and protein needed to maintain a normal red cell blood count (fifth grade).

30. Construct a mobile of the foods in an adequate breakfast. Prior to this, examine carefully the labels on breakfast cereal packages.

31. Try some food experiments. For ideas see Ethel Austin Martin, *Nutrition Education in Action*. New York: Holt, Rinehart, and Winston, 1966.

4. Dental Health

Desirable Outcomes (Primary Level)
To develop favorable attitudes toward caring for the mouth and teeth through habitually practicing good dental hygiene.

To acquaint children with the dental health teacher, the dentist, and dental equipment, thereby establishing a happy relationship and overcoming any fear of dental personnel.

To develop the necessary skills pertaining to proper and regular brushing of teeth and rinsing of the mouth after eating.

Desirable Outcomes (Intermediate Level)
To understand that dental health is a significant part of one's total health.

To know the structure of the tooth, that sweets may be harmful, that crooked teeth can be straightened, that selected foods are important, and that there are different kinds of teeth.

To understand the causes of toothache and the need for immediate treatment, that diseases in the body may be related to diseased teeth, that dentifrices need to be evaluated, and that sound teeth are an aid to personal attractiveness.

Comments

About 97 per cent of all the children in the United States are affected with dental caries. Moreover, a large number have broken front teeth. This accident most frequently occurs in the eight to 11 year age group and is particularly serious inasmuch as the treatment is very difficult.[11]

So much has been said about the teeth, and so many schoolchildren over the years have been "activated" to do something about their teeth, that it may seem there is little more to say. Possibly repetition is worth while, for the records continue to indicate that tens of thousands of children have poor teeth. Poverty, ignorance, and indifference have much to do with decay statistics, but there are also many examples of parents, who have adequate finances and are well edu-

cated, whose children's teeth are no better than those of the average schoolchild.

The makeup of a thorough dental program consists of dental information for the general public, including educational material for civic groups, a patient education program in the dentists' offices, and a dental health program for schools. These three means of improving dental health have a strong bearing on classroom activity. Every child who learns that the dentist is his friend and why he is becomes a walking dental health educator when he enters his home at the end of the school day. Parents often "move" under the pressure of their children's candid remarks. Procrastination and even indifference are sometimes put aside when the child urges his parents to take him to the dentist "because the teacher says so." Literature distributed in the schools in the afternoon sometimes finds its mark in the family kitchen or across the dinner table that evening.

[11] Lewis, Thompson M. "Current Dental Concepts," *Journal of School Health*, 32:324–327, October 1962.

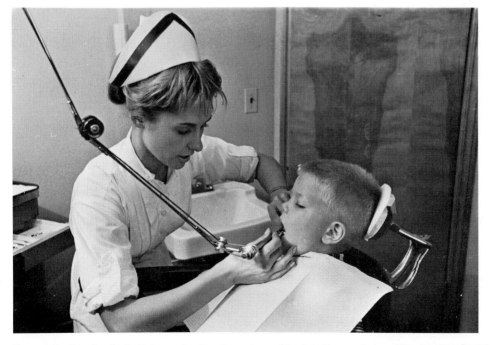

Figure 8–5   Cleaning the teeth is an educational experience. (Reprinted by permission of The American Dental Association.)

Most state health departments, as well as the American Dental Association and the numerous companies that make dentifrices, are very willing to make available for the teacher's use a variety of teaching aids, brochures, and suggested learning experiences. The majority of these are good when used in the right way. It must be remembered that some elementary schoolchildren have heard about tooth decay and have drawn pictures about teeth for several years. Yet tooth decay is present today as much as it ever was. One might ask what is wrong with the effort. For one thing, the effort has been a weak one. For another, when it has been made it has not been made *vital*. There has been too much talk and not enough action. Experiences have not been lifelike; the problem has not been brought home to the students or parents in a real and personal way. In short, much of the so-called dental health education has been like water running off the back of the proverbial duck. It simply has not been effective.

Children's experiences have to be challenging. Most children like a challenge. Taking advantage of this understanding of children, the teacher gets young Robert interested in tooth decay by telling him that many centuries ago the Chinese built a wall across the northern part of their country. This wall was built for defense, and so well was it built that it stands today. If there had been any weak parts in its structure, it would have long since crumbled. Man is still building defenses (name some) and he puts the best material available into his structural defenses. So the interest is developed in the fact that good food builds strong teeth. But this is only the beginning. The activities to follow must be so stimulating that something more than a recognition of facts takes place. Perhaps keeping a daily record of foods that help the teeth

grow strong and bright would be vital, especially if the pupil knows that he is trusted to keep his own record and that he alone can build his own defenses. This may inspire him to develop self-control in an attempt to build his body into a veritable Wall of China with no weak nutritional blocks in his makeup.

Suggested Activities

PRIMARY LEVEL

1. Ask the class to tell what they know about teeth. How the teeth chew food, how they help in talking, and how they look.

2. During story hour read an interesting story of adventure that deals with the teeth. One example would be *Little Red Sky*, the story of a real Indian boy who did as many observing boys and girls do — watched the squirrels cracking nuts with their teeth.[12]

3. Talk about toothbrushes. Are some better than others? Have a few samples of new and well worn brushes on hand to look over.[13] Discuss proper care of the brush.

4. Teach about teeth in an incidental way, especially when a child loses a baby tooth or has just returned from a trip to the dentist.

5. Bring animal and human teeth to class. The local meat market may have teeth and the local dentist will be happy to loan teeth. Bring a live cat and dog to class so that the teeth of pets may be seen. Or show pictures of the teeth of different animals.

6. Demonstrate and practice proper toothbrushing. Recent studies, reported by the American Dental Association, show that a total of one hour of instruction (in four sessions) usu-

---

[12] Distributed free by the makers of Arm and Hammer Baking Soda, Church and Dwight Co., 70 Pine St., New York, N.Y. 10005.

[13] For a primary grade story of toothbrushes, see C. B. Woofter, and Don E. Harley. *The Adventures of Toby Brite and Bobby*. Minneapolis: C. B. Donald Co. (free).

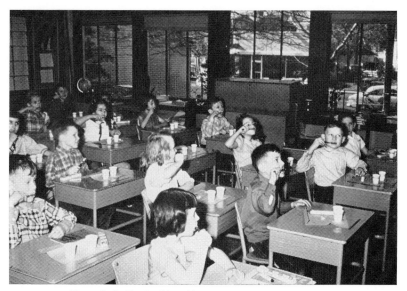

Figure 8–6 The toothbrushing drill—a pleasant experience.

ally is adequate. Drills may be executed by the whole group right in the classroom. This is easy when below-cost toothbrushing kits are available. The Procter and Gamble Company, Cincinnati, Ohio, 45201, supplies excellent classroom kits at a modest cost. They include dental floss and an hour-glass type timer. This program is provided for the third grade level only. A free publication with full instructions for a toothbrushing drill is available from the American Dental Association entitled, *You Can Teach Tooth-brushing.* The Division of Dental Hygiene, Ohio Department of Health, distributes (free) an excellent booklet, *School Toothbrushing Program.*

7. Discuss reasons for considering the dentist as a friend. Write the statements formulated by the class on the board. These may be copied later on a ditto sheet for each pupil to carry home. This may, on occasion, alert the parents to take their child to the dentist right away instead of waiting until there is toothache or other complaint. The heading for such a ditto sheet might read:

"Hello" says the friendly dentist.

"I like to help you take care of your teeth. Come to visit me."

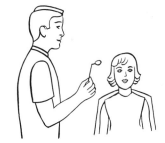

8. Have each child look into a well-lighted mirror to see if his mouth is clean and to see what the dentist did or can do for him.

9. Demonstrate decay in an apple. Start with two sound apples. Break the skin of one and place both on the window ledge for daily observation. After a few days observe what has occurred. Compare this to tooth decay when a "break" in the tooth occurs.

10. Use   mimetics   and   creative

rhythms. Mother Goose rhymes may be played to music with dental health folks substituted for other people. A song, a poem, an idea—even a happy tooth—suggests a movement for imaginative children. The words to the familiar *Farmer in the Dell* may be easily modified so that the farmer "takes a wife," "the wife takes a child," "the child takes a dentist," "the dentist takes the tooth," and "the tooth stands alone."

11. Use music. Sing about brushing and keeping the teeth clean. An excellent source of songs, complete with music and score, may be obtained free and in quantity from Proctor & Gamble: "Beware Take Care"—a catching story dealing with brushing, found in the booklet, *Tom Visits the Dentist*.

12. Mimeograph a chart such as the accompanying one on 8 inch × 11 inch paper: *(see below)*
Post the charts in class. Every time the pupil brushes his teeth—breakfast (B), lunch (L), or dinner (D)—he may color the proper square. He may use different colors (first grade).

13. Make clay models of the teeth, bring in pictures showing happy smiles, use films and exhibits; in short, do more than talk about teeth.

14. Have all classmembers take the "Tablet-test." Procter and Gamble distributes free two little tablets containing a harmless coloring agent. The pupils first brush their teeth the way

BRUSH UP ON YOUR BRUSHING

TAKE THIS ● TABLET-TEST ●

they always do. They then chew one tablet letting it dissolve in the mouth. They swish the solution around in the mouth, then rinse the mouth. When they look in a mirror the children will see red areas here and there indicating harmful, decay-producing deposits that were missed in brushing. Rebrushing, of course, will remove the stains. Also, along with the tablets, each pupil gets a set of seven rules with brushing instructions—drawings entitled, "Handy Guide to Good Toothbrushing" (third grade).

15. Plan a "Dental Health Week" program and invite the parents. Special attention may be focused on teeth through films, exhibits, posters, essays, and short, pupil-made plays.

16. Keep a daily record of toothbrushing in the home.

17. Plan a "Bunny Party"—fix and eat raw fruits and vegetables in class.

18. Build a "Health Train"—fill it with pictures of foods necessary for good dental health.

19. Encourage parents to supervise the brushing of teeth at home. Consider sending an information letter to the parents. See Figure 8-7.

Sunday	Monday	Tuesday	Wednesday
B			
L			
D			

SCHOOL DISTRICT OF CHELTENHAM TOWNSHIP
Elkins Park, Pennsylvania

March, 1968

Dear Mother and Dad:

When you and I were youngsters (back in the olden days, as
our children say), we and our parents accepted as fact that teeth
will inevitably decay. In recent decades, however, dental research has made great strides. We know now that most tooth decay
is caused by carbohydrates (starches and sweets), which are not
brushed from the teeth. The starchy foods are changed into a
sugar in the mouth, and within fifteen minutes the sugar (by
action of the mouth bacteria) is changed into acid. This acid,
unless the teeth are brushed after eating, is what causes most
cavities.

The children in our Cheltenham Township Public Schools are
being taught three important safeguards against dental caries
(tooth decay):

1. Brush right after eating.

   a. If you can't brush (after lunch, for instance),
      rinse your mouth or eat one of nature's tooth-
      brushes, such as raw, crisp apple, carrot or
      celery.

2. Try to get the raw vegetable and fruit snack habit.

   a. Watch the use of sweets and sodas and gum, etc.

3. Visit your dentist regularly.

If all of us work together - you in the home and we here at
school - perhaps we will hear more frequently the happy cry, "Hey,
look - no cavities!"

Sincerely,

Champy, the Cheltenham Good Health Cub
Margaret D. Johnson, Dental Hygienist
Robert R. Goodhart, D.D.S., School Dentist

Figure 8-7 Parents can help educate for health too.

INTERMEDIATE LEVEL

1. Examine the wall chart showing a sound tooth. Refer early to three factors associated with tooth decay: nutrition, brushing, and individual differences (hardness of teeth and hereditary strengths or weaknesses). This last factor is important. There will always be people, exceptional cases, who eat poorly and appear to have good teeth. Children see them and often draw erroneous conclusions. Thus these exceptions, together with other examples of variation need discussion in the classroom.

.2. Have a student committee visit a local dentist and report back to the class with their findings regarding tooth decay, extractions, dental tools, filling materials, and anesthetics.

3. Make tooth powder. Have the class members mix one part of salt to three parts of baking soda. Put a few drops of wintergreen extract into this to give it a pleasant smell. Let it dry, then try it out. Everyone may comment. Perhaps the group will want more wintergreen added to a new batch of powder, or another flavor may be desired.

4. Show pictures of crooked teeth, diseased teeth, and bright, clean, sound teeth. Learn the parts of the teeth. Investigate the functions of the joints and heart for the purpose of associating disease in these areas with infected teeth. Show how decayed teeth are bathed by the blood stream so that one's total efficiency may be reduced through poor teeth.

5. Teach dental health in connection with a study of foods and nutrition. Emphasize experiences dealing with bone building foods.

6. Formulate and record by way of tape recorder a list of reasons why teeth are important and how teeth should be cared for. Play back the tape and appraise it in terms of its effectiveness in changing habits. Encourage suggestions for shortening the recording and making it appealing.

Compare it to radio and television advertisements for dentifrices and foods.

7. Collect toothbrush and dentifrice advertisements; study the claims made. Gather information to determine whether the claims are reasonable and accurate.

8. Prepare, as a group, such snacks as apple slices, dried fruit, celery, carrot sticks, and nuts that can be eaten between meals. Talk about how satisfying they are to the appetite and the values of each kind of snack. Note how celery and carrot sticks help keep the teeth clean (fourth grade).

9. Have a dentist or dental hygienist come to class. Have a panel of students on hand to ask questions. From such an interview the class should find that the dentist does at least the following important things: he makes a complete health inventory and dental history; he cleans and scales the teeth; he x-rays every tooth, locating the cavities no matter how small; he detects abnormal conditions of the gums or mouth; and he gives a full explanation of his treatment plan, number of visits, and proposed fees.

10. Stress the relationship of good grooming, appearance, and pleasant breath to success both in school and in the community. For upper grade pupils this approach may hold more interest and shape more attitudes than the approach through foods, disease, and body physiology.

11. Hang the Norman Rockwell poster, "Look, Mom — No Cavities!" where all can see it. This is published and distributed free by Procter and Gamble Co. This is a superb picture of a freckled face girl holding up a dental slip from her school. It reads "Teeth in excellent condition. *No new cavities* since last examination."

12. Using small pocket mirrors, one for each row of pupils, have each child look at his own teeth and try to answer the questions, "How do our teeth work?" "What work do the different

shaped teeth do?" "Do my teeth meet evenly when I close my mouth?"

13. Make wax impressions of the teeth. Using household preserving wax, 2 inches × 2 inches and ¼ inch thick (molds may be made in class to this size from heavy aluminum foil). For further hints on this project secure a copy of the free booklet, *The Way to Smile* from Procter and Gamble Co.

14. Find out how much sugar is in many of the popular foods. There is more than a casual relationship between excessive sugar consumption and dental decay. Most children hear about this at an early age, but they do little about it because of other more impressive factors. Discuss these other factors; the pupils will know what they are.

There is a substantial amount of sugar in most popular foods. For example:

		sugar
Coca-Cola	6 oz. bottle	4⅓ tsp.
root beer	10 oz. bottle	4½ tsp.
candy bar	1–5 oz.	5–10 tsp.
angel food cake	4 oz. piece	7 tsp.
ice cream sundae	1	7 tsp.
cherry pie	1 slice	10 tsp.

15. Make and display a diorama of a dentist's office. Use pipecleaner figures.

16. Post this sign at the front of the classroom:

> PAUL REVERE MADE FALSE TEETH FOR GEORGE WASHINGTON AND ADVERTISED HIS PRACTICE IN THE *BOSTON GAZETTE* IN 1786! WHAT ELSE CAN YOU FIND ABOUT THE EARLY PRACTICE OF DENTISTRY?

(See the book by Esther Forbes, *Paul Revere and the World He Lived In.* Boston: Houghton-Mifflin Co.)

17. Include dental words in spelling lessons. Fourth and fifth grade pupils should be able to spell words such as:

erupt	enamel	fluoride
cuspid	pulp	abscess
bicuspid	decay	malocclusion
calcium	tartar	orthodontist
molar	bacteria	
permanent	Novocain	

18. Do not overlook the opportunity to point out that water fluoridation is a classic example of the public health approach to dental disease control (sixth grade). Over three decades of brilliant research have shown that the community may reduce the dental caries attack by over 60 per cent by fluoridating the water supply.

19. Distribute a 10-inch piece of dental floss to each pupil. Have class practice using the floss to clean the

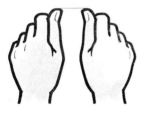

For upper teeth

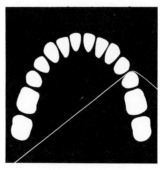

MOVE FLOSS GENTLY BACK AND FORTH BETWEEN TEETH

(Courtesy of Johnson & Johnson leaflet: *How to Use Dental Floss.*)

area between the teeth. A leaflet suitable for grade four or above may be obtained (free) from Johnson & Johnson. It is entitled *How to Use Dental Floss.*

5. Body Structure and Operation

Desirable Outcomes (Primary Level)

To develop an understanding of the structure of the body as a basis for healthful living; to have a simple understanding and appreciation of how the various systems of the body work together.

To develop an appreciation of the relationship between good health and personality; good health and appearance.

To encourage optimum posture in sitting, standing, and walking.

Desirable Outcomes (Intermediate Level)

To understand the functions of the organs and systems of the body; to know that sound structure is a prerequisite to proper functioning.

To have an understanding of how exercise and recreation tends to relax tensions caused by strong emotions and overambitious living; to know that the nerves, muscles, and glands of internal secretion work together.

To develop an appreciation for the process of normal growth.

To understand some relationships between posture and disease and defects.

To acquire and use understandable scientific terms concerning the human body and its functions.

To develop an increased understanding of the special senses, and to acquire proper habits of care and respect for the eyes, ears, nose, and mouth.

Comments

According to Abraham Maslow, one of the characteristics of a healthy,

self-actualizing person (his term for maturity reaching toward the fulfillment of the individual) is that he has an understanding and appreciation of his body which lead to less actual body consciousness and greater use of the body *as an extension of his whole personality.*[14] If this is true, then educators for years have been missing an opportunity to influence human effectiveness through a study of the physical self.

A study of the body structure and its function is a fundamental one. It is a biological topic that should be carried on as soon as the class is ready for it.

Primary graders require very little reference to body function. Short general answers to questions of "why" usually suffice, but the upper grade pupils very often want a detailed reason. This is the time to bring in elementary anatomy and physiology — not in a cut and dried approach, but with familiar examples and choice references to personal well-being and appearance. In fact, in many cases boys and girls are impressed more with how they look to others and feel on special occasions than they are with the circulation of blood or the physiology behind good sight and hearing.

Children of all ages tend to be interested in their posture and their general body mechanics if the topic is presented in terms of personal growth and well-being. Measuring growth in the classroom by checking height against the wall and weight on the scales seldom fails to ferret out a number of excellent questions, especially in grades one to three. Here the teacher has an opportunity to demonstrate good standing posture, to discuss ligaments, tendons, and muscles that maintain this posture, and to relate this function to sound nutrition, adequate sleep, and freedom

---

[14] Maslow, Abraham. *Motivation and Personality.* New York: Harper and Row, 1960, p. 196.

from disease organisms. It may readily be shown that poor eating and fatigue cause many things, that postural attitudes tell much about a person's mental health and self-respect.

Upper grade children will be especially fascinated by a study of how the foot works, the nature of the longitudinal and metatarsal arches, why the policeman is called a "flatfoot," why sneakers are not advisable for use on hard pavements, the benefits of good shoes and foot exercises, why top rate athletes practice proper foot hygiene, and how overweight can cause pain in the feet. Of course, merely lecturing to a class about the position of the feet in walking or how they should stand or sit will not in itself change the body mechanics of many children. In fact, talking is not enough. In every class one finds a child whose poor posture represents a kind of rebellion against nagging parents and teachers who have overpreached on this topic. Postural changes are brought about when children hear, see, and *feel* what optimum posture is. Bring a mirror to class. Have boys and girls take a side view look at themselves. Have them back up against a flat wall and with their hand feel how much space there is between the hollow of the back and the wall. Let them "stand tall" and walk away from the wall to the mirror so that they can reinforce the way they feel with what they *see*. The same thing may be done with a plumb line dropped from the classroom ceiling, or a straight window pole. That is, have a pupil put his shoulder against the hanging plumb line or vertical window pole and see if he is on a straight line "between heaven and earth." If he is, the line will fall through the tip of the ear, the center of the shoulder, the hip joint, the knee, and through the outside ankle bone. Once this is checked on one person, half the class will want to try. Posture education can be very

interesting if the teacher supplies a number of practical experiments.

It is important to note that when postural defects are discovered early in the grades, there is a much better chance of doing something about them. Defects that are permitted to continue, due to indifference and ignorance, tend to get worse. It is increasingly true that in many cases postural abnormalities are symptomatic of some other disease, defect, or disturbance. For example, immediate postural exercises for round shoulders may be the wrong thing, for the condition might be due to chronic fatigue or malnutrition. This should be corrected first so that the energy will be available for remedial exercises later on. In the case of the tall girl who is seen stooping a bit while talking with a number of friends, it may be that her defect is due strictly to an intense desire to "keep up with the Joneses" by lowering the body to the level of her shorter friends. Such an illustration is rich in instructional ideas. Tall children should know that many a tall person has a kind of upright bearing and grace in movement that is the envy of others.

Included in this particular topic of structure and function is the care of the special senses. Primary grade children need to discuss in detail how to protect their eyes and ears. They should understand the relationship of light and glare to seeing and eye comfort, and they should know how eyeglasses work and how to watch television. Intermediate classes should have a simple understanding of how the eyes and ears work as well as how to take proper care of them. Fifth and sixth graders almost always show interest in a large size model of the eyeball or ear, especially if the parts as shown are immediately related to abnormalities shared by members of the class. For example, nearsightedness (myopia) or farsightedness (hyperopia) are readily explained. A simple eyeball sketch on the blackboard showing a convex or concave lens which is used to correct the particular difficulty will be effective. This is especially true if it is used with actual eyeglasses which the children are permitted to examine. The flexibility of an eyeball can be demonstrated by noting the properties of a hard boiled egg. A Snellen Test chart, employed to measure simple visual acuity or accommodation, can be used in the classroom both as a screening instrument and a teaching device. Some reference should be made, when the special senses are being investigated, to the relationship between safe driving and optimum seeing and hearing. Good eyesight has much to do with per-

sonal safety—riding bicycles, crossing streets, and reading roadside signs and markers. The question of how blind and deaf boys and girls behave and how they feel is one that provokes discussion. If possible, this topic should be dramatized by a visitor to the classroom, a special story, or a trip to insure that the care of the special senses will be of vital concern.

The body structure and its operation simply cannot be taught in terms of systems, processes, and mechanics to elementary school children. It has to be taught quite personally with pertinent questions being answered as they are raised by the class. Good teaching motivates the questions the teacher knows to be important. Most children want to know sooner or later

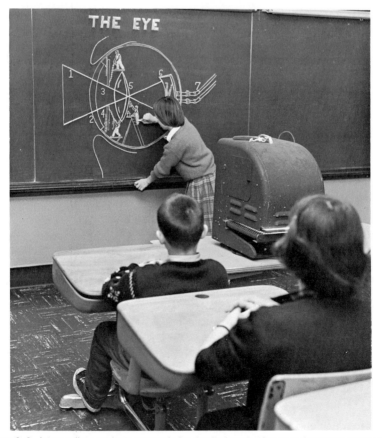

Figure 8–8 Intermediate students are ready for detailed work. (Courtesy Cincinnati Public Schools.)

what they look like with the skin off and why their bodies function as they do. They want to know how the heart beats and what it sounds like, why they perspire in summer, how the arms move, and a hundred other such practical questions. Without the teacher's moralizing, the class can be shown that the body, in the words of the poet, is the "temple of the soul" and the "organ of the will." It is, by simple statement, an amazing machine with intricacies so numerous that man has not yet figured out all of its actions. Finally, and this is significant, children will not treat the body as a fine instrument until they learn to appreciate it for what it is. Every learning activity provides an opportunity for the development of appreciations, but it takes careful planning to select those activities and experiences that will develop the most appreciations.

Suggested Activities
PRIMARY LEVEL

1. Post baby photographs around the classroom. A set that shows development through the years is most valuable. Pictures of babies, children, and young people may be cut from magazines and brought to class by the pupils. These can be graduated in such a way as to depict the story of a steady growth.

2. Bring pictures of machines to class and discuss similarity to body functions. Feel arm and finger bones and shoulder and hip joints and see how they move. Choose a pupil to bend, twist, and straighten his backbone to show that the spine is made up of many little bones (second grade).

3. Measure each child for height and weight at intervals. Tie this activity in with body growth. Refer to the growth of the hair, fingernails, and toenails. An excellent "How Tall" wall chart for measuring height is put out by the Travelers Insurance Co., Hartford, Connecticut (free). It is hung on a

wall or door, 2½ feet above the floor. The names of the children may be written in at the head of the height column. Each time a measurement is made, add the date near the height mark. Seven charts will service a class of 28 pupils.

4. Using this growth measuring activity show the relationship of height to standing posture, stress standing tall without affecting a braced type of posture. Illustrate this by dropping a string plumb line from the ceiling of the classroom. The line should run approximately through the tip of the ear, the center of the shoulder, the hip joint, the knees, and the outside ankle bone. Let each class member try this. (A window pole held vertically may be substituted for the plumb line.)

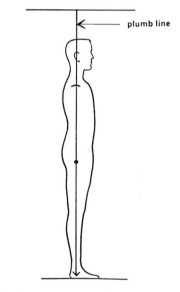

5. Play a game of posture relay. The object of the relay race is to walk fast to the other end of the classroom while balancing a blackboard eraser on the head. Show the class that this calls for straight posture.

6. Discuss sitting, writing, reading, and sleeping postures. Have the class dramatize various examples of good and poor posture. This keeps the situation humorous but serious enough to foster appreciation.

7. Emphasize good posture occasionally throughout the day while the students are reading, writing, or engaging in other class activities. Look for the tall child who stoops a little to "reach down" to his or her friends. Call attention to proper standing posture while singing.

8. Listen to the beat of a heart. A stethoscope may be borrowed from the health service department so that each child can hear a heart beat. This is a good project to engage in just before visiting the school physician for a medical examination.

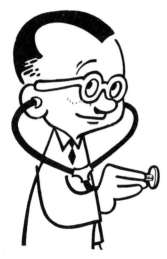

9. Compare the ears with an ordinary telephone receiver. A simple demonstration can be made with an upright telephone. This may be borrowed from a secondary school science department or the local telephone company office. First graders will be amused; third graders will want to see the telephone taken apart.

10. Identify objects by taste, odor, or sound while blindfolded. This can be carried out after the initial demonstration by making a game out of it. In a class of 28 children, four teams of seven children each may, for example, listen to a particular sound. The first child in each group guesses first. The first to give the correct answer scores a point for his team. He then moves to the end of the line. The game continues with different sensory items being introduced. This game motivates the class to want to talk about their smell, taste, and hearing and how these items work with the big sense of sight. Material to have on hand for this game might include a piece of chocolate, a spoiled orange, sour milk, or a musical record.

11. Use bellows to demonstrate breathing. Compare a sponge to the lung structure. Look at an x-ray picture of a pair of normal lungs (third grade). A school physician or local health department will usually be able to supply a no longer needed negative for classroom use and storage. Have pupils breathe in deeply, holding their hands on their sides to feel the ribs.

12. Talk about reading books which are printed in a type which is easy to read and sitting in a comfortable position while reading in order not to get tired. Examine some fine print with a reading glass or ordinary magnifying glass.

13. Appoint children to adjust the window shades and artificial lighting in the room to keep out glare and the kind of light that will fatigue or injure eyes.

14. Check sight in class by using the Snellen chart. Use it more as an object lesson than a screening device. Have children talk about their own seeing problems and what they should consider doing to correct the difficulty.

15. Measure hearing by the whisper test. Check one or two pupils at a time by quietly whispering a series of four numbers (e.g., five, six, seven, eight). Although this is a crude measure, it does serve as an object lesson in hearing to stimulate interest in the topic.

16. Let the class hear high and low vibrations to show that certain sounds are more readily heard and recognized. Use whistles, pipes, or a flute to compare with the sound of a tuba, cello string, or low note on a saxophone. One of the many records on the indi-

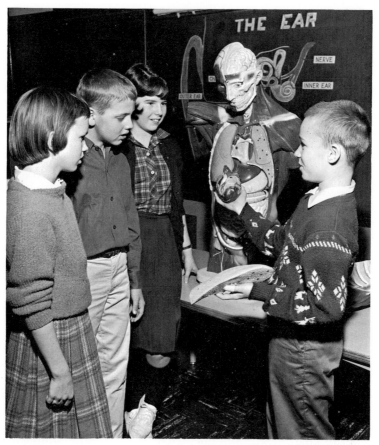

Figure 8–9 Studying the special senses. (Courtesy Cincinnati Public Schools.)

vidual instruments of the orchestra may prove helpful here.

17. Teach special senses safety. Point out that only a clean handkerchief should be used near the eyes, that one should refrain from pointing objects such as scissors, pencils, or sticks at anyone, that nothing should be put in the ear.

18. Show why it is necessary to play carefully so that the ears and eyes will not be injured. Point out that running while carrying sharp objects or glass is not a good practice. Warn pupils about shouting into ears. Make pictures of objects that may injure the eyes and ears, such as pencils, scissors, paper clips, snowballs, BB guns, slingshots, or rubber bands. Have children talk about their pictures to the class.

19. Dramatize blowing the nose properly and the need for remaining at home at the first sign of a cold.

20. Discuss ways of protecting the ears when diving and swimming or against frostbite during the winter.

21. Find out what to do in case of earaches.

22. Discuss the hearing sensitivity of various animal pets. Compare these to the human ear and its function to give us the enjoyment of music, conversation, radio, and television.

23. Make a list of pleasant sounds and unpleasant sounds. Relate these sounds to richness in living.

INTERMEDIATE LEVEL

1. Discuss growth. Of what does it consist? Look over body diagrams or

wall charts (Dennoyer-Gebhart wall charts of body systems are available in many schools). Refer briefly to the relationship of the various areas of the body, i.e., circulation to respiration, digestion to elimination. This should be brief and merely introductory in nature.

2. Make a bulletin board display showing three levels of growth: the first grader, the fifth grader, and the ninth grader. Together with the class fill in the appearances and skills usually seen at each level of growth. This may cause much thought and reflection by the pupils as they think in terms of older and younger people of their acquaintance (fourth and fifth grade project).

3. Listen to the heartbeat with a stethoscope. Study a simple diagram of the heart. Have one pupil jump up and down for 30 seconds. Then notice the increased heart action by listening again with the stethoscope. Notice also the increase in breathing. Show how the lungs perform the function of securing oxygen for the blood.

4. Locate and feel the pulse beat; relate this to the heart beat. Point out that other arteries near the surface of the body may serve as a pulse. Note the notch along the side of the chin, the artery under the upper arm, in the groin, and near the ear on the side of the head. Check these pressure points and indicate briefly how severe bleeding may be controlled by causing pressure over these points.

5. Post an open road map on the wall alongside a diagram of the body showing the road or path followed by the blood stream. Point out such items as:

a. Blood, bathing an infected tooth area, can carry germs to the lining of the heart, to another organ, or to a joint.

b. The force and rate of the heart beat has a bearing on the efficiency of the system.

c. Vigorous physical exercise calls for more oxygenated blood to be supplied to the muscles.

d. An effective brain depends as much on the blood and oxygen supply as on the muscles.

6. Show the effect of fatigue, food, rest, disease, emotions, and exercise on the pulse beat. Let the class add to this by telling their experiences. Answer the "why" questions in terms of elementary physiology.

7. Illustrate, through experiment, the relationship of physical fitness (strength and endurance) to heart efficiency. Set up a simple exercise test which is related to the rise and fall of the pulse rate.

8. Discuss the relationship of body posture to body function. Let the class point out that poor nutrition, inadequate sight or hearing, and personal feelings have a bearing on posture. Look over the "Let's See" series from the *Instructor Kit* on the human body.

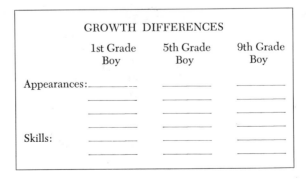

GROWTH DIFFERENCES

	1st Grade Boy	5th Grade Boy	9th Grade Boy
Appearances:	_____	_____	_____
	_____	_____	_____
	_____	_____	_____
Skills:	_____	_____	_____
	_____	_____	_____

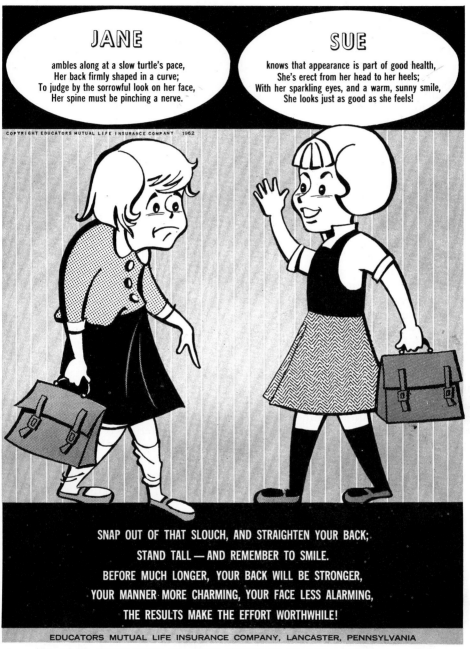

Figure 8–10 Posture posters are effective. (Courtesy Educators Mutual Life Insurance Co.)

Available from F. A. Owens Publishing Co., Dansville, N.Y.

9. Illustrate the connection between poor standing and sitting posture and general fatigue. Have two pupils stand at the front of the classroom with their left arms extended horizontally to the side. Continue with the lesson, and about five minutes later ask the two pupils where they are tired. They will mention the extended arm together with the opposite side of the body. Point out that they have expended considerable energy while in "poor posture" by trying to keep from falling away from the line of gravity. Illustrate this further by using kindergarten building blocks.

Show that there is less strain in the building block molecules when they come close to approximating the line of gravity B than there is in figure C, and that there is more stress and strain in the materials of the blocks in C. This is similar to the stress and strain in boy A who is attempting to stay on the gravitational or "fall" line. Then have several pupils walk across the classroom, illustrating a number of pronounced postural defects such as a head forward position, rounded shoulders, a high shoulder, and a hollow back curve. Relate these conditions to A and C and fatigue.

10. Discuss the mechanics of walking, sitting, and sleeping. Show the relationship of poor sleeping posture, mattresses, and beds to chronic fatigue and irritability. Further discuss the social benefits of correct posture. Practice sitting down and getting up from a chair. Demonstrate the proper way of moving a chair to seat a girl or lady.

11. Display some animal bones, which may be obtained from a meat market. Show longitudinal and cross sections.

12. Set up a long vertical mirror so children may check their own posture from the front and side views.

13. Organize a posture contest. This might resolve itself into a full elementary school assembly program. Some preparation should precede this event. Fourth, fifth, and sixth grade posture contest entrants may be checked at each of seven stations:

    a. Sitting (at a desk)
    b. Walking (across the platform)
    c. Exercises (for coordination and flexibility)
    d. Posture screen (by school nurse)
    e. Plumb line test
    f. Foot and leg alignment (by the nurse)
    g. Roaming judgment (by a judge who judges posture at all times in between the stations)

Score on the basis of 70 points for a perfect score. Many good activities and experiences may be derived from such a contest.

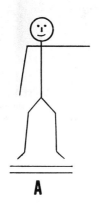

A

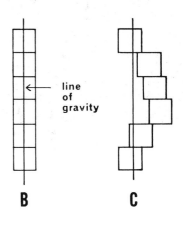

line of gravity

B   **C**

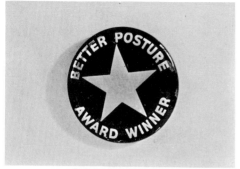

Posture Award Button

14. Talk about good foot health. Secure an animal's foot or the bones of a leg and foot from the local meat market. Show a cow's knee joint. Have a leg and foot of a chicken on hand to show how muscles and ligaments are associated in the human foot. Explain the longitudinal and metatarsal arches and the relationship of their functional efficiency to gait, shoes, and posture.

15. Measure a footprint angle with the protractor (fifth grade activity). Supply each child with a piece of brown paper, a ruler, pencil, and protractor. Have each child step on a damp towel and then stand on the brown paper. Do the same for each foot. Before the paper dries, draw lines A–B and C–D. Measure the angle formed by these lines:

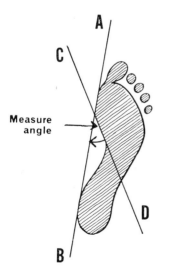

This is a project that will promote all kinds of foot questions. What is a good arch? What is a flat foot? Why should policemen sometimes do foot exercises while standing on the corner? Are sneakers and moccasins harmful to the feet? How should the heels wear down on the shoes? How should we walk? Is pigeon-toed walking harmful or helpful?

16. Make a large, simple diagram or picture that shows the component parts of the human eye. Compare the eye to a camera. Discuss the rods and cones of the retina and their relationship to good nutrition, disease, and body poisons. The eye of a sheep is especially useful for classroom use.

17. Smear a drop of blood on a glass slide and examine it through a microscope to observe the structure and arrangement of blood cells.

18. Collect and display pictures that depict people from all walks of life taking part in various work and play activities in which good eyesight, good hearing, and a fine sense of balance are necessary. Supplement the display with pictures that show how certain handicaps and inadequacies can be compensated for by the use of such devices as braces, hearing aids, artificial limbs, and eyeglasses.

19. Tell stories to illustrate how the emotions affect the body. Show how stress items such as fear, anger, jealousy, hate, and worry increase the pulse rate and make people tense. Read a particularly exciting and suspense-filled story or show a movie along these lines. Stop the class at the critical moment to have them notice their heart and respiration rates.

20. Try introducing the topic of eyesight in a startling way:

DO YOU KNOW
That there are more blind people in the city of Calcutta than in the whole of Canada!

```
┌─────────────────────────────────────────────────┐
│           HOW LARGE IS THE HEART ?              │
│                                                 │
│   BOY'S HEART        =    A FIST                │
│   RABBIT'S HEART     =    AN EGG                │
│   DOG'S HEART        =    A TENNIS BALL         │
│   GIRAFFE'S HEART    =    A BASKETBALL          │
└─────────────────────────────────────────────────┘
```

21. Tell the story of Thomas Edison and his hearing problem.

22. Introduce the subject of the heart with a large drawing of a giraffe standing next to a basketball. Have the class try guessing the heart size of a giraffe.

23. Demonstrate the use of an audiometer by the nurse.

24. Draw and label parts of the respiratory system. Follow this with demonstration of how mouth-to-mouth breathing is administered to a person in need of artificial respiration. Leaflets for class distribution are available from Johnson & Johnson (free).

6. Prevention and Control of Disease

Desirable Outcomes (Primary Level)

To understand the necessity for proper healthful practices concerning himself and others. To develop favorable attitudes toward the school physician and nurse and their equipment, thereby overcoming any fear of medical personnel.

To develop an appreciation for people engaged in protecting one's personal health and the health of the community.

To acquire habits which will protect the individual and others from common diseases and illnesses.

Desirable Outcomes (Intermediate Level)

To understand the specific role of germs in disease, that some are harmful, others are harmless, and some are helpful.

To know how germs may be spread, and their relationship to common communicable diseases.

To understand how the body defenses react to disease, and that scientists are laboring to obtain more information about disease.

To acquire habits of staying home when ill, of keeping immunizations up to date, of covering coughs and sneezes, of keeping appointments with physicians and dentists, of practicing cleanliness in the preparation, serving, and storage of food.

To appreciate the disease prevention value of professional health workers in the community.

To understand and accept the personal responsibility for promoting school and community health.

Comments

Disease prevention and control has more than a slight bearing on the lives of schoolchildren of all ages. Illustrations of this are everywhere, and disease experiences come to every pupil. This fact should do at least one thing for the teacher; it should contribute significantly to the pupil interest level.

Teaching the concept that germs cause disease and that disease can be prevented through the control of germs may seem like uphill work in the elementary grades. Yet children have been successfully taught that micro-organisms are everywhere and can be controlled. But because they are not completely controlled, they cause such things as upper respiratory infections sometimes leading to hearing impairment, pneumonia, colds, and stomach and intestinal upsets. "Strep" germs alone can cause sore throats, tooth decay, and heart damage. Today, some of these germs can "come alive" in the classroom through the use of special slides, films, filmstrips, overhead transparencies and powerful microscopes.

An especially effective film, entitled *Spot Prevention* (color, sound, 13½ minutes), designed to show the chase and capture of the measles "germ," is available for showing to children in kindergarten through second grade. It is distributed by the U.S. Public Health Service, Audiovisual Facility, Atlanta, Georgia 30333.

As far as the primary grade children are concerned, the prevention and control of disease might well come under the area of personal cleanliness and appearance. Certainly disease control is related to one's personal habits of cleanliness. Children in the first three grades are quite capable of understanding this, especially if the subject is treated lightly and tied in directly with such routine health practices as covering the mouth when coughing, washing the hands before eating and after going to the bathroom, drinking properly from the drinking fountain, keeping away from others when ill, and staying at home when ill.

During the primary grades the teacher is especially concerned with day-to-day signs and symptoms of infectious diseases and defects. She is alert to note deviations from normal health and performance. She has an excellent opportunity to make clear to her pupils that they should remain at home when ill, and not place too great a premium on perfect attendance. Third grade pupils, for example, may be interested in preparing a note to

their parents encouraging them to make careful observation of their children before sending them to school. Third graders are also interested in the first stages of the common communicable diseases such as measles and chickenpox, immunization and vaccination, and simple first aid procedures. Upper graders, of course, may want to talk about specific immunization for whooping cough, tetanus, typhoid, and diphtheria, and smallpox vaccinations (see Chapter 5).

Health teaching in the primary grades deals principally with helping children develop practices which will protect them and others from common diseases and from most illnesses. The kindergarten child or first grader may find the school an entirely new environment, one which presents new problems and new learning opportunities in health in relation to other people. At home a family hand towel may hang near the kitchen sink, while at school such a practice would not be permitted. Occasionally a child is not completely happy or at ease in the classroom and may develop such habits as rubbing the eyes, sucking the thumb or fingers, or chewing on pencils. There is always the chance that disease may be spread by bringing the objects or fingers in contact with someone else. Such occurrences in the classroom provide the opportunity for teaching proper health practices. It is not necessary that young children know in detail why these behaviors are harmful, but they do need to learn and appreciate that they are undesirable.

As one grows older and must accept additional responsibility, the topic of disease control and its prevention takes on greater meaning. At the intermediate level it offers discussion possibilities greater than the topic of cleanliness and personal appearance. An effort is now made to use scientific knowledge and give decisive answers to "why" certain practices are helpful or harmful. Children show interest in scientific materials. The mystery surrounding bacteria, and why some kinds are difficult to see even with powerful microscopes, and such questions as whether or not bacteria are useful arouse much comment. Experiences dealing with the wonders of natural and man-made objects are almost always worthwhile health activities.

It would almost be a mistake to miss an opportunity to present real case studies to a fifth or sixth grade class. Two case studies, such as the following, could be used to initiate a unit and provide immediate kindling of interest and discussion:[15]

CASE 1 – Seventeen persons aboard a ship became ill within 8 hours after eating a noon meal. Nausea, vomiting, cramps, and diarrhea were the symptoms. Macaroni had been cooked prior to the meal, and chopped pimentos, lettuce, boiled eggs, mayonnaise, and mustard were hand-mixed by two mess cooks. One of those cooks had several minor cuts on two fingers. These finger cuts yielded Staphylococcus aureus, the same kind of bacteria found in the salad.
PREVENTION. – Never use your hands to mix foods when clean sanitized utensils can be used! Never work with food when you have infected cuts because the germs causing the infection may be a source of foodborne illness!
CASE 2 – One hundred and fifty-five persons became ill with severe diarrhea and stomach pains. The suspect meal, roast beef and gravy, had been eaten by 170 persons. This beef and gravy had been prepared the day before and allowed to cool in open trays without refrigeration for 22 hours. Clostridium perfringens organisms were found in the beef and gravy.
PREVENTION. – Potentially hazardous (readily perishable) foods should be thoroughly cooked and then either

kept hot (140° F. or above), or cold (refrigerated to 45° F. or below) until serving.

When upper elementary grade schoolchildren review the long and stimulating record of medicine and hygiene practices, there is a good opportunity to impress them with the historical emphasis on disease prevention and control. The control efforts came first, for people were plagued with sicknesses. Even today, in countries like Egypt, some 80 per cent of the population is disease-ridden. Problems of control are of first importance, followed quickly by prevention techniques. The first project is to save the life of the afflicted, then set out to prevent the disease in others. It is suggested, therefore, that intermediate graders take a look back through the pages of history and see what has gone on in the past. Superstitions, magic, and witchcraft in primitive society, the worship of special gods during the early days of Egypt, Greece, and Rome, and the slow transition from alchemy and astrology to the science of chemistry and astronomy are items that challenge the imagination of eager fourth, fifth, and sixth grade pupils. This becomes even more stimulating when present day superstitions, quackery, misconceptions, and ignorance are compared with a period two thousand years ago. In fact, most children would be amazed to know that the Roman aqueduct water system was superior to many of the homemade devices in our land today, and that disease control through sanitation, isolation, and quarantine was better in ancient Hebrew civilizations than it is in the backlands of the United States and in the greater part of the world today.

Suggested Activities
PRIMARY LEVEL
1. Consider germs from a general point of view. Ask if all germs are harmful. Talk about helpful little

---

[15] From You Can Prevent Foodborne Illness. U.S. Public Health Service, Publication No. 1105, Washington, D.C. 20201.

germs that give cheese its wonderful flavor. If possible, emphasize this point by giving each child a little cube of milk cheese to eat on a small cracker. Talk about the yeast that makes bread rise and the germs helpful in turning apple juice into vinegar. Ask how many children have tasted apple cider. Follow this discussion with some information on harmful germs that make canned fruit spoil and milk and cream turn sour. Continue by relating germs to disease — the common cold and sore throat.

2. Ask someone to tell the class what measles, chickenpox, or some other common communicable disease is like. Why do people feel sick when they have a disease? What are some of the ways to keep germs away from the body? Emphasize cleanliness, injections by the doctor, vaccinations, good food, rest, and sleep.

3. Post on the board an enlarged picture of the common housefly. Discuss other disease-carrying insects and rodents. West of Colorado, rats, squirrels, and rabbits spread more disease germs than in the East. Examine a fly under a magnifying glass. Note the hairs. Discuss how flies spread disease.

4. Build a simple exhibit of items about the house that help people control disease germs. A number of items, including a garbage can, a trash basket, a refrigerator, a clean toilet bowl, a bath tub, or a garden hose, may be made from cardboard (third grade).

5. For one week keep a record of the people who have been absent, taking notice of the reasons people are not in school. Emphasize improved health, not improved attendance.

6. Call attention occasionally to an opened box of clean paper tissues on the corner of a classroom table.

7. Stress personal cleanliness and its relationship to the transmission of diseases. Call attention as often as needed to the manner in which germs travel between boys and girls:

    a. By coughing and sneezing

    b. By dirty hands and fingers of one person touching those of another

    c. By picking up and eating food that has fallen on the floor or sidewalk

    d. By failing to refuse food that has been bitten into by another person

    e. By sharing individual cups, glasses, and straws

    f. By coming to school with a bad cold

8. Call on a cub scout to describe his part in a cleanliness campaign.

9. Have the class find how the early American settlers kept clean in such settlements as Jamestown or Plymouth.

10. Make a list of all the housekeeping chores engaged in by the mother or maid to help keep the home clean. Then have each pupil choose a chore and illustrate it in mimetic form, or the chores may be selected by the class members as a topic for a drawing.

11. Engage in pupil-teacher planning of ways to keep the school washroom clean.

12. Demonstrate how to use the soap dispenser and towels.

13. Build a model hospital on a small classroom table. Dress several dolls as the doctor, nurse, and patient. Have a garage where a toy ambulance is ready and waiting. A total class project can be planned by having the children, voluntarily or by assignment, secure the necessary items.

14. Keep a record of the classroom temperature. Learn to read the thermometer and know the optimum room temperature.

15. Talk over the danger of swimming in crowded pools, dirty water, and polluted streams.

16. View the colored movie film, *How to Catch a Cold*. It may be obtained on a free loan basis from Kimberly-Clark Corporation (Kleenex) or Associated Films, Inc. Following the movie discuss the 2000 year old problem, the common cold.

17. Hang an attractive sign from the

ceiling which may readily be seen by all pupils:

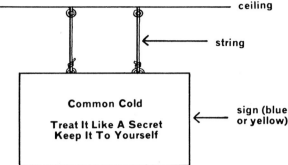

Point out that colds are related not only to cleanliness, but also to getting overtired, wet, or chilled, balanced diets, sleep and rest, and fresh air and exercise.

18. Hold a clinical thermometer up for all pupils to see. Ask questions. Do you have a thermometer at home? Is it an oral or rectal thermometer? What does it tell? Should we encourage our parents to get a thermometer if they do not already have one?

19. Ask how many children have screens on doors and windows at home. How many pupils have flies and mosquitoes in the home? How may they be eliminated besides having effective screening?

20. Ask the question, "How fresh is fresh?" Is there any difference in the food value of canned, fresh, or frozen fruits and vegetables? Point out that because of modern refrigeration and transportation, fresh fruits and vegetables are not superior in food value to commercially canned and frozen foods; it is all a matter of preference and taste. Food values will be lost if the homemaker overcooks these fruits and vegetables.

21. Discuss how dishwashing affects the family health. The commonplace food utensil is a potential carrier of many infectious diseases. Discuss hand washing, proper rinsing of dishes, hot water, soap, detergents, drying, and machine washed dishes (third grade). The machine washed

dishes are the cleanest, according to the research results available from the American Public Health Association.

22. Make posters to illustrate ways in which children can avoid infection, supplying appropriate captions for each poster, for example:
   a. "Catch That Sneeze" (a child may be shown coughing or sneezing into a disposable tissue).
   b. "Cut the Apple to Share It" (indicate the danger that can result from several persons taking bites from a single article of food).
   c. "Use Your Own" (show a child drying his face with his own towel or combing his hair with his own comb).

23. Discuss the ways in which people live around the globe. They have special ways for living in hot, dry deserts; in hot, wet jungles; and in snow covered lands.

24. Talk over the problem of drinking water supply while traveling or camping. Demonstrate how to purify water for drinking.

INTERMEDIATE LEVEL

1. Prepare immunization record forms for parents to complete and keep at home. An excellent sample form may be obtained from the U.S. Public Health Service, Washington, D.C. 20402. Have pupils enlarge these forms and discuss their meaning.

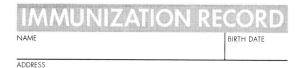

IMMUNIZATION	YEAR SERIES COMPLETED	YEAR BOOSTERS RECEIVED			
		1	2	3	4
D. T. P.					D.T.
POLIO					
SMALLPOX					
MEASLES					
OTHER					

U.S. DEPARTMENT OF HEALTH, EDUCATION, AND WELFARE / Public Health Service

GUIDE FOR FUTURE IMMUNIZATION

THIS IS A GENERAL GUIDE ONLY. See your doctor or health department for your own schedule of immunizations.

D. T. P. Diphtheria, Tetanus (Lockjaw), and Pertussis (Whooping Cough) should be repeated at 18 months and 5 years of age.

D. T.* (Diphtheria-Tetanus), after age 8.

T.* (Tetanus)

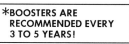

SMALLPOX*

POLIO See your doctor about boosters.

2. Discuss the community rules and regulations concerning garbage and rubbish disposal. Bring a copy of these rules to class.

3. Visit a community incinerator, garbage disposal plant, pumping station, or pasteurization plant.

4. Collect newspaper clippings concerning communicable diseases, community sanitation and cleanliness; and magazine advertisements having to do with health protection, cleanliness, and disease. Post these accounts and compare the number of magazine advertisements with the number of advertisements used for other topics. The soap and beauty ads alone will be quite plentiful.

5. Experiment with bacteria. Show that the germs "like" a warm, moist, and dark atmosphere in order to thrive and multiply.

a. Crush several dried beans. Place half of the beans in each of two containers. Cover with water. Store one of the containers in a warm, dark place and the other one on the classroom sill. After several days note the results.

b. Secure two apples. Peel one and place it in a dark, moist, and warm place; leave the other exposed to the air and sunlight on the teacher's desk. Note the results in a few days.

c. Indicate how the human skin acts as an envelope somewhat like the apple skin to protect the body.

6. Using a magnifying glass, study the molds that have grown on stale bread, fruit, or other material. Point

out that there are other bacteria so small that only a microscope can magnify them enough for the human eye to see. Bring a microscope to class. Let each child use it. Talk about Leeuwenhoek's discovery of the microscope.

7. Spell and be able to use correctly such words as:

contagious	bacteria	scientists
disease	dangerous	laboratory
harmless	superstition	infection
sterilize	microscope	immune
pasteurize	health	ferment
quarantine	science	illness

8. Read the poem, *Strictly Germproof*, by Arthur Guiterman.

9. Show the ways in which drinking water differs. Illustrate the passage of water through stones and sand. Have a committee of several persons build a stone and sand model for class use: pour muddy water in at the top of the box; see how much cleaner it is when it comes out at the bottom.

10. Learn the differences between acute and chronic illness.

11. Study local rules about dogs and rabies immunization.

12. Inquire about raw milk. What are the dangers in drinking it? What is meant by tuberculin tested cattle? How does this compare with pasteurization in terms of health protection?

13. Read excerpts from the stimulating books by Hans Zinsser, *Rats, Lice, and History*. Here is a man who did a great deal of research and writing on typhus fever and wrote a best-seller. Follow this reading by discussing head lice. What are nits? What are graybacks? How may lice be controlled? Name other small insects and animals responsible for carrying disease.

14. Discuss illnesses attributed to meats. Point out such things as the following:

    a. Meat killed in the woods is not always properly refrigerated in time.

    b. To prevent spoilage of meats a farmer sometimes coats it liberally with salt. Notice how salty country hams taste.

    c. Look for the federal or state inspection stamp on meat that has been processed under favorable conditions.

    d. Many animals are capable of carrying undulant fever and diarrhea to people. Swine spread hookworm, tapeworm, and muscle worms (trichinosis). All animals may spread tuberculosis.

    e. The first meat inspections were made by early Egyptians and Israelites. Mohammedan food regulations today are similar to those of years

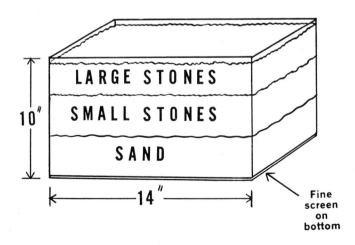

LARGE STONES

SMALL STONES

SAND

10"

14"

Fine screen on bottom

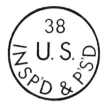

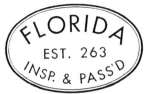

ago. Meat inspections by the Federal Government began in 1890.

15. If at all possible, visit a meat-packing plant and see what takes place in the way of inspections, cleaning, and refrigeration. Post two large stamps of approval.

16. Talk over illnesses attributed to foods, poisons, and chemicals.

17. Assign library research reports on the stories of the lives of such scientists as Koch, Jenner, Pasteur, Reed, and Salk.

18. Ask a restaurant owner or any food handler to come and speak to the class on the rules and regulations for protecting the public from spoiled foods and inadequate sanitary practices.

19. Bring to class a number of labels from canned and packaged foods to show that the government inspects the food products before allowing them to be placed on the market. Discuss the United States Government's Department of Agriculture and the Pure Food and Drug Act.

20. Experiment with the growth of bacteria. Sterilize several jar covers and glass lids. Make a gelatin solution and pour it into the jar covers, covering with the glass lids until the gelatin becomes solid. Then do the following:

   a. Remove a glass lid and have a child with a cold cough or sneeze over the gelatin. With other covers use such items as human hair, a penny, or dust from a window sill.

   b. Place the plates in a warm, dark place for a couple of days.

   c. Using a magnifying glass or microscope, study the con-taminated covers and compare them with a non-contaminated cover.

21. Discuss cancer. Show the American Cancer Society film *From One Cell*. Discuss how cancer spreads. Illustrate uncontrolled growth in plants (galls). Plants can be induced to develop cancer-like growths by applying chemicals. Encourage school laboratory or home experimentation: Paint the stems of growing tomato, castor bean, or sunflower plants with diluted tar or with a solution of ammonia in water. Irregular masses will form on the stems.

22. Discuss whether the children's parents have regular medical examinations and their attitude toward this health practice.

7. Safety and First Aid

Desirable Outcomes (Primary Level)

To understand and be able to practice such items as the following:

Crossing the street safely.

Using the safest route from home to school.

Ability to give name, address, name of school, and name of parents.

Ability to get on and off the bus safely and behave safely when riding on buses, cars, and trains.

Walk in the right places and run in the right places.

Knowledge of what to do in cases of illness or injury to self or a companion. Understand the importance of proper care of open cuts and abrasions. Know enough to report accidents and emergencies to an adult.

Use swings, slides, and other playground equipment properly.

Recognition of the need for keeping

buildings, walks, gymnasiums, and playgrounds safe.

Ability to use and properly store such items as saws, scissors, hoes, rakes, pins, needles, and other school-home equipment.

Know that one should not accept rides with strangers.

Acceptance of responsibility for helping protect younger children.

Ability to act properly in case of fire and practice simple rules of fire prevention.

Proper attitude toward bicycle safety.

Proper attitude toward teasing pets and playing with strange animals.

Ability to practice safety at home as well as at school.

Desirable Outcomes (Intermediate Level)

To understand and put into practice such items as:

Sound home and school safety practices.

Crossing streets at intersections, obeying traffic signals, lights, and traffic rules.

Safety in free play situations.

Knowing and practicing safety in using a bicycle, the school bus, and all forms of public transportation, tools, electricity, and fire apparatus, playground game equipment according to regulations, and in flying kites where there are no power lines and no danger from automobile traffic.

Being responsible for his own safety and for the safety of others.

First aid skills required to administer first aid for slight injuries, such as sprains, fainting, insect, dog, or snake bites, burns, blisters, nosebleed.

Safety precautions needed while swimming, fishing, boating, canoeing, and water skiing.

Knowledge of harmful substances.

Comments

As indicated in Chapters 1 and 7 the magnitude of the accident problem to-day is reflected in the figures of the National Safety Council. According to this source, accidents to children outrank all other causes of death — killing more children between the ages of five and 14 years than cancer, congenital malformations, pneumonia, and poliomyelitis combined.

The need for safety education continues to increase despite the slight decline in child deaths and injuries. And there is some evidence, as a result of careful investigation, that safety education is being dealt with somewhat inadequately. The elementary reading books, for instance, appear to be weak in this respect.

Certainly the school, where half the accidents to children occur, has a definite responsibility in the area of safety instruction. Teachers must be cognizant that young people usually seek adventure and excitement. This is as it should be, for it is through adventure, challenging experiences, and bold activities that young people grow and develop their personalities. Frequently, however, children become absorbed in their classwork or in their play and forget to exercise precautions essential for their personal protection and the protection of other children around them. It is the little things sometimes that cause the greatest trouble and alert the teacher to a health teaching need. For example, among the non-hospitalized accidents to youngsters, injuries caused by cutting and piercing instruments and those involving bicycles exceed even the accidents due to motor vehicles. Falls in and about the school occur continually. Rabid dogs bite and sometimes disfigure children. Firearms explode at the wrong time. Drownings occur in every community where there is a body of water. Primary grade children become victims of their curiosity when it comes to poisons. The newly formed poison centers in one state alone handled 470 cases of poisoning in a recent year. There were 48 cases of children drinking kerosene, 40 eat-

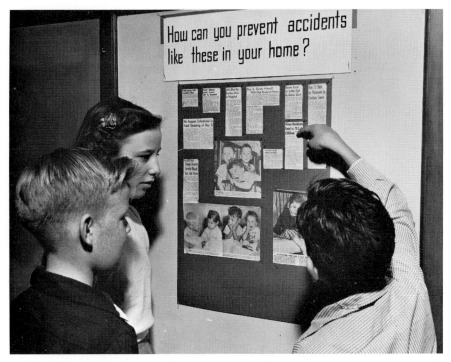

Figure 8–11   Hazards are everywhere. (Courtesy Safety and Youth Services Branch, Los Angeles Schools, California.)

ing roach tablets, and 92 eating too many aspirins. These are items the school can do something about. In this respect, an excellent teaching guide is available from the Division of Accident Prevention, U.S. Public Health Service. It is entitled *Teaching Poison Prevention in Kindergartens and Primary Grades.*

The experiences for this topic, as in all major health topics, must be sufficiently vital to stimulate pupil curiosity and eventual appreciation; they must be real. More than one author, in discussing the prevention of child accidents, has pointed to the educational value of minor painful experiences in teaching young children to respect but not to fear those things and forces in their environment which have the power to do them harm as well as good. Although children must be protected from major hazards, they should be allowed to discover that hot things burn, sharp things cut, and that water in the air passages is not com-

fortable. This may seem like an extreme type of learning by experience, but properly handled it can be effective.

In the lower grades safety is taught informally on a day-to-day basis. Little attention is given to first aid except to relate injuries to the function of the physician, nurse, and parents. Safety and first aid are taught in a more organized fashion in the intermediate grades, and there is considerable merit in the practice of teaching safety when the occasion demands it. After children have become safety conscious, it may be more effective for them to get the practical part of their education in safety as they engage in the activities of the playground, gymnasium, workshop, classroom, and on field trips. Many times during the school week the classroom teacher will find occasion to emphasize and clarify safety concepts. Excitement-loving fifth and sixth grade boys and girls are sometimes repelled by the idea that being

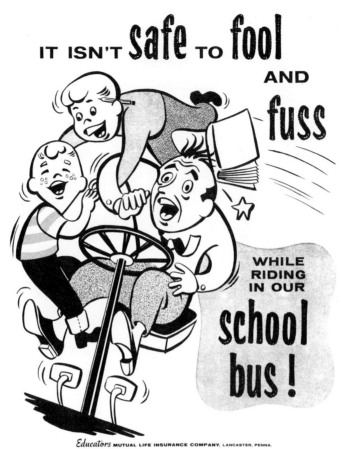

Figure 8–12   Free safety education materials. (Courtesy Educators Mutual Life Insurance Co.)

safe means avoiding all risks, but they may be intrigued with the idea that it takes smartness to recognize and appraise risks, and good judgment and skill to overcome them. Almost anything may be accomplished either in a hazardous or a comparatively safe manner. In class discussions teachers can help their pupils to realize that what counts in accident prevention is the ability to anticipate risks and the willingness to prepare to meet them with clear thinking and skill.

Teaching first aid to boys and girls permits the teacher to strengthen attitudes concerning how a person should react to emergency situations. Injury and sickness should be dealt with calmly and with an air of confidence.

The teacher herself should have some training in first aid and be familiar with first aid supplies and the emergency practices in her school. She should also be able to capitalize on the curiosity aroused by individual first aid occurrences in the classroom. Taking advantage of interest by holding a group discussion on a topic growing out of an emergency situation is good teaching. As an example, an appropriate time to consider the control of bleeding and the precautions which should be taken to prevent it is when a pupil cuts his finger and requires immediate first aid. Likewise, when a child gets a blister or burns himself there is an opportunity to make safety education a vital subject in the health curriculum. A helpful booklet, *Teaching Safety in the Elementary School*, by Peter Yost, is available for the classroom teacher. It may be obtained from the Department of Classroom Teachers, N.E.A., Washington, D.C. 20036. Another excellent classroom teaching aid is the programmed instruction manual, *First Aid*, developed for sixth grade use by Behavioral Research Laboratories and distributed as a public service by Johnson & Johnson.

Considerable instructional assistance is available to any teacher who requests it from the National Safety Council. The materials are informative and are carefully designed to create and maintain student interest in personal health and safety. The Council periodically distributes leaflets illustrating desirable experiences in elementary safety education. Teachers who want to meet real needs:

1. Make an analysis of the temporary and permanent hazards in the student's environment.
2. Make an analysis of the hazards connected with the pupil's activities.
3. Study the records collected through the usual student accident reporting system.
4. Study the hazards associated with the various seasons and with such special days as Fourth of July, Halloween, and Christmas.
5. Carefully consider individual student abilities, limitations, and difficulties.

Thus proper safety programs provide for many experiences in the classroom involving textbooks, audiovisual aids, and pupil-made materials. They also involve experience with school equipment, school buses, emergency drill, physical education activities, and such other major motivation items as junior safety councils, safety patrols, safety committees, monitors, and bicycle clubs.

It should also be pointed out that *Safety Magazine* is a periodical of high caliber which is worth reading each month for new ways and means of making this topic more effective with children.

No study of safety would be complete without referring to bicycle safety. The need for bicycle safety education is emphasized by the fact that three out of four youngsters between the ages of six and 15 ride a bicycle. There are more than 20 million bicycles on American streets and highways. Every 19 minutes, day and night, a cyclist is injured; every 21 hours a cyclist is killed by an automobile. It is recommended that all communities establish a sound procedure for testing, registering, and licensing bicycles. Four recommended practices, which the schoolteacher should know about, are as follows:

1. Test all bicycle owners for knowledge of traffic rules and regulations and skill in riding.
2. Inspect all bicycles for mechanical operation.
3. Register and license all bicycles.
4. Teach bicycle safety in the elementary school health program.

There used to be a time when primary grade children did not get very far away from home on a tricycle, wagon, or scooter. Today, in virtually every community children of all ages, even very young children, are seen riding two-wheel vehicles across main streets, over seeded lawns, on busy sidewalks, and anywhere they see fit to ride. The implication for health teaching is clear. Bicycle safety must be taught from grade one through the sixth grade. It must be taught with enough variety of activities and experiences to make it live in the minds of the boys and girls.

Numerous communities, working through the schools, have developed quite satisfactory bicycle safety programs. In Hamden, Connecticut, for example, a standard bicycle safety test

BICYCLE SAFETY TEST RECORD

Name of Pupil	Initial of Inspector
Written Test	
Mechanical Condition	
Test #1—Balance	
Test #2—Obstacle Course	
Test #3—Precision	
Test #4—Braking	
Test #5—Maneuvering	
Test #6—Hand Signals	
Certificate	

HAMDEN PUBLIC SCHOOLS
BICYCLE OPERATOR'S CERTIFICATE

This is to certify that

PUPIL'S NAME	SCHOOL

has passed an examination on Rules of the Road for bicycle riders and has passed the Bicycle Riding Test.

Matthew Barberi

SUPERVISOR OF PHYSICAL AND HEALTH EDUCATION	PRINCIPAL

record is kept on boys and girls. Once the examination is passed a wallet-size card is issued.

The experience of the Oklahoma City schools demonstrates how the combined efforts of several groups of people can be brought to bear on bicycle safety problems with effective results. With the excellent cooperation of teachers, administrators, parents, police, bicycle dealers, and local safety council personnel, it was possible to draw up a plan consisting of a city bicycle code and a safety education curriculum.[16] A "bicycle clinic" was also established in which bicycles could be inspected and skill tests given to determine a pupil's ability to control the bicycle in close quarters.

The suggested activities which follow on safety and first aid, instead of being grouped together, have been set up in categories. This is because safety embraces so many phases of the school and community environment. The categories are home and community safety, bicycle safety, school safety, playground and gymnasium safety, and first aid. Of course, some items overlap and tend to apply to more than one category. Bicycle safety, for instance, could easily have been incorporated under the home and community area or under school safety. However, because bicycle safety is such a major problem, the activities and experiences are treated separately.

Fire safety might well be treated as a separate topic. It is included here as an item under home and community and school safety. With over a million fires a year, 11,000 fatalities (one third of them children), it becomes necessary to prepare lessons in fire prevention, many of which can be integrated with classes in history, science, and social studies. In this connection, the most thorough publication — filled from cover to cover with top teaching activities — is the teaching manual for

elementary schools, *Fire Prevention and Safety* (1961), distributed by the Hartford Fire Insurance Company. This is the same organization which began the Junior Fire Marshal program in 1947 as a year-round activity. Their "Junior Fire Marshal Song" is well written and is printed in full in the manual. The list of topics in this publication is more than sufficient to care for the teaching needs of any classroom teacher or health and safety specialist. It may be obtained free of charge. Significant fire safety materials for classroom use may also be obtained for a small cost from the American Insurance Association in New York and the National Fire Protection Association in Boston.

Suggested Activities

HOME AND COMMUNITY SAFETY—
PRIMARY LEVEL

1. Fires can be dangerous. Prepare an ordinary fire on the playground. Show that any child may put it out by pouring sand or water on it. Stress that children should not build fires by themselves.

2. In the winter, appoint several pupils to put sand or ashes on icy steps or pavement. Show young pupils how this reduces the danger of slipping. Show also how calcium chloride melts and helps break up ice.

3. Make an exhibit of familiar items which have rough surfaces to reduce the danger of slipping. This exhibit might include sport shoes, automobile tires, tires with snow treads, bicycle tires, rubber gloves, rubber backed throw rugs or mats.

4. Post the following poem on the board:

> In the street I'll never play
>
> I have no arms to give away.
>
> I have no legs that I can spare,
>
> To keep them all I must take care.

---

[16] Gilliland, Lonnie. "Schools, Children, Bikes," *Safety Education*, 3:16–19, February 1967.

Discuss the causes of street accidents: not looking in either direction, running after a ball, dashing from behind parked cars, crossing the street diagonally or in the middle of the block (third grade).

5. Draw an imaginary street with intersections on the classroom floor. Use the children as buses and automobiles, a traffic officer, and people. Teach how to cross the street safely and obey signals (kindergarten or first grade).

6. Build with blocks. Make streets and sidewalks; place people, cars, and buses.

7. Use the sand table to build a community complete with streets, playgrounds, and houses. Put in traffic lights and stop signs. Use small toys for community equipment such as bulldozers, derricks, trucks, police cars, fire engines. Build an airport on the outskirts of the town. Use twigs and sticks as trees and telephone poles.

8. Make a stop and go sign for class use. Place a small inexpensive flashlight behind each piece of colored paper. Have the class practice operating and responding to the light changes.

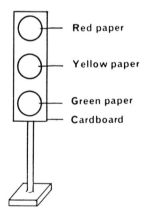

9. Visit such nearby places as the fire station, public playgrounds, railway stations, parks. Combine community health with safety education.

10. Play a game such as "grab bag game." Produce a big bag filled with various items. Have students draw from the bag pictures of pins, scissors, matches, nails, and sharp instruments, and tell how each should be taken care of.

11. Show that haste causes accidents in the community. Scatter children about a small open room. Have one pupil run as fast as he can from one end of the room to the other, attempting to dodge his friends. Note how easy it would be to have a fall.

12. Build a model of a house that is open on one side, or borrow a large doll house for class demonstration of the relationship of space to accidents (third grade). Falls and poisonings may be traced to the unwise use of space. With the model show:

Small objects left on stairs
An open window on second floor
An open basement door
Medicines left where toddlers can "try" them
Electric toaster partly plugged into outlet
Ladder against the house
Milk bottles sitting on window sill
Bubbling coffee pot on edge of stove (with model of small baby standing under it)

13. Discuss "Our Friend the Fireman." Read or tell stories about brave firemen. Have children check off a list of fire hazards in their homes.

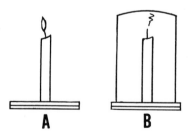

14. Demonstrate that a candle will not burn after it has used all the air under the glass jar which is put over it. Point out that if clothes catch fire, the fire can be smothered by wrapping the person in a rug (third grade).

15. Integrate the sound of a real siren with music. Compose a song about firemen and fire prevention. Secure "The Junior Fire Marshal Song" from the Hartford Fire Insurance Company.

16. Organize a fire brigade with the following duties:[17]

    a. Inspect the school premises. Gather up papers and other waste materials and put them into metal containers. Watch for anything that might cause fires and report the condition to the teacher.

    b. Confiscate matches brought to school by boys and girls. Emphasize the need for thinking of others.

17. Have the class list ways in which falls may be prevented. Here are some examples:

    Keep toys where they belong
    Keep rugs straight
    Ask grownups to reach things on high shelves
    Keep shoelaces tied
    Do not play on window sills and porch railings

18. Visit a drug store. Have the pharmacist point out poison labels and caution children regarding tasting substances they know nothing about (third grade).

HOME AND COMMUNITY SAFETY— INTERMEDIATE LEVEL

1. Make a class survey of the community agencies for recreation. Discuss the facilities available and some of the hazards involved in their use.

2. Study the beaches and swimming pools with an eye to sanitation, supervision, safety devices, and the presence of lifeguards, and inform children about these conditions. The

---

[17] Especially useful safety ideas may be obtained from the National Safety Council. A very good coverage of the topic is also contained in some state courses of study. Texas and Maine are noteworthy examples.

suggestions prepared by the American Red Cross may be quite helpful.

3. Build a model of a safe well, showing that it should be dug properly, lined, and covered to protect the water from pollution; a model of the local inspection and purification plant might also be made by a committee of about three who would arrange to visit the plant manager and make sketches.

4. Encourage wide discussion on safety in the use of fire. Point out that over 2000 children die each year in home fires. Discuss lighted cigarettes, bonfires, electrical appliances, candles, gasoline and kerosene, rubbish, defective chimneys, stoves, fireplaces, and furnaces. Display the poster, *Don't Give Fire a Place to Start*. It may be obtained from National Fire Prevention Association. Order copies of the comic strip booklet, *Is This Your Home?* for all class members. This well prepared story (in color) may be obtained from the American Insurance Association (Safety Department).

5. Have a student demonstrate how to roll over and over on the floor in case the clothing is on fire. Have another pupil demonstrate how to wrap someone in a rug, blanket, or coat. "Never run. Inform an older person at once or turn in the alarm and wait for the firemen at the alarm box."

6. Demonstrate through group action such fire fighting methods as the bucket brigade and the volunteer system. Follow this with a description of the way the big city system is operated.

7. Invite the local fire chief or director of public safety to visit the class.

8. Have a pupil roller-skate into the class, preferably at a most inopportune time. Discuss roller-skating safety.

9. Have a pupil bring his pet dog or cat to a class. Talk about safe practices in handling animals and about

avoiding strange dogs. Discuss rabies and, if appropriate (in the southern states), talk over animal hookworm.

10. Inquire about the meaning of pedestrian safety. Cover such topics as:

Being alert on sidewalks and streets
Avoiding jay walking
Avoiding ride hitching on moving vehicles
Bicycle safety
Walking on the highway

11. Plan a clean-up campaign in each home. Let the class hear some of the plans.

12. Check the daily paper for one week for accidents of all kinds. Note types of accidents and age classification.

13. Either organize a school safety council or consider ways of improving the one in existence (sixth grade).

14. Secure a list of city ordinances which pertain to public safety. Study these to find what they are all about.

15. Have the school or local electrician discuss and exhibit different electrical tools and household appliances. This activity will be more valuable if pupils are assigned the task of bringing a small electrical appliance to class themselves.

16. With the help of a local conservation officer or fish and game club representative, plan a lesson on firearms safety. This will be particularly meaningful in a vast area of the United States. Consider firearms in the woods, in the home, and on the range. This is generally a fascinating and extremely practical topic that falls under five major headings:[18]

Knowledge of guns
Proper gun handling
Good shooting
The hunter's responsibility
Essentials of safe hunting

---

[18] A Plan to Safeguard New Hampshire Youth. *Firearms Safety Education.* Concord, New Hampshire: State Department of Education, 1954, p. 4.

How is your
CONSCIENCE?

Some of our younger citizens saw you when you Jay-Walked... They imitate and learn from older citizens.

Were you a
GOOD EXAMPLE?

distributed
in the interest of Public Safety

LAKEWOOD SAFETY COUNCIL

17. Discuss "the grownups." Do they always set a good example?

Display in front of the class the poster on page 230.

Tell the class that this is a reproduction of a jay-walking ticket actually distributed in Lakewood, Ohio. Discuss its implications (fifth or sixth grades).

18. Study the ways poison is identified on medicine bottles, insect powder, and similar items. Follow this with a list of the poisonous materials commonly found at home. Some of these items might easily be brought to class.

19. Study industrial safety measures in such curriculum units as aviation, the newspaper, sound communication, and in studies of all units based on cultures.

20. Discover the hazards of pesticides. They are potentially dangerous both in diluted and concentrated form. Accidental swallowing by children has

┌─────────────────────────────────────┐
│ READ THE LABEL!   │
│ FOLLOW DIRECTIONS!   │
└─────────────────────────────────────┘

been responsible for most deaths from pesticides.

BICYCLE SAFETY—PRIMARY LEVEL

1. Display a large poster of a bicycle with lines going to all significant parts.[19]

2. Talk about bicycle safety aids. Discuss the *bell or horn* as an important signaling device which should be used to warn of approach. Discuss the *headlight,* so essential for safe bicycling at night. Stress, however, that night riding should be held to a minimum. Illustrate how the *reflector* brightens when a headlight beam hits it and how it serves as a warning signal

_____

[19] Excellent posters may be obtained free from the Bicycle Institute of America and Employers Mutuals of Wausau.

to protect *you* from unforeseen dangers. Show how the *basket* or *carrier* keeps the hands free for the proper control of the wheel. The Bicycle Institute of America will furnish an excellent four-color poster which wisely illustrates these bicycle aids.

3. Practice giving hand signals. Have several class members illustrate these by riding a bicycle on the playground for all to observe:

    a. Left arm *pointed up* for turning to the right.

    b. Left arm *straight out* for turning to the left.

    c. Left arm *pointed down* for slowing up or stopping.

Posters in green and orange on bicycle hand signals may be obtained free from Bicycle Institute of America.

4. Bring a bicycle into class. Stand it on a table where all pupils can see it

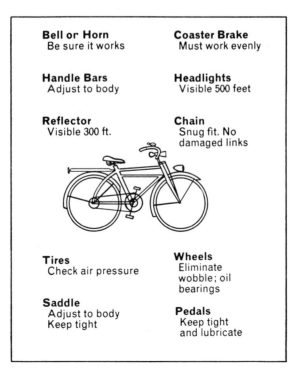

Bell or Horn
Be sure it works

Coaster Brake
Must work evenly

Handle Bars
Adjust to body

Headlights
Visible 500 feet

Reflector
Visible 300 ft.

Chain
Snug fit. No damaged links

Tires
Check air pressure

Wheels
Eliminate wobble; oil bearings

Saddle
Adjust to body
Keep tight

Pedals
Keep tight and lubricate

clearly. Discuss "How to care for your bicycle." Include the saddle, wheels, brake, handle grips, reflector, chain, pedals, warning devices, level of handle bars, fork bearings, light, spokes, tire pressure, and tire valves (third grade).

5. Have class members demonstrate the method of getting on a bicycle, the means of guiding it, applying the brake and coming to a stop, and parking the bicycle (first or second grade).

6. Discuss using the horn or bell. Do not use the horn or bell as a brake.

7. Encourage pupils to send for safety materials from state motor vehicle departments and other sources. Materials designed to assist those working with bicycle safety are available from:

    a. American Automobile Association

Traffic Engineering and Safety Department
1712 G Street, N.W.
Washington, D.C. 20006

    b. Bicycle Institute of America
122 E. 42nd Street
New York, New York 10017

    c. Insurance Institute for Highway Safety
1725 DeSales Street, N.W.
Washington, D.C. 20036

    d. National Safety Council
425 N. Michigan Avenue
Chicago, Illinois 60611

8. Have the class draw and color road markers. The ones illustrated are used in most states. Check on local variations by contacting the traffic police.

9. Make a list of all the sidewalk vehicles owned by members of the class. Discuss how to ride these, especially the tricycle.

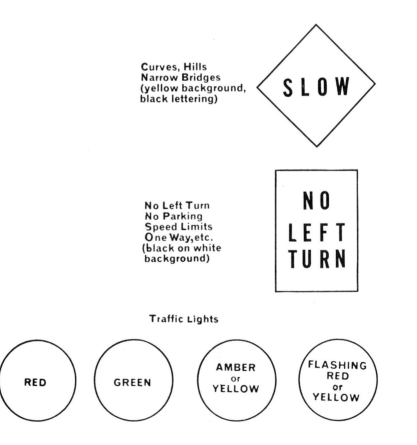

Curves, Hills
Narrow Bridges
(yellow background,
black lettering)

SLOW

No Left Turn
No Parking
Speed Limits
One Way, etc.
(black on white
background)

NO
LEFT
TURN

Traffic Lights

RED   GREEN   AMBER or YELLOW   FLASHING RED or YELLOW

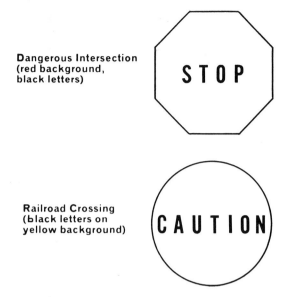

Dangerous Intersection
(red background,
black letters)

Railroad Crossing
(black letters on
yellow background)

a. Ride alone on a tricycle, not double.
b. Be especially careful when there are pedestrians on the sidewalk.
c. Watch cars backing out of garage or driveway.
d. Stay on sidewalks or in own yard — streets are made for fast-moving vehicles (kindergarten or first grade).

10. With the help of the pupils, make up a safety song to some catchy tune. Example:

Tune: "Merrily We Roll Along"
I
Merrily we roll along
skate along
bike along
Merrily we sing a song
Sing a song of safety
II
Watchfully the streets we'll cross —
look both ways — and *walk across*
Happily we'll sing our song
It's fun to play safely.

While this tune is being sung, some of the children might be asked to illustrate the message.

BICYCLE SAFETY — INTERMEDIATE LEVEL

1. Administer a bicycle test at the start of this topic to see how much the class actually knows about their bicycles and how to use them.[20] The *Bicycle Safety Quiz,* distributed (free) by Aetna Life Affiliated Companies, is a good one. There are practical questions, two of which are illustrated here. (Part of the quiz appears in Chapter 12 as an evaluation instrument):

a. It is safe to learn to ride a bicycle on a busy street.
( ) True   ( ) False
b. Bicycles, like autos, should keep to the right side of the road.
( ) True   ( ) False

2. Post a readily visible list of bicycle safety rules on bulletin board. Typewritten rules on white paper pasted to a black background are easily noticed. Call attention to these rules and have the class check themselves to see how many they some-

_____

[20] This may also be used in connection with the motion picture, *Safe on Two Wheels,* distributed by the Public Education Department, Aetna Life Affiliated Companies, Hartford, Conn. 10015.

times violate. Here is a sample list of rules:

a. Observe all traffic regulations—red and green lights, one-way streets, stop signs.

b. Never hitch on other vehicles, "stunt," or race in traffic.

c. Have satisfactory signaling device to warn of approach.

d. Ride at a safe speed.

e. For night riding have a white light on front and a danger signal reflector on rear.

f. Wear white or light-colored clothes at night.

g. Give pedestrians the right of way.

h. Avoid sidewalks; otherwise use extra care.

i. Watch for car pulling out into traffic.

j. Look out for sudden opening of automobile doors.

k. Keep to the right, and ride in a single file.

l. Keep a safe distance behind all vehicles.

m. Do not carry other riders.

n. Do not carry packages that obstruct vision or prevent proper control of the cycle.

o. Slow down at street intersections; look to the right and left before crossing.

p. Check the brakes for good working condition. Keep the bicycle in perfect running order.

q. Ride in a straight line. Do not weave in or out of traffic or swerve from side to side.

r. Always use proper hand signals for turning and stopping.

s. Park the bicycle in a safe place.

3. Discuss membership in the *Safety League*. The Bicycle Institute of America sponsors this and supplies free all the necessary materials for implementing the program. Each student may receive a copy of *Helpful Hints on Bicycle Care*, a membership card, and an attractive four-color decal to place on the mudguard. The membership card in the *Safety League* also has on it a list of 12 rules for safe bicycling and a detailed picture of a bicycle showing the parts in need of constant care and inspection.

4. Invite a safety specialist or member of the police department to talk on bicycle safety, including mechanical condition of the bicycle.

5. Prepare a brief safety manual for bicyclists.

6. Organize a bike trip to a nearby park for lunch. Appoint a leader. Those who cannot go on bicycles may walk.

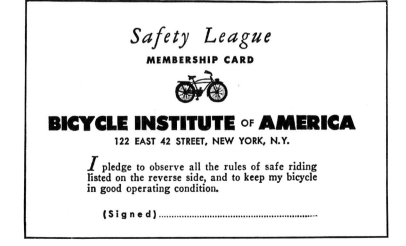

Safety League

MEMBERSHIP CARD

BICYCLE INSTITUTE OF **AMERICA**

122 EAST 42 STREET, NEW YORK, N.Y.

I pledge to observe all the rules of safe riding listed on the reverse side, and to keep my bicycle in good operating condition.

(Signed) ....

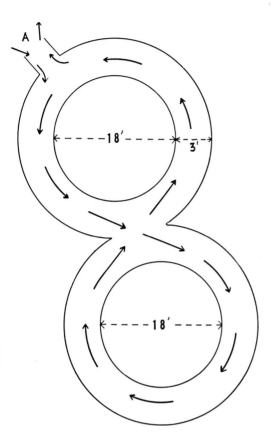

7. Prepare a bicycle skill test to be given on the school playground or play yard. Several of the pupils in the class will be especially eager to help in such a project. The following test, for example, is not hard to set up.[21]

    a. Begin at point A.

    b. Ride slowly, being careful not to touch border lines.

SCHOOL SAFETY — PRIMARY LEVEL

1. Train the class in the essentials of good fire drill. Teach the importance of a cool and immediate response, how to send in the alarm in the community (in the absence of an adult), and where to find the fire hose and extinguisher in the school. Tour the school, corridor

[21]Other interesting intermediate grade activities appear in the booklet, *Official Safety Manual*. National Child Safety Council, 125 W. Pearl St., Jackson, Mich.

by corridor, to see these locations. Follow this with the reading of *Hello, I Am Fire!* — a SPARKY fire story available from the National Fire Protection Association.

2. Talk about the safest route home from school. Early in the school term, practice crossing the street.

3. Play the little game, "Who Are You?" Line the class up in the front of the room. Appoint one pupil to ask the question of anyone he chooses, "Who are you?" The pupil selected gives his name, address, name of his school, and parents. If he does this satisfactorily, he becomes "it" next.

4. Use the school bus to practice safe behavior on a bus. Have the school bus driver speak to the pupils, especially in connection with a field trip.

5. Discuss what to do if a stranger offers a ride. Know that one should not accept rides from strangers.

6. Make simple pencil clips in order to emphasize the need to carry sharp pencils safely. To do this:

    a. Wrap a narrow strip of adhesive tape once around a pencil, about one inch down from the top.

    b. Place a paper clip on the strip and fasten the clip to the pencil with tape.

    c. It is ready to wear. Try it on the shirt pocket.

7. Organize the class on a daily basis to put away their toys and other materials when they have finished using them.

8. Discuss topics that will help the children think through the reasons for school accidents. Examples:

    a. Need to look where one is going.

    b. Need to keep to the right.

    c. Need to pay attention to what is going on.

    d. Need to *walk* in hallways and on stairs.

    e. Need to use school tools properly.

9. Practice carrying chairs in the proper manner, being certain the vision is clear. Formulate rules for sitting on a chair. In connection with chairs and chair safety, play the game, "musical chairs," or march about them.

10. Make an attractive cut-out to use with a school safety jingle. The one below, for example, could be used with third graders:

    a. Have the pupils step on a piece of colored paper. With a pencil trace the outline of the shoes.

    b. Cut out the footprints and in the space available write a safety jingle. Example:

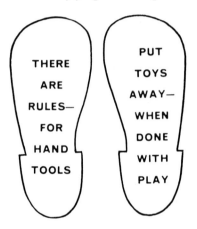

SCHOOL SAFETY — INTERMEDIATE LEVEL

1. Discuss school fire hazards. Make a survey of the school building.[22]

2. Organize the classroom for efficient fire drills.

3. Have pupils construct a cabinet for storing sharp tools, such as scissors, thumbtacks, drills.

4. Prior to an extended vacation period (Thanksgiving, Christmas),

[22] Many excellent fire safety activities for schools may be found in the manual, *Fire Prevention and Safety*, distributed free by Hartford Fire Insurance Company, Hartford, Conn. 10015. The materials distributed by the National Fire Protection Association are also superior; an excellent discussion booklet is *Take Time for Home Fire Prevention*.

make charts of safe practices to be followed during vacation activities. For example, what are the hazards to be aware of while on Christmas vacation, both indoor and outdoor?

5. Engage in safety poster construction. Each row or small group of pupils should be made responsible for a particular phase of safety; completed posters could be exhibited in the school corridor or multi-purpose room.

6. Participate in a school safety patrol. Train leaders so that everyone will eventually have a chance to be a patrolman; local traffic officials are usually available to assist the school safety patrol in setting up acceptable standards. This may well be a total elementary school project with classroom representation. Patrol standards and particulars are available from National Safety Council.

7. Describe an accident that may have happened in the school. Write down all the facts and decide what might have been done to prevent it. Compare pupil findings.

8. Discuss clothes locker safety, particularly as it applies to school corridor accidents.

9. List some of the traffic problems present in the school. Appoint a committee to take up the problems involving other classes.

10. Safety is not an isolated topic. The help of a mother or a group of mothers may be enlisted in a discussion of school, home, and community safety. The children may enjoy preparing a play or reading a report on their safety activities before a group of interested adults.

11. Investigate the relationship of the school environment to health and safety. Consider lighting, seating, stairways, lunchrooms, the auditorium, stage, and gymnasium.

12. Try "on the spot" safety messages over the school intercom system. A special event of the school day is connected to the safety message and

relayed to the students. If, for example, it is assembly day, students are reminded to pass through the halls and step down the stairs with extra care.

PLAYGROUND-GYMNASIUM SAFETY— PRIMARY LEVEL

1. Talk over the many sources of danger from playground accidents. Call attention briefly to items such as the following:[23]

    a. *General:* Broken glass, protruding nails, tin cans left on ground. Unnecessarily rough play, tripping, pushing, climbing fences, shelters, trees. Congestion of activities. Bicycle riding across the playground, especially during games. Children with contagious skin diseases mingling with others. Activities not adapted to grounds. Dogs on grounds. Pools of water remaining after rain. Need for first aid kit.

    b. *Swings:* Jumping from moving swings, running or playing between or around swings. Climbing on frame while swings are in use. Holding baby brother or sister while swinging. Improper use of swings. Other activities too near swings. Swinging too high causing chains to slap and yank. Climbing across top of frame.

    c. *Sandboxes:* Glass, cans, and broken or unbroken bottles in boxes. Throwing sand or blocks; concealing hard or sharp objects in the sand. The use of a sandbox lid or cover when box is not in use. Looking for nails working loose and splinters.

    d. *Drinking fountain:* Pushing or crowding. Molesting the drinker. Unsanitary conditions of the bubbler.

2. Appoint a swing patrol to watch other children swing; encourage safe practices.

3. Appoint a weekly clean-up squad for the play area.

4. In winter, when there is snow and ice, stress safe places to skate and slide. Point up the dangers of interfering with others. Encourage the use of targets in snowballing. Purposely set up targets and let everyone throw all the snowballs they want.

5. Sing a song of safety to a catchy, easily learned tune. For example:

Tune: "Yankee Doodle"
Oh, let's obey each safety rule
And add some for good measure
At home, at school, and on playgrounds
We'll have our share of pleasure.

Chorus
Boys and girls remember what
Safety rules are made for
Keep them all or else someday
In sorrow they'll be paid for.

---

6. Plan an outing and, after the fun and food details have been considered, talk over the safety precautions:
Provide safe transportation
Use school bus if possible
Have the school nurse go on the trip
Check the availability of a telephone
Take a first aid kit along
Consider safe cooking, water supply, provisions for shade and rest
Shelter from rain
Protection from dangers of traffic

7. Study the natural surroundings at a picnic or outing area. Give information on such matters as poison ivy, poison oak, snakes, insects, and overexposure to the sun.

8. Select from several volunteers a group of children to help mark off the danger area around swings and to warn other children about entering it while swings are being used. Con-

---

[23] List adapted from the findings of the Vermont State Board of Recreation.

sider, also, other safe practices and equipment safety rules.

9. Demonstrate the importance of proper footwear on a gymnasium floor. Stress that sneakers are cleaner than shoes, that they give better traction while shoes slide, that it is difficult to be agile and quick when wearing shoes, and that our athletic skill is improved when we wear good sneakers.

PLAYGROUND–GYMNASIUM SAFETY – INTERMEDIATE LEVEL

1. Appoint a small committee to inspect the playground or gymnasium area, its equipment, and game boundary lines. Have these people report back to the class. Point out that faulty and hazardous conditions should be remedied immediately, or the play area should be closed from further use.

2. Show boys and girls how clear rules and definite boundary lines help make a game safe.

3. Indicate the relationship between properly developed game skills and safe performance. This may be illustrated by having two boys throw a ball accurately in dodgeball or handle themselves on a dodging run in a relay-type activity.

4. Have a painting project. Gaily colored swings and slides help reduce playground injuries. In addition, the attractive colors help entice youngsters to the playground and away from the street.

    a. Slides – paint them green to counteract excessive sunlight. Paint the steps to the top of the slide yellow to draw the children's attention.

    b. See-saws – paint green, with edges painted yellow to give greater visibility and reduce chances of children running into them.

    c. Swings and swing rings – paint seats and swings yellow. Green is best for upright and overhead bars.

    d. Sandboxes – paint green.

    e. Jungle gyms – paint a cool restful blue.

    f. Trash cans – paint gray with a white star. This emphasizes neatness and encourages youngsters to help keep the playground or gymnasium area tidy.

5. Train leaders to help others, to watch for younger children, to encourage others to use gates and crossings when leaving the playground, to inspect swings, jungle gyms, and other equipment.

6. Design a "Safety Leader" emblem. Perhaps a committee of pupils and teachers could select the best looking emblem design, and a number of these could be made from felt. They could be worn on the sleeves of the safety leaders.

7. Discuss the many sources of danger on playgrounds and gymnasiums, such as:

    a. *Baseball:* Playing too near the street and chasing balls into the street. Spectators too near baseline during a game. Batting flies in too small an area. Throwing the bat after hitting the ball. Playing catch too near swings, sandboxes, and other activities. Older boys playing on an area adapted only for younger children.

    b. *Horseshoes:* Running in front of the pitcher. Careless pitching and throwing too near other activities. Pitching distance too great for control. Locating stakes where children are likely to pass between.

    c. *Gym Floor:* Unnecessary running and pushing. Interfering with others who are on equipment. Playing safe games. Wearing shoes with rubber soles in gym. Wearing quality sneakers, especially for heavy children. Safe playing facilities: Do doors open outward? Are end walls padded? Is the heat of the water in the shower room automatically controlled? Are the radiators screened or set back into the wall? Does the gym floor have a smooth, non-slip surface?

8. Show the relationship between good sportsmanship and safe play activities.

9. Make a list of safety rules for the most popular games. Example: Soft-ball: (a) The batter who throws the bat is automatically out, (b) catching behind the bat without a mask is prohibited, (c) sliding into a base is not permitted, (d) always signal that you are about to catch a fly ball so that someone else will know that you are after it and avoid a collision.

10. Review the correct use of playground equipment.

FIRST AID — PRIMARY LEVEL

1. Discuss the ways in which small children may get burned. Example:
   a. Surface burns may be caused by falling on hot radiators, touching hot stoves or electric irons or toasters.
   b. Burns may be caused by hot liquids falling off the stove, by bumping into a person with a hot substance, and by careless playing with matches.

Point out what to do when a burn occurs.

2. Sing to the tune of "Yankee Doodle":

The kitchen is no place to play

Hot stoves and pots a-boiling

If mother stumbles over you,

You'd surely get a scalding.

The kitchen is no place to play

With things as hot as blister

You might push Mom against the stove

Or even baby sister.

(From May 1948 safety flyer of the American Red Cross)

3. Stress the need for placing medicines in the proper place when through using them.

4. Show pictures or exhibit real cans of varnish, paint, kerosene, and gasoline. Give reasons for not touching or tasting these liquids.

5. Dramatize proper procedure to follow in case of an accident in the school, the house, at the beach, or on the playground. Keep calm. Call an adult. Be of help where you can.

6. Use dolls; appoint a doctor and a nurse, and dramatize caring for make-believe wounds (kindergarten or first grade).

7. Discuss accidents and emergencies that should be reported to adults.

FIRST AID — INTERMEDIATE LEVEL

1. Plan and equip a first aid cabinet for the school. Consider also the items one might need on a day-long hike or trip into the country. Local needs should be considered.

2. Read about poisonous plants. Study how to prevent poison ivy, and stress what to do if one has been exposed to it.

3. Discuss the ways of acquiring a sun tan. Refer to the dangers.

4. Demonstrate care of ordinary cuts and bruises.

5. Discuss first aid in the control of bleeding (fifth or sixth grade).

6. Practice giving artificial respiration. Blankets or heavy paper may be placed on the floor, children divided into pairs to work on each other. See the American Red Cross Water Safety or First Aid Manual for the approved manner in giving the Holger-Neilson (arm lift — back pressure) method of artificial respiration. Refer also to mouth-to-mouth breathing. (ARC Junior Life Saving material.) Complimentary copies of *The Breath of Life*, with clear drawings of how to give mouth-to-mouth breathing, may be obtained from Aetna Life Insurance Co.

7. Have the class print markers for

poison containers that should be left alone. These may be done on adhesive tape. Have the pupils take the markers home and ask their parents to put them on medicine bottles and boxes.

8. Read about poisonous snakes in the United States.

9. Discuss first aid procedures in case of internal poisoning.

10. Make a list of first aid practices that might be employed in the winter sports scene. Consider accidents while coasting, skiing, and skating. Do the same thing for summer safety. Discuss diving into unknown waters, picking strange fruit, treating sunburn, and dangers involved in using an axe or knife.

11. Prepare a list of accident prevention measures suitable for outdoor camping and woods recreation. Prepare small printed signs for a bulletin board.

8. Mental Health

Desirable Outcomes (Primary Level)

To understand what it means to be accepted by classmates and school.

To be able to adjust in part to the demands of daily living, and establish satisfactory relationships with others.

To cope with the constantly changing environment and to become gradually more emotionally stable.

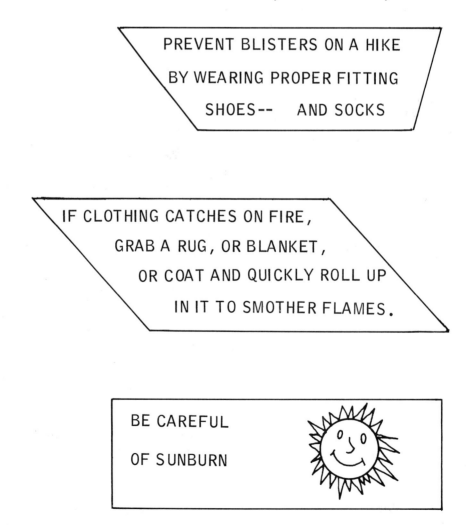

To develop a feeling of personal and over-all responsibility.

Desirable Outcomes (Intermediate Level)

To develop a personal sense of responsibility as a member of the school and community and as a member of the family.

To demonstrate specific regard and respect for the welfare of others and for oneself. To develop socially acceptable attitudes and behavior patterns. To serve sometimes as a leader and sometimes as a follower in school situations.

To enjoy working with others in play and work activities, and to realize that routine changes and unexpected failures and successes are to be taken in stride.

To understand that emotional health and personal feelings have a bearing on the way the whole body works.

Man is moving quickly ahead in his scientific exploits designed to use the atom and disembark to the surface of the moon, yet there is little evidence to indicate that the brotherhood of man is any closer today than it was a century ago. Learning to live together harmoniously is still the number one problem for the people of the world to solve. Moreover, the hospitals and physicians' offices of the country are crowded with thousands of people (vast numbers of whom are children) who are ill enough to seek the assistance of a physician, but whose illnesses are emotionally conditioned and frequently do not involve organic disease. This area of medicine (psychosomatic) is concerned with somatic symptoms (pain, rapid heart, loss of appetite, undue fatigue) and psychologically or emotionally induced reactions. Every other person today who seeks the help of a physician has emotionally induced illness. Such individuals may be classed in one way or another as emotionally immature; they are not able to face life as it really is,

and their illness serves as a measure of their vulnerability to these stresses. Unfortunately, the steadily rising tempo of American life brings on growing tensions, frustrations, and complexities.

Emotional health and mental health are the same. Everyone has emotions and values, but normal, neurotic, and psychotic people all react differently to them. The mentally healthy person is able to handle his emotions because he knows how to effectively manage himself and the situations arising in his environment.

There are few endeavors in the school curriculum of more importance then the one concerned with the development of mental health. This is admirably set forth in *Mental Health in the Schools:*[24]

> When a realistic perception of self is added to a realistic perception of the world, the possibility of effective and productive interaction is reasonably assured. The mentally healthy person's relationships with people and the world produce certain constructive consequences. Two consequences are especially significant to the school. First, the mentally healthy person perceives reality with minimal distortion and is able to communicate these perceptions effectively. Second, the possession of self-esteem contributes to intellectual functioning.

Despite the fact that sound mental health is related to the family background, the elementary school is in an excellent position to influence boys and girls toward wholesome behavior. The chief reason for this is that personalities are defined early, and children frequent the elementary grades during the most formative years. Early habits of response to teachers and classmates, to simple requests, to

---

[24] Joint Committee Report. *Mental Health in the Schools*, 32 pages, 1966. Available from Chief State School Officers (NEA), 1201 16th St., N.W., Washington, D.C. 20036.

ideas, and the like are established during these elementary school years. The needs of children and the interrelationship of these needs are impressive at this time. Mental health activities must be taught in the light of these needs; children have real feelings even if they are not aware of them at the time. Maslow suggests six groups of needs to keep in mind when teaching. These are: (a) physical needs, (b) safety needs, (c) love needs, including the need for affection, belonging, and mutuality, (d) esteem needs, including the needs for mastery, achievement, recognition, approval, and self-respect, (e) the need to solve problems and have sources of information, and (f) the need for self-realization, including the need to develop a sense of personal identity, to accomplish the tasks for which one is best fitted, and to function at a level in keeping with one's capacities.[25]

Setting up a health curriculum that includes instruction in mental health is both challenging and formidable. It simply is not easy to teach personality adjustment and wholesome participation in the classroom, although this is where the child spends most of his time outside of the home. This is the place where he is often deeply affected by his daily experience. Instruction in mental health, therefore, must permeate the *total* program. In a sense, it is not a subject at all, but a way of teaching. Curriculum cannot be divorced from method.

Since the human personality cannot be compartmentalized, every subject-matter area has experiences and activities, often too subtle to measure, which consciously and unconsciously promote mental health. Every essential skill and learning, when coupled with worthwhile feelings and attitudes, tends to build a wholesome personality. Practically all classroom and school environment activities serve as social science experiences. In the laboratory of the classroom, gymnasium, lunchroom, workshop, and playground are to be found opportunities for attaining emotional maturity. Mental health is fostered through learning the rules of sportsmanship and learning to play together in physical education. It is enhanced when pressures to succeed are relaxed a bit in arithmetic and reading. It is encouraged when scientific appreciations are deeply felt, for personal adjustment in the modern world is more than slightly related to our understanding of scientific advances. Music and art, when taught as recreational or diverting activities to be enjoyed, are rich items in the promotion of mental health. In addition, it seems true that the *way* we teach has much to do with relieving "pressures" and permitting the pupil to work up to his potential. It is interesting to note that in one study comparing pupil anxieties to intelligence, the greater mean anxiety was found in the low IQ group.[26]

In all elementary grades, the program of mental health is geared to preventing maladjustment. The teacher is in the key position for she can check the pupil on a day-to-day basis. She knows his background and can cooperate with health services and the home when cases of deviant behavior arise. Her health instruction includes the overall provision of a desirable classroom atmosphere — one that is conducive to success, security, and understanding. She realizes that mental health is built on a solid foundation and she teaches accordingly. This foundation is depicted realistically as shown in the accompanying illustration.

Instruction in mental health requires that the teacher know the pu-

[25] Maslow, A. H. "Theory of Human Motivation," *Psychological Review*, 50:370–376, 1953.

[26] Feldhuser, John F., and Klausmeir, Herbert J. "Anxiety, Intelligence, and Achievement in Children of Low, Average, and High Intelligence," *Child Development*, June 1962.

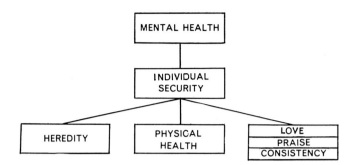

pils, not as entities in the classroom but as living personalities. The instruction, to be effective, must involve each pupil in a number of activities designed to bring out his personality. This is an ongoing process which is further enhanced by the teacher's own mental health. By example and precept she helps children make optimum adjustments in school which tend to be carried over into community living and then to adult life.

Primary grade children love movement. They love to play. In fact, they play because they must. Their running, jumping, and dodging have potential values beyond the purely physical ones. Play contributes immeasurably to personality growth. Play and game situations in the classroom, therefore, have a vital part in building mental-emotional health.

Primary grade instruction and learning activities foster and deal primarily with:

A feeling of belonging
Inspiring self-confidence
Assuming responsibility
A feeling of importance
Making decisions
Realizing limitations
Learning to profit by mistakes
Consideration for others
Making others happy
Affection
Respecting the rights of others
Etiquette
Facing up to fears
Keeping healthy
Pride in family
Getting along with others
New experiences

Intermediate grade instruction and learning activities which promote mental health deal primarily with:

Leadership and ability to follow
Assuming responsibility
Knowledge of how to act
Desirable personality traits
Worthwhile interests
Extending areas of interest
A chance to create something
Accepting oneself
Emotional controls
Interest in others
Making friends
Working together

A number of sources of substantive information and teaching ideas are available relative to the topic of mental health which are readily available to teachers. Both the Child Study Association of America and the American Medical Association have printed materials. Perhaps the most directly useful material is found in *Mental Health in the Classroom*.[27] This supplies an excellent breakdown of mental health concepts, learning experiences, and teaching materials suitable for each grade, kindergarten through college. All concepts and activities are outlined for teacher use and are set up in easy-to-read columns in terms of four categories: personality structure and development, interaction of an individual with others, socioeconomic status and its influence on mental health, and emotional climate in home and classroom.

_____

[27] This is a supplemental issue of the *Journal of School Health*, 33: 1–35, September 1963.

Suggested Activities

BOTH PRIMARY AND INTERMEDIATE LEVELS

1. Create a desirable classroom atmosphere by making the room as cheerful, attractive, and healthful as possible.

2. Observe the relationship between each child and his companions. Where a pupil avoids another, or fails to make friends, attempt to discover the cause.

3. Arrange group activities so that children showing the greatest difficulty in making friends may have a chance to participate.

4. Encourage the confident child to make friends of the timid.

5. Promote good fellowship through the art of listening and of cooperating in carrying out group ideas.

6. Develop opportunities for leadership. Group children so that all have a fair opportunity for recognition. Change groups so that leadership is not restricted to just one or two children whose leadership qualities are already developed.

7. Plan for children to share to a maximum degree in planning classroom activities. Try to give each child the feeling that he has something to contribute.

8. Provide opportunities for original effort. Avoid doing things for children which they can do themselves.

9. Give credit to pupil ideas and suggestions.

10. Challenge the pupil's creative imagination by having available a number of simple craft materials such as wood, fiber, plaster, and metal. Provide a time and place to work with these materials in an atmosphere conducive to creative work.

11. Encourage wholesome curiosity. Aid children who wish to explore and ask questions.

12. Use tests to help judge each pupil's intellectual capacity so that

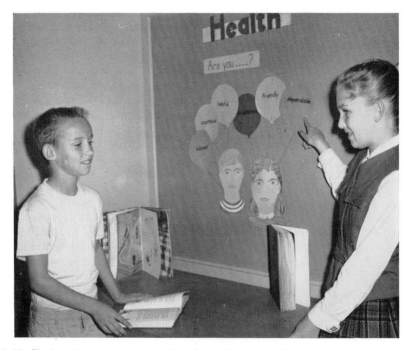

Figure 8–13 The board has been used to motivate the children. They will now use other resources for finding out more about these mental health characteristics. (Courtesy Sylvia Yellen, Alhambra City Schools, Alhambra, Calif.)

neither too much nor too little is expected of him.

13. Try to fit in at least one satisfying experience each day for each child.

14. Create a classroom atmosphere of fairness. One should see that rules and regulations are reasonable. Have only a few rules, but see that all observe them. This is also true in games played in the gymnasium or on the playground.

15. Keep the classroom atmosphere calm and serene, businesslike but unhurried.

16. Build a closer relationship between school and home.

PRIMARY LEVEL

1. Participate in showing and telling things to the class.

2. Make a preschool visit to school (kindergarten).

3. Meet and talk with school personnel such as the school custodian, the principal, or the lunch room manager.

4. Make a list of the qualities admired in other people.

5. Use every opportunity to practice using terms such as "please," and "thank you" (kindergarten or first grade).

6. Share toys and materials.

7. Send cards, pictures, or class letters to classmates who are ill.

8. Read and discuss stories which show thoughtfulness of others.

9. When a new pupil joins the class, plan several ways to make him feel at home.

10. Bring pets to class and talk about how one treats his pets.

11. Work as a group on several projects. Point out to the class what each individual has done so that everyone will appreciate the contributions of others.

12. Encourage serving on committees and taking turns as leader.

13. Let the class know why fatiguing and confining tasks are being alternated with rest periods, creative periods, or physical exercises.

14. Encourage children, especially at the start of the school year, to talk about themselves, what they like most at home, and what they think they will like around school.

15. Cooperate in keeping the room attractive.

16. Choose leaders to see that the dusting, cleaning up, and other responsibilities are carried out. Recognize good work.

17. Plan picnics and school parties. Talk about and demonstrate good manners and decide how everyone should act on the bus, on the street, in the stores, and on visits.

18. Do something about others less fortunate. Secure large scrapbooks from the ten-cent store and let the class cut colorful pictures from magazines and paste them in the books for sick children in the hospital.

19. Talk over taking turns on playground equipment.

20. Read the story *What Frightened Chicken Little?* Develop the point that the chicken scared all of the other animals by telling them the sky was falling before she found out what had really happened. What should she have done? Point out that we are usually afraid of the things we do not understand. Let the pupils tell about the times they have been afraid and what they did. This encourages them to try to understand what makes them afraid (second grade).

21. Permit pupils to talk about their families. Encourage them to tell what they do to keep their home a happy place.

22. Focus attention on something besides the pupils themselves. Get growing plants or a live pet for the classroom.

23. Keep a collection at school of something that each child cherishes.

24. Collect and post pictures of

people showing kindness, and of happy children and families.

25. Draw cartoons of various facial expressions.

INTERMEDIATE LEVEL

1. Write, tell, read, and discuss stories about emotions. Particular instances of interest may be dramatized.

2. Discuss spontaneous situations that arise to develop understanding of emotions of other children. Use interesting stories involving emotional problems to stimulate discussions on the importance of controlling our emotions.

3. Develop an understanding of how our emotions affect people physically.

4. Participate in creative activities, such as finger painting, drawing, painting, clay modeling and rhythmics, as acceptable means of expressing emotions. "Talk it out" with sympathetic listeners.

5. Send a sunshine package to someone who is ill. This may contain cards, pictures, and various objects presented by the class.

6. Share hobbies. Have pupils tell about and demonstrate their special hobby before the class (sixth grade).

7. Make up some everyday problems, and give correct and incorrect ways of solving them. Also use "open-end stories" regarding a problem, using class names.

8. Choose a class hospitality committee and set up a procedure for operation.

9. Have each class member pick out his worst habit or worst fault and tell how he hopes to overcome it.

10. Set up a question box and encourage questions concerning worries and fears of class members. "What's on Your Mind?" box precipitates some excellent discussion.

11. Hear reports on famous handicapped persons such as Keller, Edison,

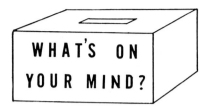

and Baruch, who have succeeded in spite of their handicaps.

12. Have several boys and girls tell how someone helped them to feel better or to gain self-confidence (sixth grade).

13. Collect newspaper clippings depicting cases of mental problems. Note, also, the numerous articles which appear in the paper and have to do with personal unhappiness. In the course of a week, check to see if news items of an unhappy nature are more or less prevalent than those of a happy nature (sixth grade).

14. Have each pupil make a list of several things he likes about (a) girls and (b) boys. Make a similar list of dislikes. Do the likes outbalance the dislikes?

15. Tie in historical and other social studies topics with such items as bigotry and prejudices.

16. Emphasize good sportsmanship and fair play. This may be done through a project on accident prevention in the school and on the playground.

17. List the characteristics of people who are able to get along well with others. Discuss famous people, their lives, achievements, and characteristics. Show the effect of a good personality as a positive force in living together harmoniously.

18. Show how fatigue or illness can make us "fussy" or irritable.

19. Talk over the fact that we all like to succeed and that everyone is good at something.

20. As a class, "adopt" a younger child who needs help. This should help encourage an awareness of, and

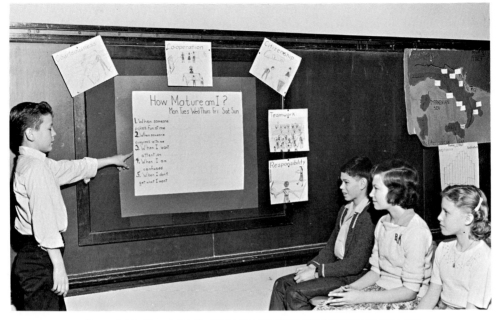

Figure 8–14   Discussing mental health. (Courtesy Cincinnati Public Schools.)

sensitivity to, the feelings and difficulties of others less fortunate.

21. Select, plan, make, and participate as project or committee members. This permits the pupils to see the other fellow's viewpoint and encourage the development of self-reliance. Identify qualities of character which may not be apparent from outward appearances.

22. Read and learn the poem *If* by Rudyard Kipling.

9. Sex and Family Living Education

Desirable Outcomes (Primary Level)

To understand the need for a happy home and to appreciate one's own place in it.

To acquire a vocabulary and a limited amount of information with which one can understand about the beginning of life and the care of the young.

Desirable Outcomes (Intermediate Level)

To understand and appreciate the role of each family member in maintaining a happy home.

To understand and appreciate the cooperative and unique contributions of both sexes to society.

To acquire wholesome sex adjustment through an understanding of how life begins, how physical growth advances, and the relationship of boy and girl behavior to social living.

Comments

It takes the organized and combined efforts of the home, school, and other community groups to educate the child of today. The well-adjusted child with the wholesome personality is generally that way because he comes from a good home—a home in which he is familiar with and actually appreciates his role in living with his parents and other children in the family. The best education for family living probably takes place in the house itself under the education of sound and sympathetic parents. Over the years, and with the vast complexities of present day society, educators have come to realize that not all homes function in a way to promote optimum family living. In fact, some of them promote anything but optimum family living. As indicated at length in Chapter 7, the school has a certain responsibility here. School people argue that if something is good for one child, it should be good for all children. Decades ago John Dewey wrote, "What the best and wisest parent wants for his own child, that must the community want for all of its children."

Much of the instruction in the grades may indirectly involve family activities. Children are frequently asked to bring items from home. They continually "bombard" the parents and older children with questions having a bearing on school happenings. Home responses to school questions have much to do with successful school learnings. The child from the well and happy family comes to class better equipped to produce than the child from a less stable home. Elementary education, therefore, is vitally concerned with the health, economic, social, cultural, and spiritual phases of family life (Figure 8–15).

Interest in sex occurs at all ages. Whether sex education is formal or informal, a part of the home life or a part of the "gang talk" on the street corner, it is of vital concern to all growing boys and girls. Knowledges and appreciations in this area are every bit as important in terms of future behavior as they are in other health areas. More and more research indicates that the school is in an excellent position to carry out a sound sex education program. Here children gain values from peer-group discussions under competent leadership which cannot be parentally duplicated.

Since attitudes are formed at an early age, it is important to start sex education at a time prior to the building up of personal inhibitions—inhibitions which tend to limit frank discussion. Foster has shown in a study of age and grade level inhibitions that children at the fifth grade level or below normally do not possess reticence toward matters of sex. He states that,

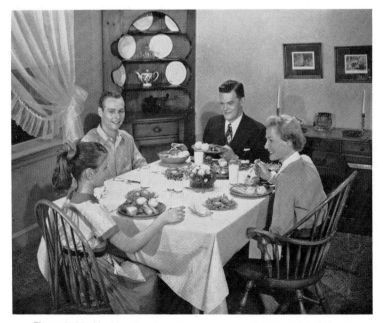

Figure 8–15   Mealtime is a happy time. (Courtesy National Dairy Council.)

"only if sex education is delayed . . . will the feeling of improperness influence his thinking since the child will have incorporated all of the fears and incorrect thoughts of his peers and perhaps his family. . . . It is better to be a year early in our provision of sex education during pre-adolescence than to be a day too late in adolescence."[28]

After doing continuous research relative to the feelings of people in the community, Dr. Wetherill of the San Diego City Schools concluded that every research effort elicited great interest in sex education and confidence in the schools to carry it on.

> It seemed that everyone we talked with and everything we did pointed toward approval for sex education in the schools. We could find those who questioned it, but after some briefing they always became proponents for the idea. We discovered that disapproval came only from people who did not understand the purpose of a program of sex education. Certain people we thought would certainly be against it were often those who were really the most enlightened and had the best attitudes toward sex, especially if they thought someone had the courage to try to improve attitudes toward it.[29]

The success of the San Diego program of sex education, since it began in 1937, is due in part to good public relations. There was an informed public over the years, and at no time did the 128 schools get too far ahead.[30]

It is evident that there need be no apprehension about having sex in-

struction at any grade level. There are, however, a number of fundamental considerations in setting up the program. Prior to getting under way, one should secure the approval of the school principal. And since this is a topic in which most parents and members of the clergy are quite interested, it is well to secure the support of the community. In many places this has been successfully accomplished through the efforts of the local elementary school Parent-Teachers Association. It is becoming common practice to invite parents to the school to witness pilot programs in operation. For several years the fifth-grade parents in the Evanston, Illinois schools have been encouraged to sit in with their children as the reproductive unit is covered. Although primary grade teachers need very little extra preparation to instruct in this area, it is not uncommon to find in-service training programs designed to improve both primary and intermediate grade teaching. In fact, carefully selected and well-prepared teachers increase support and cooperation of the public in this program. This has been successfully demonstrated in the Bedford Public Schools (Mass.) in which the Center for Sex and Family Living Education has explored this teaching area for some time.

The question of what to teach and how to teach it is the next consideration. Everyday classroom experiences are suitable for integrating information about the beginning of life and the care of the young. At an early age children are curious about life in all of its many manifestations—how it originates, how it grows, and how it perpetuates itself. Children's questions are generally not difficult to answer, but they do require that the teacher have the ability to answer them honestly, unemotionally, and accurately. Instruction must be conducted with dignity and discretion. Sex is a life

---

[28] Foster, Greg R. "Sex Information vs. Sex Education: Implications for School Health," *Journal of School Health,* 37:248–250, May 1967.

[29] Wetherill, G. G. "Accepting Responsibility for Sex Education," *Journal of School Health,* 30:107–110, March 1960.

[30] Wetherill, G. G. "Sex Education in the Public Schools," *Journal of School Health,* 31: 235–239, September 1961.

function that is normal, clean, respectable, and admirable. Here are some guiding principles to follow:[31]

Sex education in schools should be integrated with the total health education program at all grade levels. It should not be singled out for separate or undue emphasis.

Example on the part of parents and teachers is far more effective than precept.

Sex education should be couched in terms easily understood by the child and should make use of examples within his experience.

Sex information should not be forced upon the uninterested child but should be adapted to his maturity level at each stage of growth.

Sex should be presented in a dignified vocabulary.

Sex should be taught positively by showing its nobility in terms of creative drive and family happiness rather than negatively through the enumeration of horrible examples of immorality.

Sex anatomy and physiology (upper grades) should be treated as just another body system; due allowance must be made for modesty.

The many relations of sex to all phases of normal, private and public life must be discussed in an objective manner.

In the first three grades the children ask questions regarding where they came from and how boys and girls grow. The teacher endeavors to handle these questions in a matter-of-fact manner—the same manner used in introducing new units in other subjects. The best approach appears to be through human life situations as they arise and as they become important to the pupils. How a six year old boy should act when going to a girl playmate's birthday party is a human life situation and thus part of sex education. When a class is talking about kittens and puppies, some child is certain to ask, "Where did Mrs. Jones get her baby?" This is an honest question asked without emotion and no less natural than "Why do the birds sing?" or "What makes a tree grow?" To answer by saying that the stork bought the baby or to put the child off by changing the topic is hardly in keeping with good instruction. Children quickly learn that a direct answer has been avoided and that there is something embarrassing and mysterious about the topic. Therefore, the primary grader who asked about where Mrs. Jones got her baby should be simply told that it grew inside the mother's body until it was old enough to come out—just as in the case of the kittens and puppies. Children like pets and babies; they have them in their own homes, and they enjoy talking about how they look, smell, and act. This is a wholesome part of growing up. The old wives' tale about the stork bringing the baby or buying it at the hospital only causes unnecessary embarrassment in later years when the child discovers the real truth.

A very practical book, especially useful to teachers, is *What to Tell Your Children About Sex*, prepared by the Child Study Association of America. It is written in question-and-answer form, and each stage of child development from infancy through adolescence is covered in separate sections. Each of these sections discusses the kinds of questions children ask about sex, and offers many suggestions for an approach to answering these questions.[32] Here are questions

---

[31] Adapted from the Joint Committee, National Education Association and American Medical Association. *Health Education,* revised 1967. National Education Association, 1201 Sixteenth St., N.W., Washington, D.C. 20036.

[32] Child Study Association of America. *What to Tell Your Child about Sex.* New York: Arco Publishing Co., 1961.

asked most frequently by both boys and girls:

Kindergarten to Primary Age

"Where does a baby come from?"

"Why is Daddy's penis bigger than mine?"

"Does it hurt to have a baby?"

"Why can't men have babies?"

"Why do grownups have hair on their bodies?"

"Why do women have breasts?"

"How does a baby get inside the mother?"

"How does the baby breathe inside the mother?"

"Why do I have a 'belly-button'?"

"Why does the mother get so big?"

"How big is a baby when he is born?"

Intermediate Age

"What is menstruation?"

"When does menstruation begin?"

"When does menstruation end?"

"Does menstruation hurt?"

"Why do boys have 'wet dreams'?"

"How is intercourse carried out?"

"What is the male sperm like?"

"What is the female egg like?"

"How does the cell turn into a baby?"

"Why does a baby look like its parents?"

"What causes twins?"

"What causes birthmarks?"

"How is the baby born?"

It is significant to note that every one of these questions is asked by pre-adolescent children at an age when straightforward answers are effective and accepted as matter-of-fact.

Intermediate graders can ask keen questions calling for more detailed answers. Levine found that sixth and seventh graders want to know about miscarriage, abortion, and artificial insemination.[33] They ask: "Why do some girls develop before others?";

"Is something wrong with me? I like sports better than going with girls";

"Sometimes in the movies or on television, a woman tells her husband, 'We're going to have a baby!' Why didn't he know about it?" Research indicates that intermediate grade children are getting emancipated from adults earlier and earlier. Some 85 per cent of these children get their sex information from other than the home, church, or school. Oberteuffer reviews the three well-known approaches to classroom instruction: (a) through animal and plant life (the "birds, bees, and butterflies" approach); (b) through the anatomy and physiology involved; and (c) through human life situations. The best approach is through the life situations as they arise and become important. There are times when some reference to anatomy and physiology may be necessary, but as a rule this is only incidental to the solution of the problem.

Intermediate pupils need to continue their early experiences in social friendships—manners and courtesies between sexes. They need to understand the unique functions of boys and girls, men and women, in the school and at home. Early lessons in the influence of heredity and of the mental and physiological changes attendant upon growth are also valuable. In one public school in upper New York state a typical sixth grade series of lessons (with parents' permission) includes the reason for sex, anatomy of both sexes, physiology, hormones, growth patterns, menstruation, physical changes, pregnancy, masturbation, and nocturnal emissions. Specific features are used and selected books are available in the school library.[34] Here is an outline of five lessons for sixth graders from the San Diego Public Schools

[33] Levine, Milton I. "Sex Education in the Public Elementary and High School Curriculum," *Journal of School Health*, 37:30–39, January 1967.

[34] Alden, Carl B., and Blanchard, Jane. "Experiences in Giving a Course in Sex Education," *Journal of School Health*, 32:127–131, April 1962.

Teaching Monograph. Note how vital the topics are and how they develop:

LESSON 1

How we grow, differences in the growth patterns of boys and girls, responsibilities of growing up, the importance of caution with strangers, how to choose the right friends, your appearance, glands that are responsible for growth and changes in our bodies, good attitudes, and the right names of the body's organs and functions. Questions and answers.

LESSON 2

Films on animal reproduction (The Sunfish, The Snapping Turtle, Snakes Are Interesting). Questions and answers. This is a fine impersonal introduction to human reproduction; it helps boys and girls understand that in most animals a male cell and a female egg must join before a new life can begin.

LESSON 3

Read a short book or monograph on human reproduction.[35] Questions and answers.

LESSON 4

(Girls) Review the sex organs, discuss menstruation, discuss reason for body changes, sex relations, and self-control (a film may be used).[36]

LESSON 5

(Boys) Discuss glandular changes, growth of sex organs, formation of sperm, seminal emissions, masturbation, reasons for body changes, and

use of self-control. Questions and answers.

LESSON 6

Show the film Human Growth to review and clarify previous lessons and to set the stage for further discussion of such things as strengthening right attitudes toward sex and growing up, correct terminology, cell division, twins, sex determination, heredity, boy-girl relationships, moral and spiritual values. Question and answer period.

For a review of specific primary and intermediate grade sex and family living education topics and suggested concepts see Chapter 7 (p. 162). These ideas, combined with the source materials in Chapter 11, supplement the discussion here. See also Sex Education U.S.A.: A Community Approach, a filmstrip–record–manual unit designed to present the sex education curriculum, published by Guidance Associates of Harcourt, Brace, and World (1968).

There exists in Cleveland, Ohio, the now famous Cleveland Health Museum. It is unique among educational agencies in the way it has informed the community about personal and public health. Sex and family living education is the mainstay of this institution. The visitors at every age are motivated not by a love of esthetics as in an art museum or a curiosity about nature as in a natural history museum, but by a strong interest in their own physical and mental well-being. It is in this museum that sex has a unique setting, and it is in this area that the museum has made a lasting contribution over the years. Within 50 miles of Cleveland there are a large number of Ohio counties consisting of hundreds of schools that make at least one museum trip a year for a lesson on human reproduction. Elementary schoolchildren study the pictures and incomparably fine models for an ex-

---

[35] One of the finest booklets written, with colored animated drawings, is distributed by the New York State Health Department, Albany, N.Y. Entitled The Gift of Life, it has the support of Catholic, Protestant, and Hebrew clergy.

[36] The excellent filmstrip, Confidence Because–You Understand Menstruating, may be obtained free for permanent use from Personal Products Corporation, Milltown, N.J.

perience conducive to a high retention of facts in an atmosphere with a minimum of emotional trauma. So high does interest in these exhibits run, in fact, that one often finds a youngster explaining them to his parents on a Sunday afternoon following his class visit.

The famous birth series models are now available for purchase from the Cleveland Museum. These lightweight, durable polystyrene models present the growth and development of a baby sculptured in three dimensions for teaching purposes.[37] They are a superb teaching aid.

There will be times when it seems necessary to separate boys and girls, particularly in the fifth or sixth grade when a discussion of menstruation arises. As a general rule, sex instruction should be in mixed classes and the materials and methods of instruction adapted to the situation. When a topic is peculiar to a single sex, it might be more convenient to meet the sexes separately. Menstruation, for example, is so full of mystery and misconceptions that both preadolescent boys and girls should know something about it. There should be open classroom discussion regarding superstition, primitive beliefs regarding "uncleanliness" associated with menstruation, and the fear of blood. This topic is a normal part of growing children's lives. Mature attitudes begin early when the need for teaching first occurs. So we teach the life cycle and the menstrual cycle, that menstruation is normal, and we answer the question, "What is happening inside?"

Three very good films for fifth and sixth grade use are:

The Story of Menstruation. Kimberly-Clark Corporation, Neenah, Wis., color, sound, ten minutes. Delightful Disney animated film, showing causes and characteristics of menstruation.

It's Wonderful Being a Girl. Personal Products, Milltown, N.J., color, sound, 20 minutes. Tells the story of menstruation and presents a fine philosophy for being a girl.

Girl To Woman. Churchill Films, 662 N. Robertson Boulevard, Los Angeles, Calif., color, sound, 16 minutes. Shown are adolescent changes from physical growth processes to complete glandular development.

An especially useful booklet entitled *World of a Girl* is distributed (free) by the Scott Paper Company in Philadelphia. It is designed for fifth and sixth grade girls, to enable them to understand and respond wholesomely to the miraculous changes that begin their grownup life. A detailed teacher's guide is available for use with the booklet.

Another highly successful booklet for girls is *Accent on You,* distributed (free) by Tampax, Incorporated, 161 E. 42nd Street, New York, N.Y. 10017.

Chapter 11, which deals with source materials, contains a number of films useful for primary and intermediate grade pupils. For the primary grades, *Baby Animals* (McGraw-Hill Text Films), *Farm Babies and Their Mothers* (Film Associates), and *Human and Animal Beginnings* (E. C. Brown Trust Foundation) are especially well done and effective with children. For older pupils the films *Growing Up* (Coronet Films) and *The Miracle of Reproduction* (Sid Davis Productions) are noteworthy.

Suggested Activities

PRIMARY LEVEL

1. Keep a pet cat with kittens or a dog with young puppies in the classroom for several days for general observation.

2. Answer simple questions with simple answers. Give only what is sufficient to satisfy the child.

---

[37] Cleveland Health Museum, 8911 Euclid Avenue, Cleveland, Ohio 44106.

3. Visit the zoo, a health museum, or any place where baby animals may be observed and talked about.

4. Visit a local dairy farmer shortly after the birth of a calf. Children never fail to appreciate such a visit.

5. Keep a pair of canaries and observe the building of the nest and laying and hatching of eggs.

6. Raise guppies. These live-bearing fish are inexpensive and most interesting. The young may be seen inside the female late in pregnancy. Collect tadpoles or grow eggs in the spring.

7. Talk about family vacations and ways of having a good time at home.

8. Build a list of ways that children can help to make home more pleasant. Such a list should be posted with art work to illustrate this type of activity in action. A few examples of items that might appear on the list are:

Run errands willingly
Care for younger children
Come on the first call so Mother does not have to raise her voice or get angry
Help Mother with the cleaning
Hang up our clothes
Pick up our toys
Share good stories with the family

9. Talk about the effect of a happy home at mealtime, at bedtime.

10. Read a pleasant story or poem to the class about family living and good times.

We scrub the big potatoes
That Mother wants to bake
We pour the milk and water,
We cut the bread and cake.
When supper's almost ready,
We rest a little while,
And think of something funny
That will make the family smile.

INTERMEDIATE LEVEL

1. Raise tropical fish or collect caterpillars for the room terrarium. Watch the development of the cocoon.

2. Show pictures of tiny babies. Discuss special care needed for small babies. Listen to student experiences.

3. Examine charts of high grade animals such as certain breeds of cows or dogs. Study the characteristics looked for in breeding these animals. Seek help from a 4-H club leader.

4. View the Walt Disney movie film, *The Story of Menstruation*. This may be borrowed without charge from Kimberly-Clark Corporation, Neenah, Wis. This is a well-done ten minute sound and color film.

5. Study the teacher guide on menstruation and menstrual health, *From Fiction to Fact*, published by Tampax, Incorporated, New York. This is filled with excellent teaching suggestions, for boys and girls together and separately. See also the booklet, *Accent on You*, published by and distributed free by the same company.

6. Discuss (with fifth and sixth grade girls) the question of good menstrual health as a necessary part of a girl's growth into womanhood. Clear up misconceptions relative to cramps, water taboos, exercise restrictions, and the period itself. (Obtain illustrative materials from Personal Products Corp., Milltown, N. J.; Tampax Incorporated, and Kimberly-Clark Corp.)

7. Set up a question box to be used, especially during the unit on family relations. This encourages the pupils who do not feel free or comfortable enough to ask questions in class (sixth grade).

8. Develop an appreciation for the human body. Teach the intricacies and the beauty and the mechanism. Without stress, indicate the marvelous role of each sex.

9. Follow the NEA–AMA booklet, *A Story about You*, and hold a question-answer period (boys and girls).

10. Use a good up-to-date textbook to answer many of the children's questions on how the human body is made and how it functions. Stress function and its place in one's family and society.

11. Use current events at the local and state levels to provide a basis for a discussion of human relations. This should be geared to developing desirable attitudes toward being a good friend and being a good family member.

12. Discuss family vacations. Have the pupils tell what they like about their father's job. Have them add to this what they would like to do to earn a living in the future.

13. Talk over the relationship of family health to family happiness. Show also how fear, prejudice, outbursts of anger, and other similar items keep a home in a state of unpleasantness. List socially acceptable ways to counteract these feelings.

10. Community Health

Desirable Outcomes (Primary Level)

To understand how one person's health habits can affect the health of other people.

To develop positive attitudes toward maintaining and promoting community health.

To accept reasonable responsibility in keeping the school, home, and community environment neat and clean.

To be familiar with many of the community services having a bearing on his welfare.

Desirable Outcomes Intermediate Level)

To understand the health services of the community and to use them when necessary.

To understand the contributions made by doctors and dentists, and to follow their directions carefully.

To understand about having periodic dental and medical examinations.

To value the services of numerous community professional and non-professional workers.

To appreciate the need for hospital services.

To understand the contributions made to health by the garbage collectors, street cleaners, milkmen, physicians, nurses, dentists, opticians, and others.

To understand about safe sources of water supply and how the local community keeps its water supply safe for drinking.

To develop a responsibility for promoting school and community health through cooperative and independent activities.

Comments

In a sense there may be little in the way of anything new under this category of instruction, for community health is so broad in nature that it has already been referred to in some degree under such topics as Personal Cleanliness and Appearance, Dental Health, Safety and First Aid, and Sex and Family Living Education. In many elementary schools community health is taught as a separate subject matter in health. And, of course, it is taught very well as a part of a whole unit dealing with everyday life in the community.

All too often younger children feel small and insignificant. They sometimes feel as if they were truly "seen and not heard." Every now and then a teacher notes a certain apathy or lack of enthusiasm for some school-community idea. In seeking its cause she discovers an attitude that adults often possess toward their privilege to vote, namely, "What good can my single effort produce?" Needless to add, boys and girls need a chance to prove to themselves how effective their ventures may be in improving the lot of their fellow men in the community.

To make community health education meaningful, one must do more than visit the local establishments such as bakeries, water works, and garbage disposal plants. There has to be some extensive thinking and action associated with the project. Very often a problematical situation calling for investigation and preplanning is necessary to arouse the class to see the value of a particular community health item. Certainly it is hardly a treat in many school systems today to be taken on a field trip to see the local organizations, but a sixth grade visit to a readily accessible mosquito breeding water hole may challenge the class to do something about it. Such was the case in a Georgia community a few years ago. A project planned and initiated by schoolchildren blossomed into an endeavor by the whole community and greatly reduced the mosquito threat in the whole area. Even the pupil with the poorest memory would have trouble forgetting this kind of experience. And there are other activities along the same line. The report of a fifth grade committee on the cleanliness of rest rooms in local eating establishments would normally be received with a good amount of interest and enthusiasm, particularly if the report were to be followed up in some way.

Currently, the topic of pollution is a major community health concern for youth and adults alike. It is being attacked from a number of angles, chief among which is education. Moreover, elementary-age children are quite capable of understanding the problem and of carrying prevention information out into the local community. A fine discussion among fifth or sixth graders can be initiated by responding to the extreme view of a Los Angeles meteorologist:

> All civilizations will pass away, not from a sudden cataclysm like a nuclear war, but from general suffocation in its own wastes.[38]

---

[38] Berland, Theodore. "Our Dirty Sky," *Today's Health*, 44:40–42, March 1966.

When it comes to garbage and refuse disposal, clean air, and water pollution, children have a real concern. They know first-hand when the air is odorous, and they want safe water for drinking and clean water for their own boating and swimming. Thus, they are capable of getting the facts, telling the story, and influencing others to take action. Many up-to-date and informative teaching pamphlets are available each year from the U.S. Public Health Service and the U.S. Department of the Interior.

Whether community health is taught indirectly or directly, it is a potential contributor to the basic understandings sought through such educational aims as self-realization and civic responsibility. One does not fully realize himself until he feels responsible for the welfare of others in his home town. And one does not come of age in this realization until he gains a certain satisfaction from actually participating in community projects.

Suggested Activities
PRIMARY LEVEL

1. Write the following question on the board and ask for suggestions:
HOW CAN I MAKE MY TOWN A MORE PLEASANT PLACE IN WHICH TO LIVE?
Here are some of the expected answers:

> Do unto others as you would have them do unto you.
> Do not throw paper and other items out the window for someone else to pick up.
> Do not leave cans or bottles on the public beach or picnic area.
> Stay home when you have a cold.
> Use sprays such as DDT to help eliminate flies and other harmful insects.
> Help keep the house clean and sanitary.

2. Ask the class to take home the following statement to think about overnight:

HEALTH IN OUR COMMUNITY IS THE RESULT OF THE WORK OF MANY PEOPLE.

Properly carried out, this may involve parents and others in the family and, therefore, become a far more valuable experience than it may appear to be on the surface (second or third grade).

3. Read about how colds spread through a community. Many school health textbooks are quite suitable for this activity. After doing the reading, call on a pupil to tell one way to avoid a cold. Then call on another pupil to give a reason why the previous pupil's statement is true or false. Do this several times.

4. Introduce the topic of safe drinking water by showing how the microscope works and how it is used in the town or city. Prepare a slide showing plant life.

5. Show a large picture of a lake, reservoir, nearby stream, or river. Ask the class if they think it is safe to drink the water? Safe to swim in? Shortages of clean water affect the life of us all. Drinking water is becoming less and less palatable because of pollutants in the water supply. The study of water pollution is a timely topic everywhere.

6. To maintain interest in sickness in the community, discuss how sick people feel when they have to stay at home away from their good friends. Select a sick classmate to whom the children can send a "treasure chest." Build a pasteboard box to look like a pirate's treasure chest. Have the class make the items to go in it, such as gifts carved from soap, balsa wood, or clay. Flowers may be made, poems created, or letters written.

7. Talk about and illustrate with pictures and stick men drawings the various kinds of occupations in the community and how they have a bearing on one's health.

8. Plan together how elementary schoolchildren can promote good health in town or city.

9. Ask the question: "How is the life of our town affected by the extremes of weather?" Post pictures collected by pupils depicting how the different plants and animals protect themselves against bad weather. Show the effects of unusual weather conditions. How do these things affect the fire departments, police departments, public works, doctors, and nurses?

10. Have a child who has recently been to a hospital tell the class something about life there. Look for misconceptions picked up from parents and others about the way hospitals function.

11. Visit a large grocery store. Prepare for this by having each pupil bring from home the name of one relatively inexpensive item to be purchased during the class visit. This will work with over 90 per cent of the pupils bringing the necessary money to purchase a particular food product. While at the store, ask the manager to show the class how perishable foods are stored and how cleanliness is practiced.

12. Talk about safe and sanitary places to play in the community.

13. Show how disease is spread and tell why one must stay away from school, theaters, and other meeting places when he is ill. Illustrate the spread of disease by blowing on dandelion seeds. Ask the class what is wrong with this story:

> John went to the movies and was asked by the ticket collector if he was doing the right thing by being there during school hours. John replied, "It's all right, I have the measles."

14. Clean up the classroom and follow this with voluntary statements from individual pupils on how they keep their homes and yards clean.

INTERMEDIATE LEVEL

1. Receive a visitor from the local health department. Let this person tell about all the interesting jobs to be

done. (Many people are available for this. In the small city there are only a few workers, but in a city like New York there are some five thousand workers in the health department.)

2. Build a series of eight or ten models depicting *What Our Community Should Do to Keep Everyone Healthy*. Assign several pupils to each model. When they are completed, exhibit them in the school library or other appropriate place. Following are some examples of models:

    a. *Maintain health records:* Show a clerk in an office pulling out a file drawer in a file cabinet.

    b. *Collect garbage:* Show a garbage man carrying a garbage can from a house to the truck.

    c. *Control communicable diseases:* Show several homes on a street. At the door of one home depict a man hanging a "Contagious Disease" sign on the front door.

    d. *Inspect restaurants and dairies:* Show a clean restaurant with people sitting and eating at tables, or show a scene depicting dishes being washed. A dairy barn scene would also be a good choice.

    e. *Keep drinking water safe:* Show a pumping station or model of a filter system. Or simply attach a real water faucet to a large piece of plywood with a model of a hand holding a glass just below it.

3. Ask the class how much they know about their home sewage system. Where does their sewage go? Does the town or city have a sewage treatment plant? Does raw sewage or treated sewage empty into any stream or body of water? If so, what might the class do about it?

4. Discuss garbage and trash disposal, incinerators, kitchen grinders, and sanitary land fill. Show the relationship of all of this with pleasant looking areas on the outskirts of the community where there are no dumps with bad odors, flies, rats, or cockroaches.

5. Investigate why the rat is a menace to man in any community. Originate ideas relative to rats feeding on good foods (eggs, fruits, poultry, vegetables, and grains in homes and stores), starting fires by gnawing electrical wires, and spreading typhus fever.

6. Prepare posters for placement in community stores, bus stations, banks, and business establishments. Some titles which suggest a picture are:

Do Not Jaywalk in (name of town)
This Community Is What You Make It!
Treat Others Courteously
Smile—Be Friendly and Say "Hello"
Don't Eat at Unclean Eating Places and They Will Be Forced to Clean Up

7. After some work on the topic of community health, ask the pupils to write some statements in support of the sentence at the top of p. 259.

A RAT
                                      can climb
a brick wall, swim half a mile under water, walk a wire, swing from beam to beam of an old ceiling, squeeze through a hole a half-inch square, make a two-foot standing high jump or a three-foot running high jump, and learn to avoid poisons.

THE WELFARE OF THE MAJORITY IS RELATED TO THE PRACTICES OF THE MINORITY.

8. Make up some "Who Am I?" quiz questions about health heroes. For example, "I am given credit for a method of purifying milk and it is named after me."

9. Using an appropriate dictionary, look up the meaning of words such as chlorine, fluorine, filter, pasteurized, disinfected, epidemic, swab, septic tank, reservoir, homogenized, bacteriology, abscess.

10. Divide the class into "Health Inspection Committees." Assign committee members according to personal choice. Permit the separate committees to survey the community and report back to class. Topics for survey may include:

Recreational opportunities for elementary age children
Cleanliness and handwashing facilities in city eating places
Cleanliness and handwashing facilities in the school
Safety hazards in and about the city
Cleanliness of city streets

11. Discuss the various agencies in town that are working to make the town a safer and cleaner place in which to live.

12. Bring some mosquito wrigglers in water to class. Pour some oil on these and notice the results.

13. Consider some of the new homes being built in the community. Make a list of the various inspections that a new house must pass and the reasons for these.

14. What are some of the standards that owners of swimming pools, dairies, and laundries must meet? Appoint specific committees to look into this.

15. Study air pollution abatement. Use the encyclopedia to see what has been accomplished in other countries besides the United States.

11. Alcohol, Tobacco, and Drugs

Desirable Outcomes (Intermediate Level)

To understand that tobacco and alcoholic beverages do not contribute to the growth of growing boys and girls.

To understand the need for moderation in adult smoking and drinking practices as one means of preventing cardiorespiratory, digestive, and mental illness.

To understand the use of sleep promoting and pain killing drugs, and the possible hazards involved.

To appreciate the role of mental health as it has a bearing on such things as excessive smoking, alcoholism, and drug addiction.

Comments

In some schools alcohol and tobacco are scheduled for discussion in the food unit; here they may be considered in terms of the effect on growth and efficiency of the human organism. There is nothing wrong with doing this, but there is evidence to indicate that this topic is big enough to warrant separate consideration. This is more than a growth problem for children; it is something that observing children know much about, and involves people from all walks of life and circumstances.

Actually, education about alcohol, tobacco, coffee, tea, and the like is not new. In 1882 Vermont passed active legislation adding temperance teaching to the public school curriculum with "... special prominence to the effects of alcoholic drinks, stimulants, and narcotics upon the human system."[39] Four years later 18 states and the District of Columbia had essentially the same requirements.

Alcohol and tobacco education have

---

[39] As quoted in J. E. Foster, "Scientific Temperance Instruction in the Schools," *Proceedings and Addresses*. National Education Association, 1886, Salem, 1887, p. 83.

sometimes been labeled as controversial subjects. This is no longer true. Today, there is wide classroom discussion relative to the implications of drinking and smoking.

Alcohol Education. There is an increasing amount of evidence to suggest that a social change is occurring and that alcoholic beverages are becoming a part of the American culture. The Government-financed report, *Alcohol Problems: A Report to the Nation* (New York: Oxford University Press, 1967) recommends that a "deliberate effort" be made to make drinking acceptable — if practiced in moderation — almost anywhere, including at church-sponsored functions. It is pointed out, after all, that 70 per cent of all Americans drink, and that 40 per cent drink "regularly." The problem arises when drinking gets out of hand. One-third of all arrests in the United States are for public drunkenness. Thousands of persons with serious drinking problems are committed to mental institutions each year. Almost half of the automobile drivers involved in fatal accidents have had high concentrations of alcohol in their systems. The report makes it clear that the alcohol problems are more likely to be reduced through increased educational efforts — through prevention, not abstinence. Thus, the teacher's task is to bring out the factual information regarding excessive drinking and to stress responsible actions, rather than to moralize about the "evils of drink" to children whose parents probably enjoy the cocktail hour every evening.

The secret, of course, is to teach alcohol education at an early age (the maturity of the intermediate level pupil) in such a way that the readily normative drinking models, i.e., television, parents, and friends, are shown to be part of the American scene. Although research shows that the greater the number of drinking models, the more likely youngsters are to drink, it is still possible to point out

that some things are saved until one is older — just as driving the family car is saved until later years. In the "permissive society," of course, it may always be difficult to say just when one is mature enough to learn to drink moderately. Today, there appears to be no clear-cut level when adulthood begins — so children assume adult roles early. They copy adults at an earlier and earlier age. Often they seem to be trained for adulthood by exclusion from adulthood. Thus, by age 11 about 50 per cent of the boys have tasted their first drink.

Alcohol education must be acquired in relation to a particular situation; school activity must be related to life outside the school. Swimming can be dangerous, but it is taught in order to survive in the water. Drinking too can be dangerous, but it may be possible to teach how to drink safely — with personal and social responsibility. Or, as one educator put it, let us teach "survival in our cocktail culture." In this manner it may be possible in the years ahead to reduce the 6,500,000 figure of persons suffering from alcoholism.

The elementary school has a responsibility in this area chiefly because of pupil needs, that is, the "awakening interest." Fifth and sixth graders tend to become very curious about drinking. What does beer taste like? Will whiskey make you feel "funny"? How do people feel? Why do they lose control of their automobiles under the influence of alcohol? Do doctors use brandy or whiskey as a stimulant for sick people? These and a hundred similar questions are being asked today by children of this age level. Stimulants and narcotics are everywhere. Some children have been drinking tea and coffee for years. Many families have beer or wine with the evening meal. Cocktails are served in the home. People drink and drive without giving it more than a passing thought. Moreover, growing boys and girls are extremely observant of these things.

Because so many parents drink, the topic is a difficult one for the teacher to handle satisfactorily. She must not leave the impression that to take a drink is "criminal" or a mark of the "man about town." What she says must lead to abstinence during the growing years and moderation or temperance in the later years. Since a high percentage of adults drink, one should not teach that anything short of total abstinence is reprehensible. Stress the harmful effects, but point out that some people use alcohol in moderation and without any complications.

For the teacher, there exists a number of fine sources of instructional materials relative to alcohol: the Rutgers University Center for Alcohol Studies, the U.S. Public Health Service, the U.S. Office of Education, the Institute of Mental Health, Alcoholics Anonymous, and the National Council on Alcoholism.[40]

Smoking Education. There is no longer any question whether the young people who are now taking up smoking will suffer more illness and die earlier than those who do not. According to the 1967 U.S. Public Health Service publication, *The Health Consequences of Smoking,* approximately one-third of all deaths among men between the ages of 35 and 60 are "excess" deaths, in the sense that they would not have occurred as early as they did if cigarette smokers had the same death rates as non-smokers.[41] Also, there are other risks related to

chronic bronchopulmonary disease, peptic ulcers, and coronary heart disease. In the latter, the early death rate for smokers is 70 per cent higher than for non-smokers.

The findings of a number of studies are in agreement that children start experimental smoking in the intermediate grades and develop into fairly regular smokers by the eighth or ninth grade. A Cincinnati, Ohio survey indicates that 22 per cent of schoolchildren start to smoke during the age bracket of ten years and younger; 60 per cent begin between 11 and 13.[42] The pupil is more likely to smoke if his parents or his older brothers and sisters smoke and if his friends smoke. If children have low goals, little ability, and little achievement, they tend to smoke earlier.

In a society in which cigarettes are advertised, sold, and used everywhere and in which 40 per cent of the adults smoke, it is hard to educate children to the extent that they will not start to smoke. Yet, there is some evidence of progress. Not only have one-fourth of the men and one-fifth of the women smokers quit smoking, but there is evidence that fewer children start to smoke when exposed to carefully planned programs.[43] Obviously, there are exceptions to these findings because of youth's strong desire to conform and gain social confidence. A considerable amount of success was experienced in the Spokane, Washington public schools as a result of a six-year smoking education program in grades five to 12. In the fifth and sixth grades it was made very clear to pupils that the decision to smoke is im-

---

[40] An especially useful aid is the booklet, *Teaching about Alcohol in Connecticut Schools* (Bulletin No. 99, Fall, 1966, Connecticut State Department of Education, Hartford). See also, "Alcohol in Perspective," *Consumer Reports,* 32:97–99, February 1967.

[41] U.S. Department of Health, Education, and Welfare. *The Health Consequences of Smoking,* Public Health Service Publication No. 1696, Washington, D.C., 1967. See also a concise review of this publication in *Consumer Reports,* February 1968, p. 99.

[42] Streit, William K. "Students Express Views on Smoking," *Journal of School Health, 37:* 153–154, March 1967.

[43] Davis, Roy L. "Progress and Problems in Smoking...," *Journal of School Health, 37:* 121–128, March 1967. See also J. L. Schwartz, and M. Dubitzky, "Research in Student Smoking Habits and Smoking Control," *Journal of School Health,* 37:177–182, April 1967.

Results of Smoking Education Program

Spokane, Washington	Boys Who Smoked	Girls Who Smoked
1961	41.5%	14%
1967	20%	6%

portant because it is so final, and once the habit is started, many persons cannot stop even if they wish.

Throughout the nation a tremendous effort has been made to improve smoking education programs. Practically every state department of education has developed special smoking and health curriculum guides, together with resource material kits. The same can be said for hundreds of large city school systems. Legislators are acting too. The New York Senate established a concentrated five year program in 1967 to alert public schoolchildren to the potential dangers of smoking, and, about the same time, the North Dakota legislature outlawed the sale of candy cigarettes.

Helpful literature is extensive. Noteworthy curriculum guides may be obtained from states such as California, Pennsylvania, Washington, Massachusetts, New York, Arizona, Rhode Island, and Illinois. A wealth of curriculum materials are available from the American Cancer Society and the U.S. Public Health Service. The Children's Bureau in Washington distributes the pamphlet, *Why Nick the Cigarette Is Nobody's Friend,* for fourth and fifth graders and *A Light on the Subject of Smoking,* for sixth graders. The National Film Board of Canada distributes the Academy Award film, *The Drag*—a nine-minute animated film for young audiences. Elementary children seem to love the cartoon spoof film *The Huffless, Puffless Dragon,* put out by the American Cancer Society. Their filmstrip, *I'll Choose the High Road,* is also very good; and the filmstrip and discussion guide of the National Interagency Council on Smok-

ing and Health is of real value to the teacher in this health education area.

A great variety of teaching ideas relative to discussion topics, classroom experiments, and other projects appear in the teaching guide, *Smoking and Health Unit* of the Spokane Public Schools.[44] Another souce of ideas is the booklet, *Classroom-Tested Techniques for Teaching About Smoking,* distributed free by the National Clearinghouse for Smoking and Health, U.S. Public Health Service, 4040 N. Fairfax Drive, Arlington, Virginia 22203.

In the Denver, Colorado public schools a unique breathing-lung exhibit is employed to present an unusually dramatic lesson on the effects of smoking. The exhibit, which consists of two human lungs preserved by a process that permits them to simulate breathing, gives dramatic evidence of the differences between a healthy lung (elastic, flexible, pink) and a lung damaged by heavy smoking (leathery, stiff, dark). The exhibit, available throughout the state, has been used especially well with sixth grade classes.

DRUG EDUCATION

The habit-forming tendency of drugs and their poisonous effects is a proper topic for fifth and sixth grade presentation. Children should know that alcohol is classified as a narcotic rather than a stimulant. They should appreciate the great need for sleeping pills, aspirin, and pain killing substances. Information about these items should relate to the medical, economic, and social effects when they are used correctly and what is involved from both a personal and community viewpoint when they are misused.

There will be times when parents and educators wonder why it is neces-

[44] *Teaching Guide: Grades 5–12, Smoking and Health Unit,* September 1967. Publications Department, Spokane Public Schools, W. 825 Trent Ave., Spokane, Washington 99201 (price $2.50).

sary to give instruction in the more potent narcotics. They will reason that it is enough merely to refer to tobacco and alcohol in the elementary school. Yet, more and more evidence is available to indicate that the 12 year old boy or girl is ready for this level of education about drugs. Jesse Feiring Williams, in his 1952 book for the California State Department of Education, *Narcotics—The Study of a Modern Problem,* made it very clear that "instruction in the nature and effects of narcotic drugs should be started in the sixth grade and should be continued in the succeeding years as a part of the regular health instruction." In short, education on narcotics is part of the larger problem of health teaching. It relates to values in living, to confidence in oneself, to self-respect, and to the importance of developing personal traits and abilities which one is proud to possess. This is an opportune moment for young people to discover, perhaps anew, that psychological factors are vital in all health behavior—that happy, secure people have a kind of respect for themselves that does not need building up with narcotics or anything else.

Children should know about prescription drugs as well as over-the-counter drugs. Amphetamines and barbiturates can be discussed openly, first in terms of their medical use and secondly in terms of their abuse. The question of what might happen from an overdose of "pep pills" or sleeping pills should be answered with dramatic illustrations. Questions relative to smoking marihuana or "going on a trip" with LSD or some other hallucinatory drug should be discussed. News clippings such as the accompanying one may be posted on the classroom bulletin board in order to relate the drug topic to everyday living.

A very useful guide for teachers is *Drug Abuse: Escape to Nowhere.* It provides reliable information concerning drugs and offers suggestions concerning ways in which young people in the elementary school can be reached on this vital subject. It is a 1967 National Education Association publication.

Suggested Activities

1. Collect advertisements from magazines and newspapers having to do with the "benefits" of tea, coffee, cigarettes, cigars, pipe tobacco, beer, wine, cola drinks, and headache pills. Secure answers to such questions as:
   a. How much of this advertising is essentially true, and how much is misleading?
   b. How may government, medical, and health authorities be

Boy's Death Spurs Glue Warning

Medical Examiner Richard Ford pleaded Sunday that parents warn their children of the dangers of glue-sniffing.

His plea came shortly after he performed an autopsy on the body of a 12-year-old Hyde Park boy found dead in a wooded area near his home Saturday night. A plastic bag and a tube of airplane glue were found near the body.

Dr. Ford said Sunday that glue-sniffing is "a completely stupid trick. Doing this sort of thing amounts to a death warrant.

"For a small kick you run the risk of losing your life. I would advise every parent to warn his children of the danger of this.

"The amount of kick a person gets isn't equal to the risk."

used to continually evaluate the advertising?

c. What are some other sources from which people get health advice?

d. What is the action of nicotine, caffeine, and alcohol in the body?

2. Over a period of one week collect from several local newspapers clippings that have to do solely with automobile accidents in which intoxication and drinking are involved. Post these on a frequently read bulletin board. Ask for questions. Questions will arise somewhat as follows:

a. In how many feet can a driver of an automobile usually stop when traveling at 50 miles per hour (an emergency situation)? How much longer may it take when the driver has had a few drinks?

b. What disposition is generally made of cases of drunken driving in the courts?

c. How many automobile accidents involve intoxication?

3. Discuss the short film, *Alcohol and the Human Body.* This may be obtained on loan from Encyclopaedia Britannica Films.

4. Talk about alcohol and poor nutrition, length of life, social drinking, and alcoholism.

5. Invite a local druggist to appear in class and answer questions regarding habit-forming drugs, drug addiction, and the law on prescriptions. This is also a good time to discuss the sale of sleeping pills. Have the class prepare for such discussion by clipping from the newspaper items pertaining to deaths and near-deaths due to an overdose of sleeping pills.

6. Dramatize the "smoker's cough." Act out three scenes. In scene No. 1, a chain-smoker is seen going about his daily activities. In scene No. 2, he is observed arising from his bed in the morning in a fit of coughing. In scene

No. 3, his doctor is warning him to cut down his cigarette consumption because of the cough, its effect on appetite and consequent nutrition, its relationship to longevity, its effect on the heart and blood pressure, its relationship to cancer and the respiratory system.

7. Engage a small panel of community "experts" on the topic of why people smoke. In this case the "experts" may be informed class members. One may be designated as a community physician, another as a parent, and one or two others as active citizens. The panel should meet with the teacher before class in order to have several suggestions each as to why people smoke. (Examples: They enjoy it; they want to do what others do; it gives them something to do while waiting or talking; it is habit forming, and they feel a "need" for it; it keeps their weight down.)

8. Ask the direct question, "How many students have tried to smoke just for fun?" A few honest hands will be raised. Have these people tell how smoking affected them. It may have made them nauseated, even sick. Explain that medical authorities feel that smoking is of no benefit to anyone, but for growing boys and girls it is definitely harmful; one is not at one's best mentally, physically, or socially. In growing people it reduces the effectiveness of the muscle and nervous systems, may cause restlessness, dizziness, nausea, indigestion, increased heart beat, shortness of breath, and loss of appetite for good protein foods.

9. Write to the American Cancer Society for information on the effects of alcohol upon the length of life. Discuss the information received in class. Post information. Use clippings. Distribute American Cancer Society bookmarks (free).

10. Have a panel discussion on why people drink, Alcohol does many things to many people. Is drinking a

Smoking Cuts Life Span, Study Shows

cure for emotional problems? The extent of the problem: One in 16 is an alcoholic.

11. Find the meaning of such health words as:

addict	morphine
alcohol	narcotic
alcoholic beverage	nicotine
depress	opium
fermentation	stimulate
intoxication	tobacco

12. Discuss alcohol in industry: its use as a solvent in breaking down fats; its use in varnishes, polishes, paints, stains, enamels, smokeless powders, and explosives; its use in electric cables, linoleum, insecticides, disinfectants, antifreeze solutions, and thermometers.

13. Discuss alcohol in medicine: its use as a solvent in the preparation of solutions of alkaloids, oils, ether, choloroform, bromide, medicinal extracts, capsules, and surgical dressings.

14. Consider alcohol as a beverage and its effect upon the body, mind, and society. Ask the question, "What are the common effects of alcohol on the individual and society?"
Some answers:
    a. Has no essential food value except in certain circumstances, and this can be obtained in other ways.
    b. Affects the highest nerve cen-

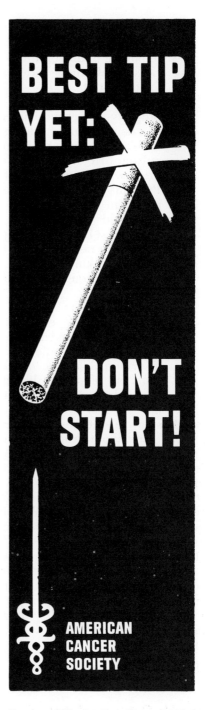

(Courtesy of The American Cancer Society.)

ters in the brain, setting free lower forms of behavior by removing brain control.

c. Lessens alertness and power to concentrate.

d. Increases hazards to life and property, lowering efficiency to a danger point for firemen, railway engineers, policemen, automobile drivers, truck drivers, and airplane pilots.

e. Prevents the highest achievement in athletics and in most fields of endeavor.

f. Reduces self-control and paralyzes the nerve centers that control walking.

g. Confuses thought and judgment.

h. Is habit-forming and may get worse, causing drinkers to waste money needed for food, clothing, and families, and is a principal cause of large numbers of people being in hospitals, mental hospitals, and prisons.

15. Display a picture of a truck accident. Talk about drugs and drinking and what "pep pills" may do. Discuss also what sedatives and tranquilizers may do to people driving automobiles long distances. The Food and Drug Administration, Washington, D.C. 20204, will supply free booklets upon request.

16. Make up a display of such items as model airplane glue, paint thinner, and carbon tetrachloride. Permit everyone to take a light sniff and read the labels. Then discuss "glue-sniffing" and its relationship to death and permanent brain damage.

12. Consumer Health

Desirable Outcomes (Intermediate Level)

To appreciate the individual role of the consumer of healthful goods and materials.

To understand that truths must be separated from half truths in order to judge whether or not to purchase a health product.

To understand that superstitions and gullibility frequently prevent people from acting wisely in the selection and use of health products.

To understand that such items as clothing, food, and medical service vary in kind and quality and that the informed consumer, by his knowledge and actions, helps keep undesirable and unscientific products out of circulation.

Comments

There are, no doubt, people who would say that there is no need for a special health topic on consumer health. They would argue that the thought and actions of the consumer are brought to a head in each of the previous eleven areas. That is to say, for example, the consumer of foods thinks of his well-being when he studies food for its vitamins and minerals, and when he purchases and prepares food. This is partially true, for we are always consumers of that which we study. Yet it seems necessary to analyze and appraise keenly that which we use from day to day in the school and community. What about the toothpastes we saw advertised? How good is the soap? Do we all really need hair tonic to succeed in life? How many people die or become very ill each year from poisonous products? How effective is a "crash" diet? Are "nagging back pains," "tired bones," and "nervous headaches" simply improved by bathing in or drinking a special product? What stand does the Federal government take? What protection is there in the community relative to qualified physicians and lawyers, well-operated hospitals, and clean eating places? What are the responsibilities of the good citizen as a consumer of health products?

Human communications and values

are at times so uncertain that at best mankind has to struggle to find out where to turn in search of truth and knowledge of the appropriate way to behave. White can be made to look black on the television screen or newspaper page. Unfortunately, advertising claims are not always based on scientific evidence. It is apparent that upper elementary school pupils must be alerted to the problems associated with properly labeled foods, false food comparison in advertising, the use of the terms "adequate," "balanced," "optional," "enriched," "low cal," and "salt free." Blood building claims are considered improper subjects for advertising, according to the American Medical Association. Quick weight-reduction schemes must also be recognized as strictly inferior to the steady loss of weight over a long term. There are many such things to be discussed in class. One frequently realizes that people hear only what other people want them to hear. Thus "educated" citizens are often ignorant. For example, in several communities in which the majority of the voters are college graduates, the issue of fluoridation of the drinking water was voted down, yet fluoridation is by far the most effective means known to man for reducing tooth decay to a significant extent.

Misconceptions abound everywhere we turn. Sutton finds them particularly common among children and youth.[45] Here are just a few that fifth and sixth grade schoolchildren subscribe to (as well as many adults):

Persons who have pimples usually have bad blood.

Taking vitamin pills will guarantee good health.

Hot food is more nutritious than cold food.

Most fat people are very healthy.

One can eat what he wants and grow thin.

Tooth powders or pastes will always cure a person's bad breath.

It is all right to use sleeping pills without a doctor's advice.

Certain medicines will prevent the common cold.

The best doctors always promise to make people healthy.

Cutting a person's hair makes it grow faster.

If you have any disease you'll always feel some pain.

A prospective mother can make the child more musical if she listens to good music.

According to the Federal Food and Drug Administration's bureau of enforcement, the most effective tool in combating quacks is publicity, particularly exposure in courts. Collecting newspaper clippings exposing quacks and false health claims is a practical project for consumer health classes. The class should know that any time the Federal government is aware that the consumer is being misled into believing that certain foods and products will prevent a disease that is difficult to treat, they will take regulatory action.

Instructing children in the particulars of Consumer Health can be one of the most fascinating tasks in health teaching. There are illustrations everywhere pertaining to all of the major health topics. From toothpaste to aspirin, from cosmetics to foods there exists a great deal of literature for the teacher to use, both for substantive information and for instructional aids. The objective is to reform the child today as a consumer and, thus, protect him against poisons in the home, show him that drugs and pills can be used safely and effectively, help him begin to see how to choose health

---

[45] Sutton, W. B. "Misconceptions About Health Among Children and Youth," *Journal of School Health*, 32:347–350, November 1962.

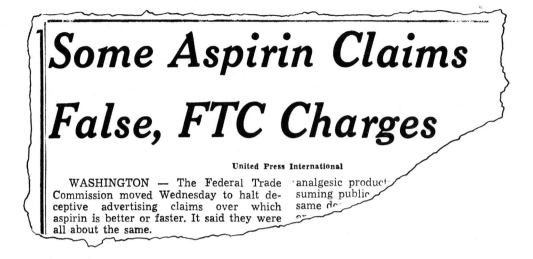

Some Aspirin Claims
False, FTC Charges

United Press International

WASHINGTON — The Federal Trade Commission moved Wednesday to halt deceptive advertising claims over which aspirin is better or faster. It said they were all about the same.

analgesic product suming public same do

---

services wisely, and steer him clear of frauds and cheats.

The task of building defenses against quackery is all the more challenging because of the numerous "half-truth" products. Much can be learned by ferreting out the truths and falsehoods. Are all toothpaste products about the same? Are all aspirin pills the same? In one year Americans gulped 450 million dollars worth of aspirin. During that time the manufacturers spent over 90 million dollars advertising which aspirin is faster, lasts longer, or upsets the stomach less. This prompted the Federal Trade Commission to warn against unfair and deceptive practices and false claims about products which are essentially the same.

The long list of "watchdog" duties carried on by such consumer protection agencies as the Food and Drug Administration, the Federal Trade Commission, and the U.S. Post Office Department can be brought to the attention of schoolchildren by obtaining excellent literature from these respective Washington agencies. Extensive lists of consumer health publications are available. Every topic has been explored. For example, if questions arise relative to cosmetics, then *Cosmetics Facts for Consumers* (FDA

Publication No. 26) is most appropriate.[46]

The FDA has *Consumer Protection* packets consisting of booklets, leaflets, and teaching suggestions suitable for use in health, science, and home economics classes. These packets (Packet A: *Foods;* Packet B: *Drugs and Cosmetics*) sell for $1.50 in the U.S. Government Printing Office.

The teaching units of the American Medical Association for all school levels are superb.[47] The sample teaching unit for the elementary schools is cleverly built around five concepts, and is complete with questions, understandings, and teaching activities:

Concept 1. Self-medication should be avoided.

Concept 2. It is important to seek sound advice concerning health care.

Concept 3. There are no special health foods.

---

[46] For a fine review of the FDA position, written in the form of four informative articles — safe food, drugs, medical quackery, and teaching materials — see "Education for Consumer Health," *Journal of Health, Physical Education, and Recreation,* February 1965.

[47] A resource for teachers: concepts and a sample teaching unit for the elementary school (1–6), *Defenses Against Quackery.* Chicago: American Medical Association, 1966.

Concept 4. There are many kinds of "doctors" who will treat us when we are ill, but some who claim to be able to treat us are not qualified or adequately prepared.

Concept 5. Diagnosis of health problems should be made by a medically trained physician, and medication should be taken under the direction of a physician.

Suggested Activities

1. Identify doctors who take care of special health problems such as eyes, feet, and teeth; also, medical specialists such as pediatricians, obstetricians, and psychiatrists. Why are there so many different kinds of specialists?

2. Americans spend over 28 billion dollars for medical care each year. The hospitals' share of this figure has more than doubled since 1929. Appoint class committees to find out why. Study the pie graphs (p. 269) and relate these to medical care.[48]

---

[48] U.S. Department of Commerce. *Survey of Current Business.* July 1966.

3. Give an overnight assignment requesting the class to make up a list of superstitions about health and disease. Suggest that they check with their parents and others in their neighborhood so that their list will be as long as possible. Make a combined list of these findings the next day. Add to the list a number of superstitions such as the following:

Onions worn around the neck prevent disease.
Aluminum cooking utensils cause cancer.
Wearing an iron ring prevents backache (rheumatism too).
Toads cause warts.
Wearing rubbers indoors will injure the eyes.
An apple a day keeps the doctor away.
People were healthier in the "good old days".
When your time comes you will die, no matter how you live.

4. Collect a variety of labels from cans and bottles and advertisements from the newspapers and magazines for class discussion. Post some of them.

5. Prepare reports on self-medication. Select the three or four best re-

DISTRIBUTION OF THE MEDICAL CARE DOLLAR
1929, 1950, 1965

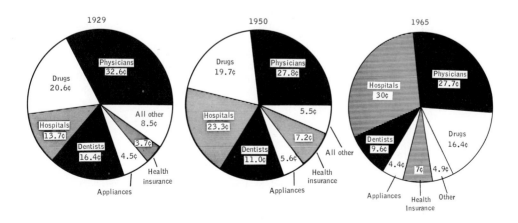

ports for panel discussion with a student leader as moderator.

6. Post on the classroom bulletin board a list of community sources where reliable health information may be obtained. Follow this up with a committee visit to each of the sources.

This will involve most of the class if properly organized.

7. Bring in an outside speaker to show how the consumer is being protected (a county health agent, local physician or health officer, or Food and Drug Administration official).

Questions for Discussion

1. The nature of the modern school is such that an imaginative teacher may set up almost any activity for her class to engage in. To insure that only the proper activities are taught, what should the teacher use as her guide?

2. To what extent do you think it is necessary to define the terms "broad" and "varied" program?

3. What seem to be the two or three significant differences between health emphasis in the primary grades and health emphasis in the intermediate grades?

4. What do you think is the potential outcome of such occasionally controversial topics as alcohol and narcotics education and sex education?

5. Prepare teaching outlines for the study of health topics using suggested teaching activities other than those appearing in this chapter.

6. How can we gain greater cooperation in closing the gap between the objectives of the school health program and what is really being accomplished?

Suggested Activities

1. Ideas for learning experiences are everywhere. Even students themselves will suggest ways and means for discovering more information relative to a particular health problem. Select a major health topic, such as nutrition or mental health, and formulate a list of learning activities which differ from the examples given in the book.

2. Carefully examine several curriculum guides pertaining to elementary school health education. (These are generally found in the college or university library with other professional education materials.) How are the specific objectives or purposes set up? Are they arranged in terms of concepts? Competencies? Outcomes? Goals? See if you can discover the rationale behind the terms used.

3. Review the research relative to smoking education. Write a short paper setting forth some of the evidences of success in the smoking education programs nationally.

4. In a sense, Consumer Health embraces all major health teaching topics. After briefly reviewing each of these topics, formulate a list of what might be called "common abuses," that is, a listing of ways in which the consumer may be put at a disadvantage through half-truth advertising and questionable products. In some areas, such as Personal Cleanliness and Appearance, there will be many illustrations.

Selected References

Anderson, C. L. *School Health Practice*, 3rd ed. St. Louis: C. V. Mosby Co., 1964, Chapter 12.
Bidwell, Corrine. "The Teacher as a Listener—An Approach to Mental Health." *Journal Of School Health*, 37:373–383, October 1967.

Bobbitt, Blanche G., and Lawrence, Trudys. "Enrichment Activities in Health Education for Intellectually Gifted Pupils, Grades One to Nine." *Journal of School Health,* 36:223–234, May 1966.

Fodor, John T., and Dalis, Gus T. *Health Instruction: Theory and Application.* Philadelphia: Lea and Febiger, 1966, Chapter 6.

Grout, Ruth E. *Health Teaching in Schools,* 5th ed. Philadelphia: W. B. Saunders Co., 1968, Chapter 8.

Irwin, Leslie, Cornacchia, Harold, and Staton, Wesley. *Health in Elementary Schools,* 2nd ed. St. Louis: C. V. Mosby Co., 1966, Chapter 12.

Lavigne, Marilyn E., and Siegel, Lillian. "Nutrition Education Involves the Total School." *Journal of School Health,* 35:101–103, March 1965.

Martin, Ethel A. *Roberts' Nutrition Work with Children.* Chicago: University of Chicago Press, 1955, Chapters 9, 11, 12, and 13.

Oberteuffer, Delbert, and Beyrer, Mary K. *School Health Education,* 4th ed. New York: Harper and Row, 1966, Chapters 4 and 5.

Report of Committee on Health Education in the Elementary and Secondary School. "Health Instruction Suggestions for Teachers." *Journal of School Health* (special edition), 34:1–80, December 1964.

Turner, C. E., Sellery, C., and Smith, Sara Loise. *School Health and Health Education,* 5th ed. St. Louis: C. V. Mosby Co., 1966, Chapters 14 and 16.

Vannier, Maryhelen. *Teaching Health in the Elementary School.* New York: Harper and Row Co., 1963.

Methods
in Health
CHAPTER 9 Instruction

In using the word, "method," as he did, the great playwright attached a reasonable degree of respect and meaning to the word. He made method stand for something sound and stable, as a contrast to something as haphazard as madness. Shakespeare's use of the word is supported by Webster's definition: method is "orderly procedure or process . . . orderly arrangement."

The Meaning of Method

The word "method" has a number of implications for people in education. In a sense, it is the very body of educational endeavor, for it involves more than objectives and curriculum. It involves the effectiveness of the program —a program in which curriculum and method cannot be divorced.

Educational method is as much the concern of the instructor as is the mastery of the subject matter used in teaching. Familiarity with this one item makes the teacher a pedagogue or educationalist, rather than simply a specialist in sociology, biology, or mathematics. In fact, it is sound methodology coupled with an understanding of subject matter, facts, and figures that makes the well-rounded instructor. The presence of one without the other produces only half a teacher; successful teaching is both an art and a science.

Historically, teaching has always been considered an art. Art and science are different and their methods contrast. Science is analytical; it breaks things up, seeks detail, and looks for causes. Art, on the other hand, is engaged in giving *meaning to experience*; it puts things together— synthesis rather than analysis. Fauré in his monumental history of art reminds us that, "Science relates fact to fact; art relates fact to life." Both science and art are regularly employed by the instructor who knows what to teach and how to teach it. The *how* is important. For example, in health teaching it means that in addition to specific skills relative to physiology, anatomy, sanitation, and world and local health problems, one must also possess an understanding of how children learn and the best methods to employ to bring this about. Methods, therefore, are ways and means selected to achieve objectives.

All methods need examination because what works with one child or group may not work as well with another child or group as long as there are bona fide individual differences; "what is one man's meat is another man's poison." Sometimes formal methods operate for the welfare of the pupils; at other times informal methods seem better. There are so many specific and worthwhile objectives in elementary school health education that it is reasonable to expect a number of methods to prove successful, depending on the local situation.

The Bases of Method

Children cannot learn except within the limits of their capacities and to the extent that they become motivated to learn. Since all education is concerned with the stimulation for learning, all instruction must be based upon accepted facts and a body of well-conceived theory about how learning takes place.

There are a number of criteria which may be applied to the various methods and instructional procedures. These include:

Methods to be Selected in Keeping with Objectives. Will the method employed promote the desired outcomes? The means determine the end, and therefore the end must determine means. This would indicate in the teaching of second grade dental health, for instance, that the degree to which pupils enjoy a toothbrushing drill will determine to some extent the carryover value of the activity. If it is taught as pure drill, it might do little to change habits and attitudes toward brushing the teeth at home. Perhaps the words of J. B. Priestley in his book, *Rain Upon Godshill,* are appropriate. "Are we not" challenges Priestley, "living too exclusively in a narrow world of how-the-trick-is-done, with too much *how* and not enough *why?*"

The Best Possible Methods to be Selected as a Means of Achieving the Goals. Simply stated, there are many methods capable of promoting achievement; some are better than others in a particular situation. Teachers who have a favorite method sometimes "ride it to death." It works, but another method might prove superior and lead to fuller values.

Methods to be Adaptable to the Kinds of Health Activities Involved. The goals of health education are broad. Each health activity presents unique challenges. Teaching community health to a sixth grade lends itself to a large group field trip, but teaching school safety to first grade pupils requires some individual attention to small groups of children.

Methods to be Selected in Relation to Space, Equipment, Time Available, and Teacher Load. Does the method under consideration have a number of limitations because of the physical environment or the abilities of the teacher? It is better to teach a unit on nutrition by the well-worn lecture method if part of the class cannot adequately observe or follow a demonstration lesson that takes place in the front of the room.

Methods to be Selected in Accordance with the Personal Skill and Interest of the Teacher. This is an important criterion. Everyone should know his strengths and weaknesses: what he can do well, or not so well, what he likes or dislikes. The teacher who honestly believes that a white rat feeding experiment would be more beneficial for her class but personally shudders at the sight of rats would ordinarily be much more effective by choosing another method of teaching the values of a sound diet.

Methods to be Selected of Interest to the Pupils. The initial interest in a topic can be seriously stifled by inappropriate methods. Children learn best when their interest is high. Extrinsic rewards, like stars or honor rolls for evidence of good health habits, should be used sparingly. As Rogers points out, "the chief motivation should be intrinsic or inherent within the task itself; otherwise children may come to expect external rewards for everything they do."[1] This does not mean that posting the result of pupil efforts is a poor practice; it simply means that interest in the activity is maintained when the method employed is fully enjoyed by the class.

Methods to be Selected in Keeping with the Skills and Abilities of the Class. Do the pupils have enough personal know-how of a certain method to profit by its application? To use a microscope successfully, for instance, involves a few techniques plus some curiosity for the world of the unseen. The whole wonderful experience of using the reliable microscope could go to waste without proper orientation in the experimental method. Similarly, a library visitation could be somewhat unproductive if little or no class planning took place beforehand.

Methods to be Selected as a Means to an End. Are some methods an end in themselves? Do teachers teach a certain way because they like it the best? Are new methods tried from time to time in a constant effort to find the most efficient way to organize a learning experience so that the finest health behavior will take place?

Methods to be Used to Allow for Individual Differences. Pupils, when given the chance to think independently about personal and community health problems, often come up with practical solutions. Learning is an individual affair. Opportunity for individual effort within the framework of the group sometimes represents the only way some pupils have an effective health learning experience.

Concepts and Discovery

Good teaching invariably concerns itself with conceptual understanding, for concepts are the ingredients for thinking. In fact, thinking actually is the process of organizing and storing concepts. In this respect, Bruner has pointed out the importance of establishing these "structures" of knowledge so that the student can find *meaningful relationships* among comprehensive ideas, rather than having to struggle with countless facts in isolation.

Simply stated, therefore, a concept is an understanding of something—a way of making meaning of things. Woodruff speaks in part of the concept activity as starting with perception, moving to register an experience, forming concepts through thinking, making a decision (choosing), and drawing conclusions.[2] Significantly, it is the *experience* itself which seems to count as the greatest single factor in conceptual learning, far outweighing mental age or vocabulary strength.

It is at this very point that the discovery idea becomes germane. Concepts are more easily formed when the student's learning is a product of his own curiosity and thinking and of his manipulation of basic facts. What he alone discovers means something.

Brecht, the playwright, substantiates

---

[1] Rogers, Dorothy. *Mental Hygiene in Elementary Education*. Boston: Houghton-Mifflin Co., 1957, p. 259.

[2] Woodruff, Asahel D. "The Use of Concepts in Teaching and Learning," *Journal of Teacher Education*, March 1964, pp. 81–97.

this method in *Galileo*. In the opening scene he shows the great Italian scientist, Galileo Galilei, in the early 1600's teaching a young boy the particulars of the movement of the earth about the sun. As he initiates the lesson there is no lecturing, no explanation; instead, Galileo asks the lad to examine his device for showing the way the planets move about the sun. "What do you see?" says the great man. "Count the bands. How many are there?" When doubting Thomases and scientists came to visit him, he taught the same way. When each would gaze into the crude telescope, Galileo would ask, "What do you see? Describe to me what you see." This not only awakened interest, but it tied the observer securely to the topic because his own *trusted senses* were involved. What he saw was real to him; it was not something someone described to him in mere words and phrases. It became a part of him and was not lightly considered and soon forgotten.

It is exactly this kind of teaching methodology that is sought by Bruner when he speaks of organizing the perceptual field around the person as center. Moreover, says Bruner, "The importance of early experience is only dimly sensed today. The evidence from animal studies indicates that virtually irreversible deficits can be produced in mammals by depriving them of opportunities that challenge their nascent capacities."[3]

Variety in Teaching Methods

Variety is more than the spice of life. It is also the spice of teaching and the spice of learning. The teacher who varies her approach to a health topic stimulates her own imagination and can often succeed where the teacher with the single approach fails. Variety bolsters interest and acts as a motiva-

[3] Bruner, Jerome S. "Education As Social Invention," *Saturday Review*, February 19, 1966, p. 70.

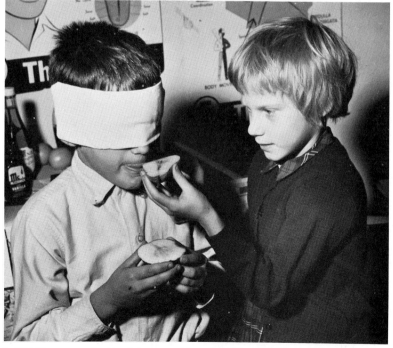

Figure 9-1 The discovery method leads to concept formation. (Courtesy Mrs. R. G. Holmes, Greenacres School, Scarsdale, N.Y.)

tion technique for learning. When all health topics are taught in a similar manner, it is difficult to maintain the interest of the class, for the element of surprise and anticipation is missing. Even a little bit of that which one pupil loves the most continues to remain high in his esteem when it is used sparingly.

Experimentation in method is to be encouraged. Varying the health teaching method is an effective way of determining how the class responds to a number of sound approaches. From this kind of experimentation successful methods are developed for the teaching of a particular health topic. One can begin to answer specific questions such as, How best to teach alcohol and narcotics? Will a white rat experiment actually put over the true meaning of vitamins? Shall I plan a demonstration? What can my pupils discover?

Conscientious teachers are generally interested in the improved method. It is sometimes believed—and always hoped for—that the discovery of a new and better method automatically results in a sudden rush to accept it. The history of education, which is not at all subtle, points out that this is far from being true. Once a new method is discovered and described, the most difficult job, that of gaining acceptance, is still undone.

The lack of immediate acceptance of a desirable method has its basis in an element of human inertia or resistance to change. People fail to appreciate that some change is inevitable. Also, some methods are more difficult to use than others. Arranging a discovery experience is frequently more time-consuming than preparing a lecture.

The versatile teacher who has several ways of approaching health topics does more than successfully teach the topic; she actually promotes a mentally hygienic situation in the classroom, for children appreciate something different, and they tend to show more real enthusiasm and genuine happiness when their teacher is flexible.

Example as Method

In addition to the specific methods employed by the teacher, the very example set by her is in itself an educational method.

I

I'd rather see a sermon
  Than hear one any day;
I'd rather one should walk with me
  Than merely show the way.
The eye's a better pupil,
  And more willing than the ear;
Fine counsel is confusing,
  But example's always clear.

II

I soon can learn to do it,
  If you'll let me see it done;
I can see your hands in action,
  But your tongue too fast may run.
And the lectures you deliver
  May be very fine and true,
But I'd rather get my lesson
  By observing what you do.
For I may misunderstand you
  And the high advice you give,
But there's no misunderstanding
  How you act and how you live!

—ANONYMOUS

We who work with youth do not need superagencies and complicated programs; we need a re-emphasis of the simple truth that the kind of people we are is infinitely more important than programs. If we give youth an example of fit living, they will want to be fit themselves. Here is the challenge:

He who would kindle another must himself be aglow.

—DRINKWATER

Growth Through Health Experiences

It is safe to say that where participation is the fullest and mere spectatorship is at a minimum, effective learning tends to be at its best. Will Durant sums this viewpoint up very nicely when he says, "The wisest of our children will not be those who merely enjoy the spectacle; it will be those who climb out of the pit upon the stage and lose themselves in action." To lose oneself in action has powerful implications. It means that the activity is total and the individual is completely wrapped up in the subject. It is a rare state, indeed, and one that most teachers hope to witness more often in their teaching careers. It is not a strange state because one cannot set a limit to which children will go to pursue the things they are truly interested in. Methods that promote experiences which fire the curiosity of youth are priceless. For curiosity, says Alexis Carrel, "is a necessity of nature, a blind impulse that obeys no rule."

Health experiences can be broad in scope or limited, formal or informal, concrete or abstract—but to be valuable, they must have meaning to the child. He alone must understand that what he is doing is worth doing. Real action is difficult to obtain. Problems have to be brought home to pupils in a personal way. Much of so-called health education is like a stream of water running on and off the back of the proverbial duck. It simply has not been very effective; it has been superficial. Facts and figures in some cases have been dispensed, but the individual pupil's health habits and attitudes have remained essentially unchanged.

All instructional methods deal with pupil experiences. Some are better than others, but all have something in common. With due respect to Rudyard Kipling and his *Just So Stories,* it might be said that methods are somewhat associated with the "six honest serving men":

> I keep six honest serving men
> (They taught me all I knew)
> Their names are What and Why
> and When
> And How and Where and Who.

When the health topic is considered and an effort is being made to find the most effective method for putting it across, one should ask:

> *What* experiences will we choose?
> *Why* will we choose them?
> *When* will we carry them out?
> *How* will we carry them out?
> *Where* will we carry them out?
> *Who* will we work with?

Each proposed teaching method may be examined and appraised in the light of these fundamental questions.

Improved Health Education Methods

The health-educated person is one who translates the understandings, attitudes, and skills learned in the classroom into his daily life. He is more than health-informed, chiefly because the teaching methods employed by his teachers encouraged him to practice desirable health behavior through many first-hand experiences. Method has made the difference, and method continues to make a difference when some of the following points are kept in mind:

1. *Present day concepts of method are far removed from the days of the teacher-dominated classroom.* Pupils memorized the body parts and recited the rules for healthful living. Repetition and memorization stifled interest, and the personal problems that pupils were really interested in went unexplained. Today, the newer concept of method in health teaching recognizes the child as a person capable of sharing in the solution of problems which concern his health. The emphasis upon the teaching of health facts has given way to an emphasis upon understandings which will improve living. Moreover, children are being taught to accept themselves for what they are, and for what they can be. They need high expectations from others which will inspire them to be the best they can be. Said Goethe:

> If you treat an individual as he is,
> he will remain as he is, but if you

treat him as if he were what he ought to be and could be, he will become what he ought to be and could be.

2. *Elementary school health instruction programs range in philosophy from those which center attention on the learning of subjects to those which emphasize the importance of developing each child to his full capacity both in his home and in his school life.* In learning subjects, considerable stress is placed on the development of skills in writing and reading about health, spelling health words, and skillfully drawing health pictures. Where schools emphasize the needs and problems of children as a basis for learning, much of the subject matter is used from broad areas such as social studies, science, and language arts.

3. *Cooperative planning of the health lesson is time-consuming, but it is well worth the effort.* Even in the kindergarten the children can and should begin to plan some of their activities. Cooperative planning for projects, units of work, parties, trips, and other classroom activities helps develop a sense of social responsibility, for children are concerned with the success of those activities which they themselves have planned. The pupil who assists in planning a class project often experiences a pleasant feeling of belonging to the group—a feeling of oneness. In health education the whole class often functions as a single group. They might be profitably engaged in planning a class round-table discussion to talk over a school health problem, studying a health technique or habit needed by the class, listening to a health story or radio program, or viewing a film. Such activities tend to create a favorable state of mental health and very often promote high morale and class spirit.

4. *Health instruction lends itself most favorably to creative activity on the part of elementary education pupils.* Learning has to be personal if it is to be used. When a pupil feels intimately involved in the learning situation, he will begin to want to use the ideas that are there for him. In this respect, there is hardly anything more personal than one's creative activity, but to be creative requires a definite setting, an atmosphere within the classroom conducive to freedom of expression. Practically all courses of study that border on some form of science present a number of opportunities for creativity. Health is no exception. Children need to be creative, but some teachers never quite see it because they cannot subordinate their adult needs or desires to those of the child.[4]

Children are creative in different degrees in different media. They may paint, draw, engage in dramatic play, express themselves through pantomime or impersonation or with puppets or other dramatic forms, may develop rhythms or dances, write music to be sung or played, or make a simple musical instrument, model with clay, weave, cook, sew, build with blocks, and write stories or poems. These and many other related forms of expression are natural to children. A number of these experiences, when carried on during health instruction, may be drawn together in such a way as to supplement each other and enrich the whole school program.

One of the greatest values of creative expression is the opportunity provided for the release from tension or frustration. The pupil may express freely the way he feels about environmental elements which cause him distress or unhappiness. Once these feelings are brought out and put into some tangible form, he may begin to relax, view them with more detachment, share them

---

[4] Lowenfield, Viktor. *Creative and Mental Growth.* New York: The Macmillan Co., 1956, p. 9.

with others, and often make some satisfactory adjustment to a situation that cannot be changed.

5. *Health is taught accurately and from a positive viewpoint.* Well-being is emphasized rather than ill health. Health is associated with happy people and more productive living. Self-responsibility for healthful living is encouraged. It is part of growing up in a democracy.

Health information must be accurate. Too much misinformation is present in most areas, and popular health advice slips freely from the mouths of people everywhere. Good health instruction teaches children how to evaluate health information and obtain reputable advice. Self-diagnosis and self-medication are discouraged.

6. *In teaching health, certain learning practices and experiences are to be avoided.* Not only are some activities ineffective, but they may be actually harmful. Avoid such things as the following:

Awarding artificial prizes for good habits of attendance in school, or promoting "healthiest child" contests.

Scheduling health education on rainy days as a substitute for physical activity, thereby punishing the pupils because it rained.

Making children overly health conscious. There are already too many neurotic adults filled with fears and worries about their health.

Using one pupil in the class as an example of a defect.

Over-using parodies or nursery rhymes and songs.

Preaching good health and promising a long life. It is better to practice healthful living oneself and be the example of the moment.

7. *In health teaching, the wise teacher uses the classroom only as a useful adjunct or tool in learning.* Simply stated, the classroom has its limitations. It might at times be referred to as an educational roadblock,

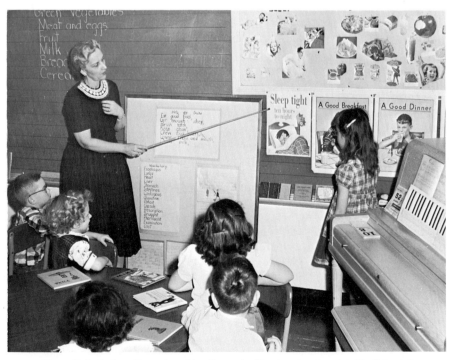

Figure 9–2 A class discussion of health words. (Courtesy Los Angeles City Schools.)

because it often places a barrier between student and teacher and frequently removes the world of books, ideas, and words from the real world. Thus the classroom at times must be vacated so that pupils may move out into the real world—to the stagnant pond near the school for mosquito life, to the playground for muscular exercise, to the city park for a study of beauty and mental health, to the local bakery or garbage disposal plant to *see* and *feel* the life and health of the community at the moment.

Most children live in communities large enough to provide an excellent laboratory setting in which to seek the solutions to problems initiated in the classroom. The manner in which one seeks the solution is the meat of the experience. Cantril says that the very process of seeking the solution may be more satisfying than the end goal achieved.[5] He is referring here to the value placed on the process of seeking and striving, the satisfactions derived from trying to determine direction or achieve a solution. It is what children mean when they exclaim, "Golly, that was fun!" or "I certainly enjoyed that game," and secretly regret that the game is over, no matter who won.

8. *Instruction in anatomy and physiology as a means of health education has its limitations.* The emphasis is controlled, for there is a tendency for pupils who have been taught with a maximum stress on anatomy and physiology to have less of an understanding of the basic health concepts than pupils taught with a minumum emphasis on these two helping sciences. This is not to say that one should omit reference to body structure and function. It is just a word of caution to those teachers who may find themselves teaching the names of bones and organs, and other similar facts

and figures, without proper concern for the use of such knowledge by the students. Several pupil-interest surveys have revealed that some of the health studies of body functions have been "dry" indeed. And one of the dryest is the lesson on the circulation of the blood. With a little preplanning by teachers and pupils, such a topic may be taught in a way to satisfy the inherent curiosity of most of the class.

Oberteuffer, in speaking about the anatomical-physiological method of teaching health has this to say:

> Anatomical detail is useful only in explanation, never, never as unrelated and extrinsic background to be taught just because someone thinks it is good to know that the duct of Wirsung is in the pancreas or that there are so many main branches off the aorta. The material is too far removed from ongoing interest, a need or a problem, and contributes only partially and then mostly by chance to the students' understanding of life. Such lifeless and meaningless teaching is responsible, in part, for the unpopularity of many hygiene courses and for the slight impact which many health books make upon the reading public.[6]

9. *Health facts brought out in the various methods of teaching are related to life situations.* This is a rewording of the old statement that knowledge is power, but it is not necessarily so without understanding. Facts are facts, and they may be learned as such, but attitudes and habits do not change unless teaching methods provide for changes. Edna St. Vincent Millay wrote a poem, *Huntsman, What Quarry?* It clearly expresses the need for something more than facts.

> Upon this gifted age, in its dark hours, rains from the sky a meteoric shower of facts. . . . they lie unques-

---

[5] Cantril, Hadley. *The Why of Man's Experience.* New York: The Macmillan Co., 1950, p. 202.

[6] Oberteuffer, Delbert, and Beyrer, Mary K. *School Health Education,* 4th ed. New York: Harper and Row, 1966, p. 106.

tioned, uncombined. Wisdom enough to leech us of our ill is daily spun, but there exists no loom to weave it into fabric.

Materials Strengthen Methods

Before engaging in a discussion of educational methods applicable to health instruction, a few points should be made to clear up any misconceptions relative to the differences between methods or techniques as such and instructional materials or aids.

Methods represent an organized way of doing something. One asks, for example, "How do we teach health?" or "By what method is the spread of disease germs best taught to primary grade school boys and girls?" Materials or aids, on the other hand, exist solely to facilitate the method. They are used to make the method more meaningful. A technique is very often successful simply because it involves the use of attractive materials. A second grade teacher, who employs a field trip to the dairy as an instructional method in the study of foods, finds that it is a good experience if her class has looked over copies of the booklet, *The Story of the Cow* (National Dairy Council) beforehand. Also, the teacher using the simple lecture method with her class will be far more effective when she illustrates her major points with cartoons or stick men drawings. These aids may have as much to do with ultimate pupil learnings as the method selected in the first place. There are times when the use of a certain aid becomes a method in itself; for example, the use of a selected textbook for mass study is a common method of putting across a concept or idea. On the other hand, browsing through a variety of books in the school library is a significant part of the library method of teaching.

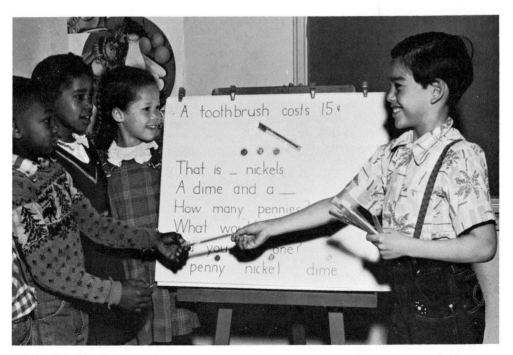

Figure 9-3 Materials strengthen methods. (Courtesy Safety and Youth Services Branch, Los Angeles Public Schools.)

It appears that there is a degree of overlapping between methods and materials, which only serves to emphasize the need for considering both when lessons are being planned. Appropriate methods, coupled with fascinating materials, do much to make health a living force in the lives of growing boys and girls.

Teaching Methods Applied to Health Education

The major techniques or methods employed in the numerous fields of education apply very well to the teaching of health in the elementary school. Some methods, of course, need modification. Others are more appropriate to the pupil age level and physical setup of the school.

It should be pointed out here that research has been carried on relative to the effect of conventional methods. Three questions asked were:

What can students learn largely by themselves?

What can students learn from explanation largely by others?

What learning requires personal interaction among students and teacher? Perhaps some health topics can best be taught according to the division of time suggested by the Trump report, i.e., 40 per cent for independent study, 40 per cent for large group instruction, and 20 per cent for small group instruction.[7]

The clever teacher may be able to apply almost any teaching method to health instruction. The following paragraphs explain the more common teaching techniques or methods with some comments relative to suitability for health teaching.

Lecture. Despite the admonitions of some people, there is little cause to condemn the lecture method. Properly applied in the grades, it can

be used to bring basic health facts to the pupils, a necessary foundation for more work to follow. It need not be dry, authoritative, uninteresting, and unstimulating—criticisms sometimes launched by students.

With the short span of interest evidenced at the elementary level, the lecture by the teacher should probably be given in the form of a chat or story, informal and yet precise. The danger is for the teacher to get too wrapped up in her topic and to overtalk to some degree. Words need action with them. Words are necessary, and they certainly have their place. However, messages repeated too often become ineffective. There is some evidence that a philosophy of "the more the better" can have undesired consequences. Frequent repetition can produce hostility toward the communicator, greater rigidity in existing attitudes, and forgetting or distortion of previously received information. No wonder children who have heard the toothbrushing lecture so often sometimes refuse to brush their teeth at all.

The health lecture must be arranged carefully with the teacher using appropriate instructional aids to put across significant points. Health methods must not fall back upon mere luck and chance, magic, exhortations, and preaching. Facts relative to vitamins or the physiological effects of alcohol on the body may be given orally, but they will probably be better retained and recalled if some discussion follows.

Class Discussion. A short lecture followed by preplanned discussion can be very effective in initiating a health unit. Discussing health information previously presented by the teacher is one way to discover the immediate and personal health needs of boys and girls. It also gives meaning to the facts. Ideas are spread about through conversation. Conversation connotes reciprocity, not monopoly.

---

[7] Trump, J. Lloyd, and Baynham, D. *Guide to Better Schools.* Chicago: Rand McNally & Co., 1961.

"Discourse," says Pope, "is the sweeter banquet of the mind."

There are a number of techniques which may be used to make the discussion more effective:

1. An overnight assignment, which requires some study or searching for ideas at home, will provoke a number of good questions the next day in class.

2. A list of questions, raised in earlier sessions and distributed prior to the discussion, helps the student who is a poor thinker. In studying teeth in the third grade, for example, questions such as these tend to generate personal curiosity:

How many teeth do I have?
When will I have all of my permanent teeth?
Will baking soda and salt clean my teeth?

3. A cloister discussion or "buzz session" where the class is divided into small groups is often productive.

One should keep in mind that all health topics are suitable for discussion. Even the subjects of vitamins, minerals, and calories, as matter-of-fact as it may seem to be, can be made quite interesting through the medium of group discussion. When teacher or pupil leadership is good, this technique is more effective.

The discussion also provides a chance for pupils to share their problems in class. Some things are elicited in discussion which may be the basis for trouble in later life. Children will often talk about their fear of the dark, the problems they have with younger brothers or sisters, or the fact that someone does not like them.

Psychologist Kurt Lewin has experimented with group discussion–decision technique in influencing attitudes and behavior. In essence it allows no one to tell a group what to do; a trained person leads discussions so that decisions come from the group itself. In one experiment, Lewin worked with two groups of women who had never eaten or cooked hearts, kidneys, or brains. The lecture method was used for one group, the discussion–decision technique for the other. Ten per cent of the former and 52 per cent of the latter subsequently used these items in their menus. Similarly, in health, a person may be influenced more by his own decision than by one he is asked or forced to accept.

Question-Answer. This is very much related to the class discussion method of teaching. Here the pupils ask questions and receive answers. The secret in using this technique is to anticipate the questions the class will ask and have vital answers ready. This may be accomplished by first initiating a certain health topic and then asking the class to prepare several questions on the topic. Once motivated, pupils will come up with a number of pertinent questions; when the pupils cannot suggest proper answers, the teacher is called upon to speak. A fifth grade class, for example, may proceed with specific questions and answers on the common cold:

Question	Answer
1. Do we know what causes a cold?	1. A virus is believed to be the culprit. Or, perhaps, several viruses.
2. Is cold weather a cause of colds?	2. No. Cold weather can't cause a common cold, but it may lower your resistance to one or aggravate an existing cold.
3. How about drafts and dampness? Won't they cause colds?	3. No. If there is no virus around, or if you are in a period of relative immunity, you could stand in ice water or in a draft for hours at a time without catching a cold.
4. What lowers resistance to a cold?	4. Poor nutrition and fatigue are believed to play a part. That's why it is wise to eat sensibly and get plenty of rest during the common-cold season.

Assignments. In studying a health topic, assignments are used to help pupils discover and solve health problems. In some health classes the group as a whole determines the assignment in the light of the problem of the moment. This is to be encouraged to some degree. There will be children, however, in need of more direct guidance who will have to have the assignment clarified by the teacher in order to eliminate confusion as to what is expected.

Effective assignments are not easy to make. They should grow from a current health topic or precede one. It is most important that they be introduced well enough in class to motivate the pupils' natural curiosity. In one elementary school class the children, as they approached the end of the school day, were talking about eyesight. One boy asked the teacher to tell him how many people wear eyeglasses. Someone else wondered how many schoolchildren wore them. The teacher then made an overnight assignment; the children were charged with

"counting noses" and finding out how many people wore eyeglasses in their neighborhoods. This assignment had meaning and did much to promote worthwhile instruction the following day.

Textbooks. Textbooks may be used so that they are classified as aids in the health instruction program. They may also be used as an effective method of health teaching.

Children cannot learn everything by experimenting or by first-hand experiences. Much is learned from reading textbooks, supplementary books, bulletins, magazines, and newspapers. Reading is sometimes condemned as a poor way to learn about health. It is often used so much that the health course degenerates into a course of reading about health. This criticism is leveled not against textbooks and reading as a method of learning, but against the *way* in which reading is used. It must not be a cut and dried approach where the teacher says, "Today we are going to study hearing. Open your books to page 36, read the first four

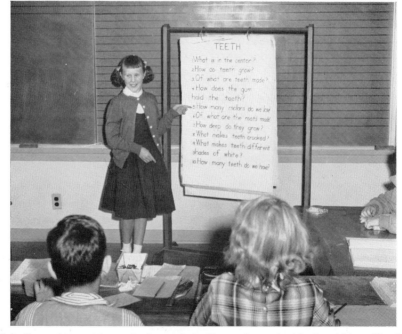

Figure 9–4 The problem-solving method may start with questions raised by the children. (Courtesy Sylvia Yellen, Alhambra City Schools, Alhambra, Calif.)

pages, and tell me what you have read." It is this kind of procedure that makes children dislike health education.

In the small elementary school where the teacher may not have enough time to prepare all of her own study materials, the textbook can be quite helpful. It should not be a crutch on the one hand or the bible of the health class on the other. It is simply used as a common tool for all children. In the case of the example of a class about to study hearing, it would be better to engage in some exploratory activity before using the textbook. Children might be asked to bring things to class which make a sound. The next day all kinds of sounds could be demonstrated in class. A violin, a flute, a drum, a ticking watch, a whisper, all stimulate interest in how the ear actually hears sounds. Someone may say, "When I had a cold I couldn't hear very well. Why didn't the sound get into my ear?" This may be the opportune time to delve into the textbook, especially if it has a particularly good picture of the ear structure.

Textbooks, therefore, are useful as guides, and reading is an important tool in learning about health. The reading is done with a specific purpose —to solve a problem, to secure more information, to learn how to do an experiment, or to answer a question. Moreover, health stories can provide nutritional material which will arouse pupil interest in studying a topic. It is excellent for individual study, and if words and pictures are carefully chosen, it can be quite effective. Words should be selected carefully. Cannon and others have pointed out that there are many "loaded" words which people react to emotionally. For an excellent discussion of this topic see the article by Johnson and Belzer.[8]

---

[8] Johnson, Warren R., and Belzer, E. G. "Language in Relation to Health," *Journal of School Health*, 32:134–138, April 1962.

For a discussion of criteria for selecting textbooks and other printed materials see Chapter 10.

Library. Because reading is more effective when it is done from several sources, the library method of teaching health holds considerable merit. Sources which supplement one another provide more information and present different points of view. It cannot be overstressed that the study of health should develop a scientific attitude in children. This means that pupils need to be open-minded, seek reliable sources for evidence, be curious, and know that there is a cause for everything. It means that pupils need a chance to appraise many health situations by experimenting and reading widely. Health reading in the library may give the pupil a clear realization that there is a real difference between materials that are read for fun and those read only for information.

The library is well suited for note taking. This may be an essential part of the research reading done for a particular health topic. With the help of the librarian, properly selected reading materials are made available, and pupils find things from books that simply cannot be discovered through observing, interviewing, and experimenting.

The elementary school library plays an important role in the entire school health program. Children need to be able to use it freely as a source of books, pamphlets, magazines, recordings, films, slides, maps, globes, reference books, atlases, dictionaries, and audio-visual projectors. The attitude of the classroom teacher toward the library usually determines how functional the library method of teaching about health becomes. The cooperative efforts of the teacher and librarian in setting up a health exhibit in the library or classroom often produce considerable pupil interest.

Problem Solving. No pupil ever becomes an improved problem solver by filling in the blanks in a workbook, by looking up the definition of something, or by just living in the same room with a cage full of white rats and a set of health textbooks. Here the ancient laws of use and disuse apply. One is better able to solve problems when he has solved previous problems — problems which mean something to him.

Solving problems is not something that takes place easily. Children have to want to find answers. They have to *discover* the problem first. They have to be disturbed, even frustrated, before they have the urge to set forth in search of health information. Motivation is involved here. In one school both the teacher and the pupils agreed that lunchroom table manners were at an all-time low. Gradually they decided that they wanted to do something about it, so they formed a club which they call "The Good Manners Club." When their classmates met the requirements, they received a certificate of achievement.

In a southern school the dietitian was invited to tell about her duties to a fourth grade class. She indicated that she was distressed at the amount of food being left on the children's plates following the noon-hour lunch period. After some discussion, the class agreed that this was a problem and that they would accept the challenge to solve it. They formulated a plan of attack, divided into small groups, and made an on-the-spot survey of the school lunchroom during the eating period. Upon returning to class and talking over the problem, it was decided that one way to solve the problem might be to organize a "Clean Plate Club." The dietitian decided to give it a try. She had buttons made, such as political candidates use, bearing the words CLEAN PLATE CLUB. All elementary teachers were given the number of buttons needed each day. Each day some buttons were recalled as occasions arose. Most teachers ate with their children and found it easy to observe the plate of each child. The

MEMBERSHIP

THE GOOD MANNERS CLUB"

(DATE)

------------------------- WAS OBSERVED AT LUNCH AND PASSED THE GOOD MANNERS

TEST SATISFACTORILY.

1 KEPT LIPS TOGETHER WHILE EATING _____

2 TOOK SMALL AMOUNTS OF FOOD AT A TIME _____

3 TALKED ABOUT PLEASANT THINGS _____

4 KEPT ELBOWS OFF THE TABLE _____

5. TALKED IN A LOW VOICE _____

6. DID NOT WASTE FOOD _____

7. HAD GOOD POSTURE _____

_____
(STUDENT JUDGE)

_____
(TEACHER)

pupils were so eager to wear the buttons that they made a real effort to eat all their food, even the food that they normally disliked. The original fourth grade problem solvers appraised the button situation and concluded, along with the dietitian, that they had successfully solved the problem.

Important health problems are usually made known with the help of the teacher. She often leads the way in discovering such items as community health hazards, causes of accidents and illnesses in school, causes of school absences, difficulties in eating, and personal unhappiness. Sometimes the problem is demonstrated by the use of a film. In one sixth grade class there had been quite a little discussion about the number of pupils who appeared to have poor posture. The teacher secured the film, *Improving Your Posture* (Coronet Instructional Films), and showed it to the class. As a result of this everyone wanted to start a posture campaign at once. A method of approach was decided upon, and the class set forth to solve the posture problem. Not only did they talk with other elementary school pupils, but they also read textbooks and supplementary readers. They made the school posture-conscious for a considerable period of time and received the praises of both the school administration and the local Parent-Teacher Association.

Problems are solved when children recognize the problems, gather pertinent data, verify and interpret the data, and present conclusions. Data may be gathered by reading, looking at pictures, viewing a film, taking a trip, experimenting, listening to a transcription, asking someone who is an authority, making a survey, and discussing the way we feel about a situation. Conclusions should be made in a general way so that they represent at least one solution to the problem.

Experiment. In many ways the experimental method of teaching health is related to problem solving. It is more formal, but it is founded on the same kind of pupil interest and is successful when there is a burning curiosity to *find out* why we act as we do, or what makes us "tick."

This method is especially stimulating to upper grade schoolchildren who are entering the adventuresome period where they rise quickly to almost any challenge to discover and explore. This is the period that Charles Kettering spoke of when he expressed his views on his own aspirations at an early age. He was always intrigued with the "why." He wanted to know "why" the black cow could eat green grass and give pure white milk. It drove him to experiment in chemistry and biology and became a moving force in initiating his famous career.

True conviction comes from testing and trying things out by oneself. Sometimes simple classroom or laboratory experiments involving the principles of food decay, moisture, or cleanliness carry more conviction than many of the elaborately printed materials and expensive films one may obtain on the topic. The really effective experimental method requires a thorough organization. This is just as true with second graders as it is with secondary school pupils. Some of the points to keep in mind when setting up a health experiment are as follows:[9]

1. Keep the experiment simple. Simple homemade equipment is often more satisfactory than the more elaborate kind.

2. Perform experiments or have them performed in such a manner as to cause children to think. Do not tell the answers or have the pupils read

---

[9] Adapted from the work of Glenn O. Blough and Albert J. Huggett, *Elementary School Science and How to Teach It*. New York: Dryden Press, 1957, p. 27.

them. Permit them to experiment and find out.

3. Plan experiments carefully and let the pupils do much of the planning. If the plan fails, the pupils have some basis for deciding why it did not work since they were the ones who made the plan.

4. Warn pupils not to make sweeping generalizations from one small experiment. Most pupil experiments do not *prove* anything. They merely help pupils answer a question or understand an idea.

5. Permit pupils to perform the experiment themselves. They should work in groups if sufficient materials are available; otherwise the experiment should be carried out where all can see it.

6. Encourage children to originate experiments in order to solve a problem. If one pupil asks the teacher what would happen if the body did not get enough calcium, with a little encouragement another pupil might suggest an animal feeding experiment (Figures 9–5, 9–6).

7. The basic purpose for performing an experiment is something much broader than just to answer the question raised. An experiment, to be worth while, should answer questions about things children see in the world about them. Too often this application to real-life situations is overlooked.

8. It is not necessary to have records of all experiments performed in the elementary school. The teacher may be guided by the idea, "Is there any reason for writing anything about this experiment?"

Children can experiment at every age. Even second graders can study moisture as it relates to colds and sore throats by holding a damp cloth over a heater and observing what happens. Third graders can watch mold appear on a crust of bread and draw valid conclusions without going into any further experimentation. Some of the health experiments that have proven

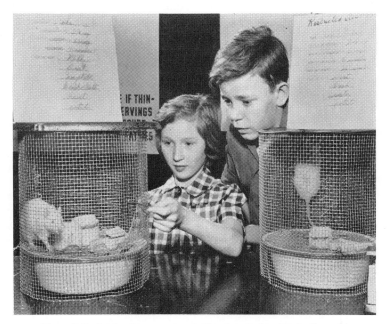

Figure 9–5 Rat feeding experiment. (Courtesy National Dairy Council.)

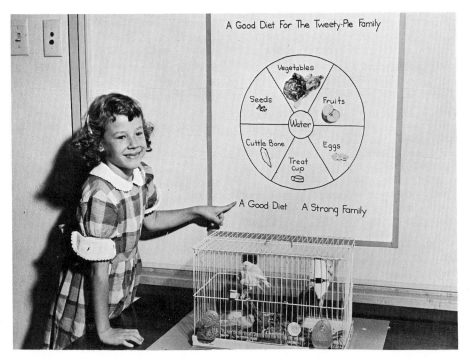

Figure 9–6   Bird feeding experiment. (Courtesy *Health Education Journal,* Los Angeles City Schools.)

especially valuable over the years include:

Animal feeding experiments to measure the effect of certain foods on growth.[10]

Individual height-weight measurements.

Decay of foods under different situations.

Analysis of the action of useful molds and bacteria in the making of vinegar and cheese.

The making of a satisfactory tooth powder.

Canning of foods.

Oxygen-consuming experiments involving the lighted candle in a glass jar over water, or done with a mouse instead of a candle.

Testing for starch and sugar in various foods.

---

[10] For a very interesting duck feeding experiment relating milk to growth, see John Bareham, "How Ducks Teach Children," *Journal of Health, Physical Education, and Recreation,* 25(4):18, April 1954.

EXPERIMENT – STARCH

DIRECTIONS FOR THE PUPIL

Problem

a. How can we test for starch in foods?

b. Do milk and the other foods listed have starch in them?

Materials

cornstarch	test tubes
baking soda	iodine
milk (dry)	dropper
sugar	test tube holders
potato	(optional)
hard-cooked egg	test tube rack
knife	(optional)

What to do

a. Place about one-half teaspoon of cornstarch in a test tube. Fill the test tube one-half full of water. Add a drop of iodine. What happens? Make the same test with baking soda. Does the same thing happen?

b. Try each of the other foods suggested under "Materials." In all cases soften the food thoroughly with water as is suggested for the cornstarch. In the case of potato and other solid foods, it is best to use scrapings. Look for any change in color in the water or on the bits of food.

What did you observe?
What do you think this experiment shows?

SUPPLEMENTARY AIDS FOR THE TEACHER'S USE

The test

When a blue color is formed with iodine, starch is present. Cornstarch, which children know as a form of starch, gives the blue color as does potato. Soda, sugar, egg whites, and milk do not.

Testing additional foods

Other foods may be brought from home to test, such as bread, oatmeal, cornmeal, ripe banana, apple, meat. The test shows best on solid foods. Omit dark-colored foods since the test is a color test. Of the above foods, only bread and cereals give the test for starch.

Equipment

Cups might be used in place of test tubes. However, children like to use test tubes, and this test offers an easy experience in handling chemical equipment. Test tubes, test tube holders, and a test tube rack might be borrowed from children's chemistry sets.

Use a tincture of about 1 per cent iodine. The test does not show well with strong iodine. It may be made weaker with alcohol or water.

Related questions and activities

Plants make starch. Where do they store their starch? Read to find out.

Do we use many foods that contain starch in our daily meals? If so, why?

What happens if you eat more food than your body uses for energy? If you are fat, name some foods of which you might eat less.

Babies, at first, use only milk in their diets. How, then, do they get what starch supplies in your food?

If a microscope is available, observe starch grains under the microscope. Drop a solution of iodine on the slide and observe again through the microscope. (Each grain of starch takes on a shiny bluish-purple appearance.)

The following animal experiment illustrates better than almost anything else the powerful motivational force inherent in a properly conceived and implemented experimental method. Throughout the experiment there is demonstrated a sustained interest of high degree. This is the report of a sixth grade experiment conducted, written up, and presented to the author by Annette Marco Penan of Jacksonville, Florida.

A RAT EXPERIMENT IN THE SIXTH GRADE

We received two white, albino, laboratory raised mice, 28 days old, from the National Dairy Council. Both were males; one weighed approximately 48 grams, the other 50 grams. They were brought to us on a Thursday morning complete with instructions regarding their care, a pair of white workman's gloves, and a gram scale.

Thursday and Friday we discussed the habits of rats, types, and differences, diseases, control, etc. We used the encyclopedias, science books, nature books, read the Pied Piper of Hamlin and played games. We compared rat ages with human ages, and made charts. Some of the boys made age comparison charts on many different types of animals—dogs, horses, elephants, etc.

The first thing I did was to go up and down the aisles and let every child touch the rats while I held them. I did not insist on everyone touching. I then explained how to pick them up so as not to frighten or bruise them, made them all promise to wear at least one glove to protect both the rat and themselves, and opened the rats' mouths and showed the little sharp teeth. The entire time I caressed and petted the little things so that all the children could see how very gentle I was with them.

For fear of injury we all decided that possibly they had been handled too much already. After each and every child came by me and touched them again, we put them back in their box and they were not handled any more that day.

As soon as they settled down (both rats and children), we began to plan. I would have liked cages but the children made different arrangements—a bird cage and the case from a record player brought from home. (I still wonder what happened to the record player, but you never in your life saw such a fancy rat cage: the top with wire, the sides painted glass, fancy food dishes, little decorated boxes for them to sleep in, etc.) We kept the rats together until Monday when we began our experiment.

We discussed what we might be able to prove, and we decided to use good and poor breakfasts. We made rules for the care and feeding as well as the handling of the rats, agreed that the children would have to bring a note from home if they wanted to take one home to care for over the weekend, and that they would give the rats only the diets we planned. We would schedule the weekend home visits after the notes arrived. I took them the first weekend to avoid confusion.

Friday, while their cage was being cleaned, the children were permitted to handle the rats themselves, and those poor little things visited on every one of 36 desks that day.

Both rats had the same diet until Monday at which time they were both weighed and measured; there was still approximately 2 grams difference in their weight. The children put the heavier one on the good diet; the other on the poor.

After being weighed, each rat was put in a separate labeled cage. The class suggested names which we voted upon, and the rats' charts read like this:

Name of rat — Mr. Kingsize
Weight of rat at beginning _____
Weight of rat at completion _____
Age of rat at beginning _____
Age of rat at completion _____
Date demonstration starts _____
Diet of rat: Whole grain bread or cereal, plus milk, plus fruit, plus bread and butter, plus egg

Name of rat — Mr. Regular
Weight of rat at beginning_____
Weight of rat at completion _____
Age of rat at beginning _____
Age of rat at completion _____
Date demonstration starts _____
Diet of rat: Sweet roll and coffee

The children brought in the food which we kept in containers. Milk and coffee were fresh every day from the lunch room.

Daily records were kept of their appearance, activity, disposition, etc. Every Monday morning they were weighed and their weight charted on a large line graph. The children kept a small graph on graph paper in their note books.

During the weeks that followed we studied about the basic foods, had posters and charts on display, made posters and charts, wrote stories, kept a diary on the daily changes in the rats, made booklets, worked arithmetic problems comparing ages, plotted weights (gains and losses), studied weights and measures, graphs (line and bar), charts, printing. The children took care of the rats — committees to clean, others to feed, others to weigh and chart, etc.

Rat cartoons appeared, booklet covers were made, the mothers came to see the progress, and children started eating good breakfasts. Other children in the school came into the room to see the rats, so we issued a weekly bulletin on the changes appearing, the weights and dispositions.

The rats performed beautifully. Mr. King-size became tremendous, developed full of mischief. Poor little Mr. Regular developed a scaly, spotted tail, feet and ears became dry and rough, hair shaggy and dull, a definite contrast to the beautiful ermine coat of Mr. Kingsize. Mr. Regular became sulky and twice I was afraid we were going to lose him, but I cheated after the children went home and I gave him a little milk and dry oatmeal and he'd perk up a little. After four weeks the contrast was great and the children were beginning to worry. Since one of the purposes had been served, the children were delighted when I suggested not continuing for the full six weeks that we had originally decided upon.

We voted to see if we should reverse the diets or to just put Mr. Regular on the same diet as Mr. Kingsize. It was unanimous that the diets *not* be reversed, so both rats then had the same diet. Within two weeks' time Mr. Regular started catching up to Mr. Kingsize and there was a sharp upsweep on the graphs. By the end of four weeks they weighed almost the same, and Mr. Regular's tail lost its scaly look, his eyes became larger and brighter, and his fur grew in thickness and became shiny. (As one of the little boys pointed out to me though, there was still a difference in their sex organs. I hadn't noticed, but there was.)

All these weeks the children had been making booklets about the experiments. We took pictures each week and then made a booklet to give to the Dairy Council containing selections from the children's booklets and pictures by the children together with the photographs.

The experiment over, and the children much more aware of the needs of a balanced diet, they became more conscious of their own growth and development. They were more alert in the mornings; only one or two ever fell asleep in class (TV late show—not lack of breakfast). Some mothers complained that they had to fix breakfast now, others were happy. One child fixed his own breakfast, but became a problem when selecting food; he insisted on buying certain items.

Any child who brought a note from home saying he could have a rat had his name put in a box. At the Christmas party we drew the names, and the rats went home with two little girls. The last week of school Mr. Regular came back to visit with us for the day. The children greeted him with great excitement—their little friend was hale and hearty. They were sorry that Mr. Kingsize had been sent to rat heaven by a neighborhood dog, but they were glad that it hadn't been Mr. Regular, who had been such a good sport and had taught them so much.

Demonstration.   Children like to be entertained; they like to see things done before their eyes, especially if there is an element of the mysterious which they do not understand. The teacher who describes some phase of the body function through skillful demonstration encourages the class to want to do it themselves.

A sixth grade health class, in studying the principles of respiration, may observe a demonstration of artificial resuscitation and follow this by a practice period in which everyone gets an opportunity to "revive" and "be revived." A first grade class, after observing the posture of the teacher who "walks tall," will want to try it themselves, and they should do so. In one primary grade the cleanliness of animals was discussed. In class the children watched a real cat clean itself with its paws. One of the pupils combed and brushed a long-haired dog. Another pupil demonstrated how

elephants in South Africa saunter down to the nearest river toward sundown and drink and bathe. This was effective.

Actually, there are three kinds of demonstrations: teacher demonstrations, individual pupil demonstrations, and group demonstrations. All three require preplanning in order to be effective. Individual and group demonstrations often promote more class interest than those performed by the teacher.

Small Group Study.   Groups of children may be formed into committees which 'work together to accomplish a common purpose. In the primary grades the word "committee" is not used. Instead, children's names such as "Tom and Sally," or "Mary and the other three girls" are used to designate groups.

The teacher guides the work of the committee or small group until it is ready to work independently. Children become members of a particular committee only because they are interested in the problem to be tackled by the group. Good committee members know what to do, ask questions, list sources of information, plan the reports, and present them to the class. One health topic may be initiated by the creation of four or five small groups who will consider the several aspects of the topic. Recent research suggests that this is a very effective teaching method which is not employed often enough.

Dramatic Play and Dramatization. To the child, play is real. It is full of meaning. Through this natural expression a wealth of learning is acquired. Mimetics and action stories are common activities in the play of growing boys and girls. One sees children imitating the cowboy, the mother, the physician, the nurse, and many other personalities from everyday life.

Dramatic play is unrestrained and unrehearsed. In the kindergarten and first grade the pupils generally prefer to play alone. Eight year olds will begin to play as a group. The teacher often finds that she has only to suggest a theme, and eager, creative children will start to dramatize it as they see fit. Because of the high pupil interest in dramatizations, the method is a good one to use in teaching health.

All seasons of the year lend themselves to dramatizations in the health line. At Thanksgiving time, for example, the story of the nutritious and tasty cranberry can be told. It is a colorful fruit to consider for stories.[11] So highly were cranberries prized by the Indian tribes in southeastern Massachusetts that they made a gift of them to the Pilgrims who cooked them into a sauce to serve with wild turkey and geese. It is believed that cranberries brightened the Pilgrims' first Thanksgiving feast in 1621. Moreover, the health-giving qualities of cranberries were recognized almost immediately, and in the early period of America's development, whenever vessels left New England's shores, they carried barrels of cranberries in the hold—not for trade but for the sailors to eat. Just as the English seamen prevented scurvy by eating limes, so American sailors ate cranberries, and in the Middle West, where scurvy was a scourge of the logging camps, cranberries were served regularly.

Health plays, created by the pupils from a classroom experience, are generally the most valuable. In discussing the maintenance of one's personal health through proper physical examinations, the class may decide to dramatize a visit to the school health service or the office of the family physician. Some health plays are acceptable for dramatizing a certain aspect of a health topic.

For many years puppets have been successfully used to put across certain

concepts in elementary education. Puppets are fascinating to the average boy and girl; they can make statements that will be remembered longer than those made by the teacher. Interest is maintained at an even higher level when the puppets are made by the members of the class.

In using puppets for health teaching, fantasy and imagination must be separated from accurate health information.

Sometimes the dramatization takes the form of an organized play. There are a number of practical ways of making the play effective:

1. Try to get as many pupils associated with the play as possible.

2. Use a small stage or platform instead of the crowded classroom if this can be arranged. Do not worry about the absence of backdrops and props; it is part of the fun, and, after all, "the play's the thing."

3. Try an arena style performance. Here the audience surrounds the actors on all four sides, adding to the intimacy of the situation and helping even the most detached pupil to feel that he is a part of the performance.

4. Simply assign children to parts and proceed to read the play without attempting to act it out. Although less effective than the acted version, this method does promote discussion.

The Health Project. This has much in common with the problem-solving method. It calls for the study of a problem which is organized by the teacher and pupils in the form of a project or task to be accomplished. It may mean experimenting or carrying on a survey, interview, or discussion in an effort to ascertain the facts applicable to the particular health question.

The first requirement in a project is to identify and define a health problem which merits study. Goals are established as in the problem-solving method, but they appear to be broader in the project method. A class project might involve several aspects of alcohol and tobacco usage, but problem-

[11] For a useful teacher's guidebook, *Cranberries, America's Native Fruit*, write to Ocean Spray Cranberries, Inc., Hanson, Mass.

solving would ordinarily represent one phase (one question) of the over-all topic.

Creative Activities. When children express themselves without restraint and without teacher control, they are usually being creative to some degree. Imaginative and creative children may develop and act upon a health topic in several ways — through dramatizations, mimetics, and creative play. These have already been referred to. Another way is through creative writing. Older children who enjoy writing are capable of treating a health problem rationally by writing about it. The outlet for this activity is through the school paper or possibly through the local newspaper.

A fascinating source of ideas and unique materials is Creative Play Things, Inc., Princeton, N.J. 08540. Here, all kinds of things pupils can work with have been developed in order to take advantage of the solid relationship between creativity, learning, and play.

Creative rhythms is another technique in teaching that is generally overlooked. Creative dance permits the child to express, communicate, and enjoy. In the process of dance-making the pupil plans, experiments, selects, and appraises a number of movements with the help of the teacher. His dance may be interpretive, such as playing the part of a "happy toothbrush," or it may be dramatic and be a part of a story danced by the whole group. Usually it is descriptive — a poem, song, or an idea is conveyed through movement — high like a cloud, low like a caterpillar, fast like a squirrel, or slow like a snowman melting in the sun.

Field Trips. The field trip, like any other experience, is planned from the earliest stage through its final evaluation and follow-up. Even before planning, the teacher attempts to find out whether the children are ready for the trip, i.e., possess the capacity and background that is needed.

In one New York school the second grade planned a trip to the zoo to observe the eating habits of animals. They asked the following questions:
    "What do we want to know?"
    "How shall we go?"
    "How shall we prepare?"
    "How shall we behave on the trip?"
    "What will we need to do?"
They decided on the following:

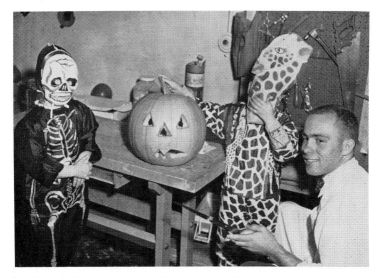

Figure 9-7   Creative activities promote interest in every season. (Courtesy Campus School, State University of New York, Oswego, N.Y.)

Talk with parents, friends, neighbors, and teachers

Obtain further information from books and other aids

Trace the route on a map of the city

Use money

Estimate time and distance

Prepare a report about the trip

Although the trip was a short-term experience, it was beneficial in terms of health instruction and in relating to other subject matter fields such as art, music, mathematics, science, language arts, and social studies.

The health area is rich in opportunities for impressive field trips. Worthwhile excursions may be taken to the dentist's office, the police department, the cannery, the bakery, the dairy, the food-processing plant, and the water works. Exercise caution because it is easy to abuse rather than use this method of instruction. Trips should be made only when there is a real reason for going. The excursion is made as an integral part of the school health lesson that is in progress. Children studying the source of a water supply and how and why it is made pure may have a natural curiosity for wells, streams, types of soil, germs, purification, and the city water works. At this stage in the topic they are ready to plan a trip to the water works to see how water is purified, what filter beds look like, how chlorine and sodium fluoride are added to the water supply to protect the health of the people, and many other items that are appropriate to consider at the time. A follow-up discussion is engaged in upon returning to the classroom; this tends to anchor the experience in the minds of the pupils. Thus "going to see" can be a most enjoyable and instructive way to learn.[12]

Construction Activities. These activities are often grossly misunderstood. This, says Macomber, "has resulted partially from lack of understanding of the basic philosophy on which this activity is based and partially from the fact that the activity has been judged by the product constructed rather than evaluated by the pupil growths resulting from the experiences."[13] After all, the appearance of the homemade simple microscope in the sixth grade or the crude milk truck made in the first grade is of little significance; *of chief concern is what has happened to the individual.*

Construction activities include everything from using the hammer and saw to build a model playground, to using paste, tape, and staples to set up a novel three-sided health exhibit. There can be as much real work involved in this method of instruction as there is in the project or problem-solving methods. Research, reading, discussion, and creative expression are background activities for the successful completion of an item under construction.

Pupil interests have much to do with method. Witty has written at length on the role of interest in child development and the need to utilize children's interests. In one study of Chicago schoolchildren it was discovered that about 92 per cent of the first and second graders said that they like to make or construct things.[14] It is possible, therefore, that teachers have underestimated the value of working with the hands.[15]

---

[12] For a practical approach to the task of arranging field trips, see Jack Zusman, "Field Trips: How to Plan and Use Them," *American Journal of Public Health*, 57:661–664, April 1967. For additional ideas send for elementary school curriculum guides in health, Jefferson Elementary School District, Dale City, California.

[13] Macomber, Freeman Glenn. *Principles of Teaching in the Elementary School.* New York: American Book Co., 1954, p. 143.

[14] Witty, Paul A. "Pupil Interests in the Elementary Grades," *Education*, 83:451–462, April 1963.

[15] Pupils must do things with their own hands. Because the potter works with his hands in shaping the clay, and because he is sensitive to the properties of the mix and its relationship to firing, color, and texture, he becomes changed as a person. He is as much transformed by his art as the clay is.

Health teaching in the primary grades permits the sandbox to be used for building grocery stores, farms, irrigation ditches, and city roads and parks. Several work tables, complete with tools, encourage the construction of models of such items as teeth from clay, toothbrush holders from wood, safety patrol emblems from tin, napkin rings from leather, metal, or wood, shower room slippers from cardboard, attractive handkerchiefs from colored pieces of cloth, and many other health related items. The object, of course, is to make sure that all constructed items are directly related to the health instruction topic.

The construction period should be fairly long. If it is too short, the actual working time is not long enough to justify the time spent in getting ready and cleaning up. Since construction activities are not done on a daily basis, it is not too long to spend 1 to 1½ hours in the primary grades and up 2 hours in the upper grades. There will be times when a health lesson is being dramatized that several pieces of furniture and other properties will be needed right away. Time spent to construct them may be especially worth while in keeping interest high at the beginning of a unit of work.

Some examples of construction activities which may be related to health teaching are:

1. Construct simple wastebaskets.

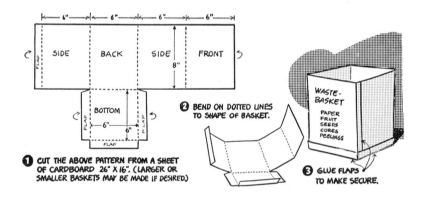

2. Build Stop and Go signals for schoolroom use and recognition.

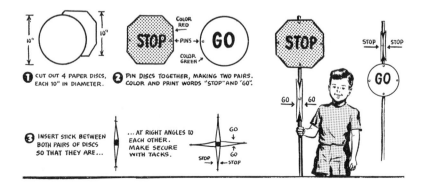

3. Make simple pencil clips to help impress children with the need for carrying pencils safely.

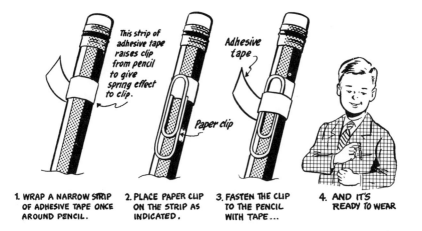

This strip of adhesive tape raises clip from pencil to give spring effect to clip.

Adhesive tape

Paper clip

1. WRAP A NARROW STRIP OF ADHESIVE TAPE ONCE AROUND PENCIL.

2. PLACE PAPER CLIP ON THE STRIP AS INDICATED.

3. FASTEN THE CLIP TO THE PENCIL WITH TAPE...

4. AND IT'S READY TO WEAR

4. Prepare "poison" labels for use at home.

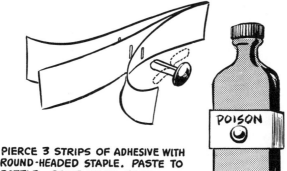

PIERCE 3 STRIPS OF ADHESIVE WITH ROUND-HEADED STAPLE. PASTE TO BOTTLE. PRINT WORD "POISON" ON ADHESIVE. THE THICK STRIP AND THE STAPLE HEAD CAN BE FELT IN THE DARK.

POISON

5. As a workship project, intermediate grade boys can make a baseball equipment rack.

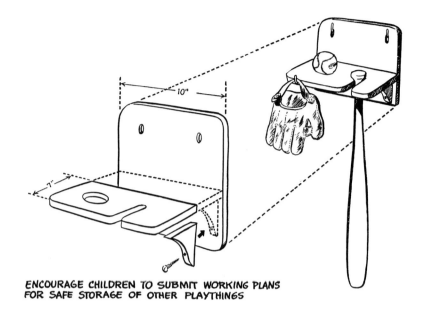

ENCOURAGE CHILDREN TO SUBMIT WORKING PLANS
FOR SAFE STORAGE OF OTHER PLAYTHINGS

Although cleverly constructed items encourage other children to try their skill and do likewise, their greatest value is obtained at the moment the individual or small group work on the particular project. There is genuine meaning to the child in a spot map built with colored pins to show the different types of accidents in the school and on the school grounds. There is value in mounting pictures, building charts and graphs, painting a picture of human anatomy, assembling a collection of foods, diagramming the local fire alarm system, putting together bird feeding trays, constructing a health museum, and dozens of similar purposeful activities.

Educational Games. The use of games to teach almost any topic adds ginger to the program. Play is to the child as work is to the man; it is full of meaning. Almost everyone knows that if something can be made to seem like play, it can be learned quickly.

Purposely making a game of something, therefore, is sound methodology.

Slow learners, say researchers, are the chief beneficiaries of games — especially when games supplement other educational programs, making real and vivid material that sometimes seems abstract in a textbook. Carlson speaks at length about how games spur enthusiasm and how many students try harder at games than in some courses.[16]

Games should be carefully planned, and the children should know what the real goals are. Games provide many opportunities for an expression of characteristics conducive to optimum social health. Properly conceived, there are many chances for each child to demonstrate cooperation, group loyalty, leadership, and fair play. Games are more than mid-morn-

[16] Carlson, Elliot. "Games in the Classroom," *Saturday Review*, April 15, 1967.

ing relief activities; they enlist mental activity, enrich the learning experience, contribute to personality growth, and help achieve classroom goals.[17]

Numerous examples can be cited showing how to use a game situation to further the learning of a particular health topic. Some illustrations follow:

1. Use a posture relay in teaching about posture. This is a regular relay race, except that the pupils running must carry a flat object such as a blackboard eraser on their heads. Point out to the class the difficulty in this feat when one does not assume a plumb-line posture.

2. Make up riddles. Divide the class into two teams. For example, in discussing the teeth, one pupil says, "I am thinking of something we should do before going to school each morning." Using her watch, the teacher notes the time it takes for the other team to guess the correct answer. Riddles are alternated between teams, with the winning team being the one that has the lowest total time.

3. To teach pedestrian safety to primary graders, have pupils draw a floor map of a busy intersection. Assign children as policemen, pedestrians, automobile drivers. Cardboard discs may be fashioned as steering wheels. Simulate normal traffic conditions.

4. Use a playhouse situation and emphasize home safety. Children play the parts of different family members.

5. A simple group game of "squat tag" may contribute to mental health, especially if the pupils realize that they are accepting the rules of the game and are having fun playing. The person being chased simply has to squat down to keep from being "It."

6. Play a game of "Health Detectives." Children report on what they have seen and heard each day that pertains to health. One child may have seen the soccer team practicing; a bicycle rider may have seen someone else riding at night without a light; one child may have noticed that children do not run up and down the stairs in the school; someone else may casually point out that Sally Jones has a runny nose — and many more.

7. Use mimetics in primary grades. When discussing pets and home safety have the class walk like cats, run like dogs, or hop like rabbits. Music may be used and rhythm developed around a theme. For example, sunflowers grow tall in the sun. As a posture activity the children may stretch high with their arms in an effort to grow high like sunflowers.

8. Identify objects by taste, odor, or sound while blindfolded. Divide the class into teams. This will help motivate the class in studying the interrelationship of the senses. Some materials to have on hand for the game might include a piece of chocolate, a spoiled orange, sour milk, or a musical record.

9. To increase the familiarity of first graders with fruits and vegetables play the game, "Upset the Fruit Basket," using the story about a farmer who brings his produce to market. Assign to the children, in pairs, names of various fruits and vegetables. Each pair must exchange places when the names are called. If the child who is "It" gets one of their seats, the one left standing must continue the story. When the storyteller says, "Upset the Fruit Basket," everyone must change places.

10. Secure copies of *Kellogg's Safari Breakfast Game* (Kellogg Co., Battle Creek, Mich.). This has been very well accepted for primary grade school usage. In this game the class is divided into four teams, the progress of which is followed on a colorful 18-inch by 15-inch wall chart. Each student keeps a record of the breakfast he has eaten each morning. Team progress (ad-

---

[17] A wide variety of unique games for kindergarten and first grade pupils may be found in Dorothy Kirk Burnett's book, *Your Preschool Child*, New York: Holt, Rinehart & Winston, 1961.

vances on the chart) is dependent on the number of team members who have eaten good breakfasts.

11. Play the game where a pupil spins a wheel made out of oaktag or heavy cardboard. It is popular in Roslyn Public Schools, New York. The wheel is divided into triangle sections. Each section contains a group of un-associated words. The pupil writes sentences using one of the words in each section.

Sample sentences:
The dentist filled my tooth.
I brush my teeth after eating.
Milk is good for my teeth.
I will eat candy only at the end of meals.

12. Ask children to bring colorful pictures of food clipped from maga-zines. Mount these illustrations on lightweight cardboard and cut to make a jig-saw puzzle.

13. Write "mixed-up" words on the chalkboard or duplicate lists and dis-tribute them to children. Let pupils unscramble the letters to make words which are names of foods. Here are examples:

iklm	milk
draeb	bread
gge	egg
epalp	apple

14. Food charades. Pupils may take

turns acting out something to do with food, such as making a cake, peeling an apple, and so on. Whoever guesses the answer has the next turn of being "It."

15. Guess the health object. Place individual pictures of health items in a large box. Have one of the pupils go to the box and draw out a picture, shield-ing it from the rest of the class. He should then describe the object. The child who guesses it is the next one to go and draw a picture from the box.

Programmed Instruction. In the best sense of the word, programmed instruction is still considered a revo-lutionary device for enriching student experiences and individualizing in-struction. As Wilbur Schramm points out, it has a potential for freeing schools from outworn theories and practices — but so far it has not realized this potential.[18]

Programmed health instruction has been employed in a number of com-munities because it provides the indi-vidual pupil with organized health in-formation which can be learned with an immediate knowledge of results.

The Behavioral Research Labora-

[18] Schramm, Wilbur. "Introduction," *Four Case Studies of Programmed Instruction.* New York: The Fund for the Advancement of Educa-tion, 1964, p. 8.

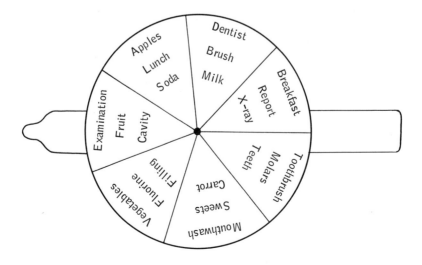

tories programmed a *First Aid* manual which Johnson & Johnson took over for distribution.[19] It has been used with thousands of students throughout the country and is designed for sixth grade use. There is a procedure for using the manual and the first aid film strip which accompanies it. A teacher's instruction manual and a test manual are also available on a complimentary basis. Students work with their own manual, and, since it is different from most workbooks, the novelty seems to appeal to children.

Other health programs which are a part of the American Health and Safety Series and are distributed by Behavioral Research Laboratories include programmed instruction titles: *Body Structure and Function, Personal Health, Nutrition, Safety,* and *Prevention of Communicable Disease.* These programmed learning experiences provide continuity between the easier and the more difficult health concepts by acquainting the pupil with the organized nature of knowledge. Because the learner can proceed at his own speed, he is not threatened by the task; he knows he is learning, and anxiety should be somewhat reduced.

An additional example of programmed instruction is the *Student's Manual on Venereal Disease,* validated with eighth grade pupils and developed by William F. Schwartz of the U.S. Public Health Service. Both the manual and the teacher's handbook may be obtained from the American Association for Health, Physical Education, and Recreation in Washington.

Miscellaneous Techniques. *Storytelling,* an age-old device, has always been a powerful way of impressing youngsters with health facts, especially if the information is accurate and the storyteller skilled in the art. Numerous good health stories are available in textbooks and supplementary readers.

The dental health stories of the American Dental Association, and the story of *You and Your Engine* of the National Livestock and Meat Board are but two examples of stories readily available for teachers. Health legends and stories on filmstrips are also available from a number of sources. Even the popular Little Golden Books are good in the health area. Children learn to listen when they are accustomed to having interesting things to hear.

The *guest speaker,* for example, the physician, dentist, policeman, or dogcatcher, is often a welcome relief in the average classroom. He brings life to the class. He is from the world of reality outside the school and is sometimes able to put across a particular health recommendation where the regular classroom teacher has difficulty.

Oral presentations have their place in health teaching. Good reports resulting from research, problem-solving, experimentation, library, and readings need to be skillfully presented to the class. Individual pupil presentations of this nature, followed by class discussion, represent a useful instruction technique.

The *anecdote* represents an interesting tale, narrative, or description of some person or event in health. It is used, for example, to give an account of the life of a man like Lister or Pasteur, or to depict the conditions present in a disease-ridden land such as Egypt or Iran.

Counseling with groups or with individuals has become one of the most successful ways of changing health behavior. In dealing less with health facts and more with individual personalities, it tends to "hit home" and bring about real changes in health habits and attitudes. It is not a classroom technique, but is one especially suited to the school setting where the teacher has a few moments here and there to talk with and guide the members of her class.

---

[19] Behavioral Research Laboratories, Box 577, Palo Alto, California, 1965.

The *student school health council* represents a fresh, interesting way to present proper health practices to the entire school. Its membership may be composed of one student delegate from each room. The group holds meetings regularly and makes plans relating to achieving certain health goals. This council idea has been very successful in Harry Stone Elementary School, Dallas, Texas. Here the pupils set up a series of weekly health messages to be broadcast over the public address system in the school. Their cooperative efforts had a bearing on the use of films, bulletin boards, and classroom discussions. The teachers and school nurse were very enthusiastic about the activities of the council.

Songs and jingles about health have been used for some time. Just how effective they are as a method of changing health practices is probably open to question, yet they appeal to children, especially in the kindergarten and first grade. In this connection the Detroit Public Schools has developed a very fine section of health songs and poems in their *1961 Curriculum Guide for Health Instruction.* Numerous nursery rhymes can be amended for health teaching purposes, provided of course that it is not overdone.

> Little Jack Horner stood on the corner
> Watching the traffic go by
> And when it had passed, he crossed at last
> And said, "What a safe boy am I!"

Children's poem books are a rich source of appropriate poems. These are easily located. So are useful songs, for every music publisher has several books dealing with music of a health nature for young people. Publishers that should not be overlooked include: Follett Publishers, John Day, Ginn & Co., ABC Music Series, G. Schirmer, Inc., Webster Publishing Company, and New Music Horizons.

The use of *student leaders* is a first-rate method of teaching. Leaders may assist in the classroom and on the playground. They may help the teacher inspect for cleanliness or form patrols for safety. The makers of Ivory Soap have some useful materials to help teachers and leaders. New leaders should be chosen as often as possible.

Examinations may be related to educational method as well as to the topic of evaluation. Primary and intermediate graders sometimes like the challenge of a test or short quiz, and use it very well as a pure and simple learning situation. Self-testing activities, where pupils measure their progress against their previous records and against the records of their classmates, are useful in health education. This is particularly true when there is no pressure to excel purely for the purpose of receiving grades.

Independent study may be employed when certain individuals show a keen interest in a health topic. It may be a short-term topic, but some phase of it is of such concern to some pupil or pupils that permission is granted to pursue the topic further to satisfy personal curiosity. This may be done without infringing on class time, and it permits the teacher to provide challenging work and study for the especially gifted child.

A *panel* is a small group of students like a committee which usually exists to ask and answer questions, and thereby thoroughly discuss some pertinent health problem. The panel discussion in health classes generally works very well if special interest topics are involved. A panel on "The Use of Tobacco" at the sixth grade level would illustrate an excellent method of culminating a unit of work in this area.

Research, even in the grades, is an effective learning technique. Almost every kind of child can find some satisfaction in "looking something up." They may learn to be thorough and carefully appraise their findings. Problem-solving and experimental methods employ various forms of research.

School surveys, interviews, and questionnaires are useful in elementary health research.

The *analysis of current events*, both in the community and the world at large, is one method that has been used for years to make geography and science stimulating. Not a day goes by that there is not some occurrence, phenomenon, or discovery taking place which has either direct or indirect health consequences. Radio, television, and local newspapers invariably refer to such news items as an improved sewer system for a nearby town, a child rushed to the hospital because he swallowed poison, a search for a rabid dog, an automobile and bicycle accident, news of a new method of aiding some disease, or another city setting up plans to fluoridate the water supply. Using current events so that they tie in with the health topic of the moment requires little extra planning and represents an easy technique to employ. From news articles may come group discussions relative to misbehavior in social situations, such as stealing, lying, fighting, or drunkenness. This is an opportunity for intermediate graders to better understand human relationships, thus leading to a better comprehension of mental health.

School-Community Activities. The day has long since passed when the school was considered a self-sufficient agency occupying a building in the center of town. Today, community life is the life of the school, and much of school life is the life of the community. Education is a two-way street. Community personnel and their accompanying ideas come into the school, and classroom health facts and figures arrive in the home to indirectly educate the parents.

There is direct learning through community experiences because they involve immediate sensory contacts with reality. It is difficult to question a properly planned and executed field trip, interview, camping excursion, work project, or survey. One raises a question only when this educational method is employed too often, or when the attending classes are not properly orientated. The following illustration of a trip to a frozen food plant gives an example of some of the activities involved in making a community trip meaningful:

FROZEN FOODS

Preparation needed by pupils:
List the varieties of frozen foods on the market today.
Discuss with parents how food is processed for the home freezer.
Explain the advantages of freezing food.
Stress safety and sanitation.
Benefits to be had from the trip:
Learn that modern methods of preservation give us fresh foods the year round.
Realize that cold as well as heat is a food preservative.
Discover that this is something which contributes to human health and happiness.
Activities suggested by the trip:
Prepare a frozen food in the classroom.
Visit a home frozen food freezer.
List products from the home garden that might be frozen.

In many schools, file cards on the particular resources are filed by the teacher so that trip information may be kept current and safety precautions may be noted. When the trip is over, the pupils make reports, and they may also write letters of thanks to the places visited.

The services of the community resources will vary in the degree to which they make a health contribution. Finding and using these resources is the teacher's job. A good place to begin is *people;* this is followed by *places* and *materials.*

People in the community who are usually willing to give assistance to health teachers include:

Health officer	Sewage disposal
School physician	plant operator
School nurse	Statistician

Public health nurse

Laboratory technician

Dentist

Health educator

Sanitary engineer

Safety director

Welfare director

Practicing physician

Hospital superintendent

Water plant operator

Social worker

Farmer

Home demonstration agent

Dairy plant operator

Places in the community that are especially helpful in health instruction include:[20]

Health department

Recreation facility

Dairy

Water purification plant

Milk pasteurization plant

Sewage disposal plant

Industrial plant

Food Freezer plant

Housing project

Fire department

Experimental station

Police department

Dental clinic

Restaurant

Laundry

City playground

Bakery

Home water supply

Home garden

Utility company

Meat packing plant

Farm

Parents, perhaps more than any other group in the community, are equipped to work closely with the schools in the program of health teaching. If there is any one modern method of teaching health, it is to get pupils to carry out at home what they have learned in the classroom. Teachers, therefore, assign homework in health that involves real action about the home, and encourages classroom-home cooperation.

Individual people can be used in many ways. They need not always visit the school to give a talk or answer questions. In Alhambra, California, community specialists come into the schools and assist in the final judging of a posture contest. The local com-munity, through announcements in the press, is made aware of the schools' posture activities.

In every community there are groups of people who are in some way interested in child welfare and school health. Sometimes an organization will actually be searching for a "project of the year." They may decide to do something like financing an eyeglasses program of purchasing prophylactic tablets for a rheumatic fever campaign. As an example of what happened in one locality, the following was reported to the author:[21]

> The Junior Woman's Club in our city furnishes both brushes and holders for the children in Grades 2, 3, and 4. Each room is also furnished a rack for the brushes. At the beginning of the school term, a committee from the Club distributes the brushes and demonstrates in each room the correct method of brushing the teeth. The teacher supervises the brushing during the rest period after lunch each day. This play has been in operation for two years. Next year we hope to include the 5th and 6th grades.

Correlation and Integration of Health Instruction

There is an interrelationship between direct teaching, correlation, and integration. It is difficult to say that one is better than the other, for all three methods of instruction may be used in health instruction.

There is a distinct difference between correlation and integration. *Correlation involves the use of other areas within the curriculum by which health material is taught.* Health, therefore, is correlated with physical education, science, and social studies. It may also be correlated with additional areas such as art, arithmetic, and English. In the elementary classroom,

---

[20] For a useful list of voluntary, professional, and commercial organizations see Chapter 11.

[21] From Mrs. Rebel Rhoden, elementary classroom teacher, Ocala, Fla.

in which there is less formality and the teacher has her own pupils most of the day, it is not difficult to relate the materials in one subject matter discussion to that of another. True correlation means that the teacher, when thinking of English, must plan for some health teaching in the English lesson. The same is true for other lessons. In discussing ventilation and heating in the sixth grade science period, some definite reference to the personal and community health aspects of the topic would be provided. In social studies the teacher purposely plans to talk about health conditions and the practice of bloodletting during the colonization days at Plymouth and Jamestown. Likewise, health is correlated with physical education games, stunts, and dances by definitely organizing the time available so that specific reference may be made to such items as playground safety, exercise, food, rest, and personal cleanliness. There are many opportunities for correlating health teaching with art through the preparation of posters and charts relating to health problems under study and in the making of puppets to dramatize an idea.

It may be seen that almost any school activity can be correlated with health. In the primary grades the study of foods can be a romantic one touching on many fields. And to be successful it *should* touch on many fields:

Social Studies
  History of foods
  Eating habits over the world
  Food preparation for the party
Art
  Discussing and arranging flowers for table
  Making place mats
  Poster drawing
  Foods modeled from clay
Arithmetic
  Counting: "How many will eat with me?"
  Building number vocabulary: quart of milk, one-half slice of toast, pound of butter

  Concept of time: time needed to eat breakfast
Science
  How foods grow
  The effect of climate and weather on foods
  Animal experiments with foods
Physical Education
  Food and energy for play
  Rest and recreation
  Overeating and undereating
Reading
  Health textbooks
  Charts and posters about good foods
  Captions under food ads in magazines and newspapers

Good health instruction helps make correlation a two-way process. Not only is health taught through English, but proper speech, writing, and spelling are taught through health activities. An example of this kind of cooperation is illustrated by the story of what happened in one elementary school. The teacher of a third grade class felt that the parents were not always aware of what meals were served in the school cafeteria. So the class copied the cafeteria menu for the next day as part of their writing lesson. This was taken home to the family. The children were encouraged to use their best handwriting so that their parents would really know what they were going to have to eat. Another example from the English area involves the use of the school library. Health assignments require familiarity with books, card catalogs, encyclopedias, and guides. The pupil not only discovers information about a health topic, but he also improves his concept of the use of basic library tools.

There are several excellent sources of ideas relative to correlating health instruction with other subject matter areas. The free booklets listed here are among the finest, for they help the teacher see many avenues through which health can be made a vital subject in the curriculum.

Teacher's Idea Booklet (General Mills). Shows how nutrition may be taught

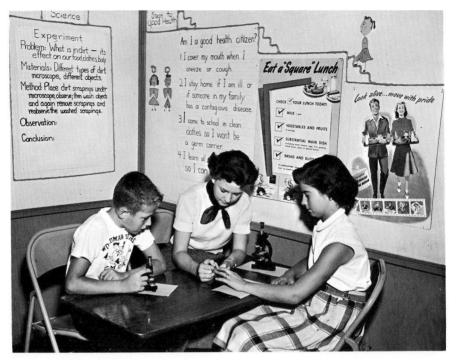

Figure 9–8   Examining fingernail dirt under the microscope. (Courtesy *Health Education Journal,* Los Angeles City Schools.)

through Language Arts, Social Studies, Science, Mathematics, and Art. A digest rich in ideas from previous booklets.

Our Bread and Butter in Pioneer Days and Today (National Dairy Council). Shows the relationship of people to their environment for fourth grade boys and girls. Thoroughly correlates listening, speaking, reading, writing, and music with health. Special methods and current resources are listed.

Health from Field and Orchard (United Fresh Fruit and Vegetable Association). An intermediate grade approach to fruits and vegetables with colored photographs.

Integration involves an organization of learning experiences around a central objective. It differs from correlation by relating parts to the whole. The "whole" can be anything. A well-integrated bicycle, for instance, is one in which all parts—wheels, chain, nuts, bolts, seat, handlebars, fenders— fit perfectly together to afford the rider a safe and pleasant journey. By the same token, a well-integrated child is

one who has been exposed to the hundreds of educational stimuli and has emerged to take his place in society as a "whole" person. He is like a giant mosaic—all the unique parts make a complete being. This may be accomplished by the well-integrated curriculum, one which is balanced and refined, and embraces many areas of instruction.

Instruction in the lower grades is very often based on centering the attention of pupils on broad topics rather than dividing the school time into periods for different subject matter areas. Here, arithmetic, art, spelling, social studies, science, and health are interrelated as part of a broad learning experience. As an example, third grade children in Baltimore studied housing problems. A dilapidated old house being rejuvenated according to the Baltimore Plan was dramatized by the children. They acted the parts of germs, trash, garbage, and mice, and declared that this was no longer a home for them. In the same school there were other examples of integration. One second grade study was built around the quality of Baltimore's water supply. Health aspects were considered with social study aspects. Moreover, the choice of words and ease in speaking gave proof to the observer that these lower grade children understood the importance of good water.

The fully developed, well-integrated school health program obviously involves many persons and things. The traditional classroom will hardly serve its purpose, for many things need to be done which will involve the entire school atmosphere.

No subject in the elementary curriculum can long remain divorced from the total program. An overlapping of topics is necessary in order to give appropriate meaning to the various pieces of information. As it is, too many children know a great many health facts but fail to see their usefulness in the world they live in. This may be due to the fact that we live in an integrated or whole society, but we often continue to formally study the parts without in any way relating them to the whole. This is somewhat true at all educational levels. It has only been in recent years that physiology and psychology have been examined together with the resulting emphasis today on psychosomatic phenomena in general behavior.

Questions for Discussion

1. What seems to be the essential difference between correlation and integration of health materials?

2. Does there appear to be any one educational method of instruction that works more effectively than others in the teaching of health at the elementary school level? Explain.

3. What essentially is the philosophy behind the statement that the health instruction program should be "broad and varied"?

4. Differentiate between an integrated experience and an integrated curriculum.

5. Suppose your fourth grade was studying an integrated unit on "Early America." Suggest a list of health learnings pertaining to this kind of a unit.

6. To what extent does the teacher's personality and aptitude for teaching influence the choice of educational method employed in health instruction?

Suggested Activities

1. The discovery method of teaching has received a fair amount of publicity in recent years. Prepare some material to initiate a unit on dental health in which the discovery method is used. How does this relate to the problem-solving method? Is there any degree of certainty that the discovery method will produce changes in health behavior?

2. Read an article or two about innovation in teaching methods. Are there ways of teaching that literally "turn kids on"? The Borton reference seems to convey the message that there are. List the essential points set forth in the article you review; follow this up with your comments.

3. According to several sources, programmed instruction, as a method of learning, has yet to reach its potential. Review three or four articles having to do with this topic and summarize the reasons why programmed learning is slow in taking hold.

4. Visit an elementary school classroom and observe the teaching method being used by the instructor. After the class is dismissed, ask the teacher *why* the particular method was chosen. Ask also if the method has replaced another method or has been changed at any time during the last year or two. In short, are teachers flexible in the use of methods?

5. Design an experiment to appraise the effects of three different teaching methods on the acquisition of knowledge. The health topic and methods selected may be of your own choosing.

Selected References

Anderson, C. L. *School Health Practice*, 4th ed. St. Louis: C. V. Mosby Co., 1968, Chapter 12.

Blough, Glenn, and Schwartz, J. *Elementary Science and How to Teach It*. New York: Holt, Rinehart and Winston, 1964.

Borton, Terry. "What Turns Kids On?" *Saturday Review*, April 15, 1967, pp. 72–75.

Bruner, Jerome. *Toward a Theory of Instruction*. Cambridge, Mass.: Harvard University Press, 1966.

Greenslade, Margaret. "Textbook Content in Controversial Areas." *Journal of School Health*, 31:288–290, November 1961.

Humphrey, James H., Johnson, Warren R., and Moore, Virginia D. *Elementary School Health Education*. New York: Harper and Bros., 1962, pp. 221–360.

Jarvis, Oscar T., and Wootton, Lutian R. *The Transitional Elementary School and Its Curriculum*. Dubuque, Iowa: W. C. Brown Co., 1966.

LaSalle, Dorothy, and Geer, Gladys, *Health Instruction for Today's Schools*. Englewood Cliffs, N.J.: Prentice-Hall, Inc., 1963, Chapter 5.

Mendelsohn, Harold, "Which Shall It Be: Mass Education or Mass Persuasion for Health?" *American Journal of Public Health*, 52:131–137, January 1968.

Schneider, Robert E. *Methods and Materials of Health Education*, 2nd ed. Philadelphia: W. B. Saunders Co., 1964.

Wagner, Guy, Alexander, Mildred, and Hosier, Max. "Let's Put Instructional Games to Work." *Education*, 77:293–295, January 1957.

Weatherford, Margie Herron. "The Planned Field Trip–An Exciting Experience." *Safety*, 1:8–11, February 1966.

Material
Aids in
CHAPTER **10** ## Health Teaching

*Thinking directly in terms of color,
tones, images, is a different operation
technically from thinking in words....
If all meanings could be adequately expressed by words, the arts of painting
and music would not exist. There are
values and meanings that can be expressed only by immediately visible and
audible qualities and to ask what they
mean in the sense of something that can
be put into words is to deny their dis-
tinctive existence.*

—JOHN DEWEY
Art as Expression

This is a chapter about the use of materials in health teaching—materials that do not depend primarily upon reading to convey their meaning. It is based upon the principle that *all* health instruction can be measurably improved by the use of such materials because they help make the learning experience memorable. The word *all* is used because health materials, when used intelligently, promote the most effective kind of learning.

It is not uncommon to hear the modern elementary school criticized because children spend much of their time working with a multitude of materials. It is a well accepted fact that education is more than just exposing a learner to information. Somehow he must be involved in the process by taking part in it. He has to *do* something *with* something. And because it is purposeful activity, he feels, listens, smells, and acquires health concepts *through the use of material things.* Homer once said, "Greater glory hath no man than that which he wins with his own feet and hands." Therefore, we may say that children learn some from what they hear, more

309

from what they see and hear, and most from what they do. If something appeals to a child because he has heard or read about it, he usually wants to "try it out," "feel it," and "work it"—himself. He seeks a rich, full-bodied experience that is the bedrock of all education. It is the unabridged version of life itself—commonly referred to as "something you can sink your teeth into." This alone is reason enough for the existence of good instructional materials and the continuous search for better ones.

The Nature of Instructional Materials

Instructional materials, by definition, exist to aid in the instructional program. They are not a substitute for good teaching—they are only a supplementary item. They are *aids,* and as such are a bona fide part of educational method. They are treated separately only because of their importance and because they are sometimes abused—used in a questionable manner. They are never a program "crutch." If their use is not purposeful and does not prove expeditious in learning, they have no place in the program. If they are essentially entertaining rather than fruitful in effecting predetermined health behavior, they should be relegated to the entertainment hour and no longer used to promote health.

Since all material substances which children manipulate are generally seen or heard, it is not uncommon to speak of instructional materials or teaching aids as *audio-visual* in nature. Only a purely deaf and sightless child would respond to materials in any other way. And, of course, one must not underestimate the effect of such senses as smell and feeling in making lasting impressions on youth.

As a whole, audio-visual materials are well supported by research. When properly used in the teaching situation

they accomplish the following:

They supply a concrete basis for conceptual thinking and hence reduce meaningless word-responses of students.

They have a high degree of interest for students.

They make learning more permanent.

They offer a reality of experience which stimulates self-activity on the part of pupils.

They develop a continuity of thought; this is especially true of motion pictures.

They contribute to growth of meaning and hence to vocabulary development.

They provide experiences not easily obtained through other materials and contribute to the efficiency, depth, and variety of learning.

The Teacher and New Media

There are many exciting opportunities which today's new teaching media present to alert teachers. Unfortunately, good ideas relative to methods and teaching aids are slow to spread. The research department of the Ford Foundation reports that there is a time lag of about 25 years between the time a new idea in education is advanced and the time it is universally accepted.

Such media as overhead transparencies, educational television, and programmed instructional materials have something to offer if used to supplement other techniques and aids.

Associated with programmed instruction are so called teaching machines. A teaching machine is a device, mechanical or electronic, through which self-instruction materials are fed to the pupil. It indicates continuously whether or not a pupil comes up with the right answers. The answers are not disclosed until the pupil responds. Pupils have been found to respond remarkably well despite the fact that they performed poorly under traditional teaching methods. In time, programmed materials may lead to a complete reappraisal of tests. However, to date they have not been widely accepted.

The Proper Use of Health Teaching Materials

The numerous teaching aids and instructional materials, regardless of type or worth, cannot take the place of the teacher. It is the teacher who determines the opportune time for each type of instructional material and who guides pupils in the use of these learning aids. It is the teacher who selects the health materials because they are needed by the child in a particular learning situation. Materials used in this way become an integral part of instruction and perform a special function in achieving health goals.

Whether teaching aids are success-

ful or not depends upon preplanning and effective usage. There are a number of criteria for evaluating instructional materials:

Are they closely related to the children's current activities and interests?

Are they suited to the maturity levels of pupils using them?

Are they selected and used with a specific purpose in mind?

Are they durable and safe to use with children?

Do they present accurate information?

Are they well constructed?

Do they encourage pupil participation?

Are they accessible?

It is interesting to note when considering the proper use of instructional materials that Comenius, in his *Orbis Pictus* (a book of "sense objects" numbered to tie in with English and Latin words), warned his students about making pictures and other materials

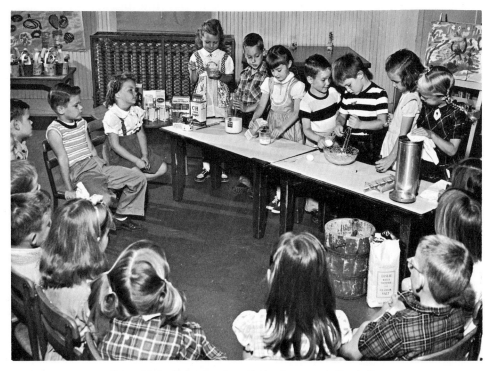

Figure 10–1   Materials galore. Making ice cream in Grade One.

the main part of education. Materials were to be used chiefly to avoid verbalistic teaching. They were not to be an end in themselves.

Edgar Dale stresses eight ways of evaluating these materials.[1] They may be readily applied to the general use of all health teaching materials:

"Do the materials give a true picture of the ideas they present?" Not every child is impressed to the same degree by the exhibit he sees or the recording he listens to. It is altogether possible for an idea to be overshadowed by the nature of the materials used. For example, to a city child the small poster picture of a cow would go unrecognized; this has happened.

There are other items of importance relative to the distortion of the truth. For example, because of an effective toothbrushing drill in a dental health class, it might be possible to give some pupils the idea that toothbrushing is far superior to a good diet in the growth and maintenance of healthy teeth. In the study of foods, there is always that chance that someone will "go overboard" for cereal breakfasts, dark bread, raw carrots, or blackstrap molasses, because the display cards or colored charts were so convincing. Also, a sixth grade class may view a film on mental health and conclude that almost everyone is mentally ill. The immature trick of generalizing from limited information is ever present, and it takes very little sometimes to cause errors to blossom into full bloom.

"Do they contribute meaningful content to the topic under study?" The only way to really answer this question in a health class is to evaluate the results of teaching. Do the pupils know any more about the topic? Are habits improved and attitudes

changed because of the materials used? We say that "a picture is worth ten thousand words," but is just any picture that effective? One may have an elaborate and highly authentic display of alcohol and tobacco pictures, pamphlets, and other supplementary materials, but it may not alter behavior any more than a movie or a talk by the school nurse. Probably the chief reason more television is not used in schools is not because sets and programs are difficult to obtain; it is because, in the minds of some people, there is a question whether television is a highly effective educational aid.

"Is the material appropriate for the age, intelligence, and experience of the learners?" One of the common mistakes of inexperienced teachers is to use materials with the wrong age group. A cancer film that appears interesting to the teacher may leave her primary grade class "cold." A lesson on the making of tooth powder may insult the intelligence of an upper grader, yet be most appropriate for the second grade boy and girl. Certain health textbooks are difficult when used alone, but supplemented with other materials, they become usable. To a class that has never used flash cards, they may be confusing, especially if concerned with something like vitamin and mineral food graphs.

The appropriateness of materials is best determined by ascertaining the common custom and practice in their use. Many school systems today employ personnel to manage a materials center and to be of service to teachers. These people have the evidence and the educational listings; they make it their business to know which teaching aids are satisfactory for a certain grade level. Beyond this, some experimentation by the teacher is necessary.

"Is the physical condition of the materials satisfactory?" Few things can detract more from a teaching aid

---

[1] Dale, Edgar. *Audio-Visual Methods in Teaching.* New York: Dryden Press, revised 1964.

than untidiness and uncleanliness. A broken working model of the eye, a dirty graph, a grimy poster, or a film with a noisy sound track can hurt the teaching lesson measurably. Health teaching exhibits, drawings, and models should be fresh and almost sparkling in appearance. An old posture picture that has been used for years might well be thrown away before the negative concomitant learnings associated with it overshadow the purpose of the lesson.

"*Is there a teacher's guide available to provide help in effective use of the materials?*" More and more teaching aids are being produced commercially, and they are made available to teachers complete with instructions for their optimum usage. This is especially true when it comes to films, filmstrips, recordings, textbooks, and supplementary readers. Ideally, every teacher should preview materials before she ever uses them. A good guide can provide a detailed understanding of the items being used and offer numerous practical suggestions. Time is at a premium today; there may be little time to experiment with a certain model or film—only time to read what others have previously done with it.

One of the finest sources of teaching aids may be found in the teacher's guides distributed with the health reading books of several of the larger book publishers.[2] These guides are often as well prepared as the texts they are made to accompany. Ginn and Company, for example, publishes a series of books, teacher's guides, and aids that by themselves constitute a complete health instruction program. These, or any other guides, should not be followed rigidly. A flexible approach is necessary to focus some attention on local health instruction needs.

"*Do they make students better thinkers, critical-minded?*" Because children usually enjoy moving pictures, it is not difficult for them to be lulled into accepting and believing something that they might otherwise challenge if they had examined it critically. Dale brings this point out when he says:[3]

> Since we are trying to develop maturity in thinking, we must reject instructional materials which make students more dependent, less mature. In short, we must ask whether a certain field trip, film, model, or television program will promote sound thinking or discourage it. Bear this in mind when you next watch a motion picture or television drama. Does it give you deeper insight into the behavior of the main characters or false ideas of why they acted as they did?

Most materials tend to sell themselves. The poster holds our immediate attention, the exhibit seldom raises our doubts as to its veracity, and a clever felt board may be capable of convincing many children that white is black, or at least a dirty gray. Simply stated, this means that all materials tend to have a fair degree of attractiveness to youngsters. One must, therefore, assume a reasonable amount of responsibility for their use; unexamined and unappraised materials should not be used.

"*Do they tend to improve human relations?*" Children learn to live together harmoniously not only by studying about it in social studies and other subject matter areas, but also by practicing it as they live together in the school. Human relations is a continuous process. It is a kind of health education that is most desir-

---

[2] Notably Scott, Foresman, & Co., Lyons & Carnahan, Laidlaw Brothers, Bobbs-Merrill Co., 3M Co., and Ginn & Company.

[3] Reprinted from *Audio-Visual Methods in Teaching*, rev. ed., p. 83, by Edgar Dale, by permission of Dryden Press. Copyright 1956 by Dryden Press.

able and often comes about as a concomitant learning in the everyday activities of the pupils. The use of a wide variety of materials in teaching health tends to pave the way for cooperative effort, sharing of ideas and objects, and understanding the skills and feelings of the other fellow.

"Is the material worth the time, expense, and effort involved?" This, of course, is the culminating question. In every educational endeavor it becomes necessary sooner or later to appraise fully the expended efforts of teachers. It is at such a time as this that the criteria of economy is applied. Just how costly, in terms of time and money, is the project? In a third grade class studying cleanliness, is it better to draw posters for a poster contest than to view a ten-minute film on some phase of community sanitation? In a fifth grade class studying the relationship of food to personal vigor, is a rat-feeding experiment worth all the time it takes to feed the animals, clean the cages, keep the records, and secure the food?

Much research remains to be done with teaching materials in order to ascertain which ones are most effective in favorably changing pupil behavior. It is a bit difficult to do this, for it is always difficult to hold the teaching factor constant while evaluating the effect of the specific material aids. It is not impossible for a superior teacher with inferior teaching aids to produce pupil results similar to those of an inferior teacher employing superior aids. Other things being equal, it is possible to show that some aids are far superior to others. In the Pittsburgh public schools, for instance, the use of a film was found to be the most successful way of teaching the pertinent facts of diet early in childhood.[4] This

conclusion was reached after many aids had been tried.

Varieties of Teaching Aids in Health Education

There are few fields of educational endeavor that are as fertile for the use of teaching aids as health education. Health has a biological, sociological, psychological, and philosophical basis that cuts across all areas of effort. It is concerned with total human welfare: mind, body, and spirit. Because of this, practically every known teaching aid can in some way be used in the health instruction program. But school time is at a premium; one must be scientific in the use of methods and supplementary aids. This chapter will be concerned only with those material aids that have proven useful in elementary school teaching. These include:

Books	Mirrors
Pamphlets	Workbooks
Bulletin boards	Writing pads
Chalkboards	Comic strip drawings
Posters	Collections
Cartoons	Copy equipment
Sketches	Radio
Stick drawings	Television
Charts	Phonograph
Tables	recordings
Maps	Guides and
Flash cards	workbooks
Mobiles	Models
Puppets	Exhibits
Graphs	Specimens
Museums	Tape recordings
Flat pictures	Motion picture films
Photographs	Filmstrips
Magazine and	Slides
newspaper	Opaque projection
clippings	Overhead projection
Flannel boards	Songs and poems
Magnetic boards	

Variety in the use of these material aids is as important as varying the method of teaching from time to time. Children welcome a change, and since some pupils prefer one aid to another, it is only fair to everyone to be flexible

---

[4] The film used: *Bill's Better Breakfast Puppet Show* (25 min., 16 mm., color), the Cereal Institute. Recommended for kindergarten through fourth grade.

in the use of the various materials. By the same token, some material aids are better than others at a particular grade level. To children who cannot read, a typical poster may be less effective than a flat photograph. A colored slide, for instance, may do a better job of depicting the relationship of food colors to one's appetite than almost any other available means.

Numerous errors are committed in the name of variety. Care must be taken not to forget eye and ear appeal nor lose sight of the fact that materials should be pertinent to the health lesson. Also, materials should be free from objectionable commercial advertisements.

Materials Available to the Classroom Teacher

The following materials are not easily made in class and should be available to the teacher:

Essential in Health Teaching
Catalogs of films
Catalogs of equipment
Card file of films
Model boards
Bulletin boards
Chalkboard
Picture file
Filmstrip projector and filmstrips
Motion picture projector
Portable screen
Overhead projector
Record player

Desirable in Health Teaching
Daylight projection screen
Camera (bl. & wh. and 35 mm. color)
Movie camera
Opaque projector
Tape recorder
Public address system
Slide projector and 35 mm. slides

In the larger elementary schools in which there are satisfactory materials centers the average classroom teacher will have little trouble securing the necessary aids. In fact, by selecting from the "Desirable" list, she will be able to experiment somewhat with other items. She may try out a tape recorder in class or borrow a 35 mm. camera and take her own pictures of the pupils in action to be shown on the slide projector at a later date. The "Essential" list should be standard equipment even in the small two-room schoolhouse.

Sources of Instructional Materials

The classroom teacher, possibly more than any other teacher, needs a working knowledge in instructional materials. Selecting, preparing, and utilizing these materials has become almost a science. This chapter will do little more than scratch the surface. The teacher in most areas will have to become proficient by virtue of her own efforts and experimentation. And in the special area of health teaching, a trial and error approach will prove helpful in weeding out ineffective teaching aids that do not appeal to the pupils or that fail to impress the teacher. This last point is worth dwelling on, for there are several ways to "skin a cat" and each teacher has her favorite way. Where photographs may appeal to one teacher, another may dislike bothering with them and find success in the use of stick drawings.

It is no small task to find new techniques and clever materials for putting across a particular health lesson. The teacher who discovers and uses several instructional aids successfully is apt to continue to do so. Skill in the use of these materials will depend upon the teacher's background, interest, and energy. It will also relate to a great extent to her professional zeal. If she is intent on doing the best possible job of teaching—health or anything else—she will investigate all available educational materials. She might do well to look beyond the education field to business, sales promotion, and advertising. Hard-headed men of finance have products to sell. What materials do they use? How do they use them? Look over a sample of everyday magazines. Study the ads to find new approaches in selling and promotions. Can anything be gleaned from such an advertisement that may help in preparation of health instruction materials? Why was the ad attractive to you? Was it the topic? The layout? The colors? Or was it so directly personal that you could not help looking at it?

The teacher with an open mind, who is searching for new ideas and sources of information on the selection, preparation, and use of audio-visual materials, will find most of the following sources helpful:

Printed Materials

Aids to Learning, grades one to eight, a project of Creative Playthings, Inc., Princeton, N.J., 1960.

Audio-Visual Methods in Teaching, rev. ed., by Edgar Dale, New York: Dryden Press, 1964. A complete treatment of the topic of graphics.

Educator's Grade Guide to Free Curriculum Materials, edited by Patricia H. Suttles, and published annually by Educator's Progress Service, Randolph, Wisconsin.

Educational Media Index, a project of the Educational Media Council, New York, McGraw-Hill Book Co., 1964. Contains a vast range of materials; volumes 1 and 2 refer to health and safety materials for kindergarten through sixth grade.

Free and Inexpensive Learning Materials, published annually by George Peabody College for Teachers, Nashville, Tenn.

Guide Book Describing Pamphlets, Posters, and Films on Health and Disease, published periodically by the Maryland State Department of Health, Baltimore, Md.

1001 Valuable Things You Can Get Free, by Thelma Weisinger, published periodically by Bantam Books, Inc.,

New York, N.Y. Contains an extensive list of materials that are bona fide give-aways.

Sources of Free Pictures, edited by Merton B. Osborn and Bruce Miller, published periodically by Bruce Miller Publications, Riverside, California.

Sources of Information on Educational Media, edited by John R. Molstad of Education Media Council in cooperation with U.S. Office of Health, Education, and Welfare, Washington, D.C. (available from U.S. Government Printing Office).

Vertical File Index, published monthly with an annual cumulative volume by R. R. Bowker Co., New York, N.Y. Lists free and inexpensive materials from private and public sources.

Periodicals

Audio-Visual Instruction. Washington, D. C.: Department of Audio-Visual Instruction, 1201 Sixteenth Street, N.W. Nine issues.

Educational Screen and Audio-Visual Guide. Chicago: 2000 Lincoln Park West. Ten issues.

EFLA Film Review Digest. New York: Educational Film Library Association, 345 E. 46th Street. Eight issues.

Journal of Health, Physical Education, and Recreation. Washington, D. C.: American Association for Health, Physical Education, and Recreation, 1201 Sixteenth Street, N.W. Nine issues. Each issue contains an audio-visual section.

Journal of School Health. Kent, Ohio: The American School Health Association, 515 E. Main Street. Ten issues. Each issue contains a section entitled, "New Teaching Aids."

Junior Scholastic. New York: Scholastic Magazines, 33 West 42nd Street. A weekly for grades six to eight. Features material on plays, short stories, science, health, radio, TV, records, personal guidance, and hobbies.

AUDIO–VISUAL MATERIALS IN HEALTH INSTRUCTION

Health may be taught very well by the usual oral and written methods of instruction. But it may be taught better and reach more pupils when it is enriched with audio-visual aids. Sensory experiences are to health and safety concepts as food is to the hungry animal; they reach deeply and make a noticeable impression.

Of the dozens of techniques and aids being used in the elementary schools, some are more common than others. A brief discussion of each follows this paragraph. It begins with the more spectacular projected materials involving motion, sound, electricity, and electronics, and moves to the older and more elemental forms of non-projected materials. One cannot accurately say that a certain material aid is superior to another without qualifying the statement in terms of the objectives. If, for example, the class objective is to understand how cold germs are spread and if they have read about cold germs and discussed them, it is time to get closer to the topic. This may be done by drawing a sketch or diagram of the spread of germs when a person sneezes, by looking at germs under the microscope, or by viewing a moving picture. To say that one material aid is better than the other depends upon a number of variables—variables such as the teacher's ability and the make-up of the class. Each classroom teacher will have to determine to what extent the following material aids can be successfully used in her classes of health instruction.

Motion Pictures, Filmstrips, Slides, Opaque Projector, Overhead Projector

Effective use of films and film projectors requires a degree of skill. First, there is an immediate skill that one must possess that cannot be obtained merely by reading about it. Motion pictures, filmstrips, and slides need to be handled, examined, and run through appropriate machines, if the teacher is to be skillful in the use of this kind of teaching material. There is no other way.

Secondly, the effective use of this kind of material requires skill in planning. Where a film is shown without introduction and follow-up discussion, the chances are it will not long be remembered. Health films, slides, filmstrips, photographs, and similar aids have, generally speaking, one or two definite functions. They are objective in introducing a health subject, supporting it, or in summarizing what has taken place. Rarely, if ever, can a film or slide be the "whole show" by itself.

1. Motion Pictures. In one breath we can say that the use of motion pictures to convey health messages is almost as badly abused as the use of pamphlets; they cannot stand alone in putting messages across. In the next breath, however, we can state with certainty that motion pictures may well be one of the finest mediums for presenting health ideas in readily acceptable terms. Why the extreme difference in these two statements? The answer lies in planning.

When good planning takes place, health interest and health understanding increase. Specifically, health education instructional films are planned to reach certain goals. They may be used:

As an introduction to a unit to stimulate interest or give an overview.

In the direct teaching of a health lesson, i.e., to help develop an idea or attitude, to convey certain facts, or to help solve or correct certain problems.

As a review or summary of previous learnings.

a. The *preliminary steps* are:

Familiarize yourself with the film before showing it.

Make a list of the important points in the film that you want the audience to understand and remember.

Prepare some thought-provoking questions which will stimulate discussions.

Introduce the film to the class, bringing out the points you want them to look for.

b. The *presentation* is a challenge:

The viewing distance of the farthest seat from the screen is approximately six times the width of the picture for pupils in the front row.

The room should be effectively darkened.

Acoustics are better when the room is filled with people or has many drapes to muffle reverberations.

Room ventilation should not be overlooked.

The projectionist must know how to maintain and care for the machine.

Before the showing, check cords, lamps, reels, position of speaker, amplifier, and film gates.

Test run and focus picture.

In starting the picture dim the room lights, turn on the motor, then the lamp, check focus, increase volume, and adjust the tone respectively.

During the showing check the loops, volume, and frames, and stay with the operation until the film is over.

In ending the picture turn off the lamp, fade the volume, turn on room lights, turn off motor respectively.

Following the showing rewind the film, clean film channels, put all parts in their proper places, get film ready for return to film library, and make out required records.

c. The *follow-up* "sets" the experience:

Review with the class the main points of the film.

Clear up any existing questions concerning the film.

Ask the class questions (oral or written) for the purpose of evaluating the film and its effectiveness.

Repeat film showing if time permits and some points appear to need re-emphasis.

Engage in follow-up activities, i.e., tests, papers, drawings, demonstrations, experiments, as necessary to insure a practical understanding of the topic.

d. The *evaluation* is as important as any of the above points. Standard evaluation forms may be obtained from the Educational Film Library Association, Inc. Teacher-made forms for elementary classroom appraisal should include answers to a number of questions. The following questions are adapted from a report by the American Association for Health, Physical Education, and Recreation:

Evaluate the film by placing a check in the appropriate space.

Yes No

___ ___ 1. Was the film interesting?

___ ___ 2. Was the material well selected?

___ ___ 3. Were the topics covered adequately?

___ ___ 4. Was the material authentic in content and appearance?

___ ___ 5. Was the material arranged in proper sequence?

___ ___ 6. Were the correct details stressed?

___ ___ 7. Was the acting natural and convincing?

___ ___ 8. Were the pictorial and sound elements well integrated?

___ ___ 9. Was the introduction well executed?

___ ___ 10. Was the conclusion well executed?

___ ___ 11. Was the narrative quality good?

___ ___ 12. Were the objectives of the film clear?

___ ___ 13. Is the motion picture medium the best one for the treatment of the particular topic?

___ ___ 14. Is it up to date?

___ ___ 15. Is it a good source of information?

___ ___ 16. Would it help to develop attitudes and understandings for the indicated age level?

___ ___ 17. Does it compel emotional and mental participation?

___ ___ 18. Rate the following technical qualities:

	Good	Fair	Poor
Photography	___	___	___
Sound	___	___	___
Music	___	___	___
Voice	___	___	___
Perspective	___	___	___

19. In view of the above items, I would rate this film as:

_____Excellent _____Good
_____Fair _____Poor

If the teacher of health will carefully consider all that has been said thus far about motion pictures, she will have only one thing left to do and that is to become familiar with the large number and variety of health films appropriate for the primary and intermediate grade levels. Such a list would more than fill this book. Also the lists of producers and distributors are continually being revised. For a wide coverage of current sources consult the following:

The Blue Book of Audio-Visual Materials, Chicago: Educational Screen, 64 East Lake Street. Included here are films, filmstrips, slides, and recordings.

Educator's Guide to Free Films, Educator's Guide to Free Film Strips, Educator's Guide to Free Transcriptions, Tapes and Scripts, Randolph, Wisconsin: Educator's Progress Service. An annually

revised guide with title index, subject classification, brief descriptions, and cross references.

Film Evaluation Guide, New York: Educational Film Library Association, 1965.

Public Health Service Film Catalog, Washington, D.C.: U.S. Public Health Service, U.S. Government Printing Office, annual.

Visual Materials in Safety Education, Supplement II. Washington, D.C.: National Commission on Safety Education, 1201 16th Street, N.W. A bibliography. (Revised periodically.)

U.S. Government Films for Public Educational Use, compiled for the U.S. Dept. of Health, Education, and Welfare and published by the Government Printing Office, Washington, D.C., annual.

It sometimes makes a good project to produce a health film at school. The teacher who can operate a movie camera and knows something about the composition of pictures can often make an 8 mm. or 16 mm. colored film that may be used from year to year. A good homemade film does not outgrow its usefulness very soon. Future classes enjoy seeing their older friends in the moving picture, and the class that makes the film has a wonderful opportunity to integrate the health message with other subject matter areas. In writing the script, the various scenes are tied in closely with the narration. This, like everything else in the aids line, takes conscientious planning, but it can be quite worth while for there is a tremendous range of health problems which can be approached by this teaching technique. Some examples of films produced by classes include first aid to the injured child, boating safety, swimming safety, garbage disposal, shopping for safe vegetables and fruits. Even a simple on-the-spot movie of a field trip to the dairy or of a group of happy youngsters surrounding an animal feeding demonstration can be a motivating device for children that follow. Also, a good amount of fun may be had in filming the bicycle skills of several children riding about the school playground. Ideas for a local film could come from viewing a short commercial film such as the excellent 11 minute color film, *Rules of the Road,* distributed free by Employers Mutuals of Wausau.

2. Filmstrips. Much that has already been said about the selection, presentation, and evaluation of movie films can be applied to the utilization of filmstrips (slide films).

Filmstrips are a very convenient technique of showing a series of still pictures. They are mounted on a continuous strip of 35 mm. film and vary in length from 18 frames to several times that number. The film is threaded through the filmstrip projector and engaged with the teeth of a sprocket wheel. A knob connected with the sprocket wheel makes it possible to advance the filmstrip, frame by frame, as needed.

The advantages of filmstrips for elementary health teaching are:

They are lightweight and easy to handle in the classroom. The projector is simple enough for a primary grade pupil to operate.

They are relatively inexpensive — one of the cheapest projected visual aids.

They are available in vivid colors.

They may be obtained for use with a sound recording.

There is a wide variety to choose from in health.

Body functions and specific health implications can be effectively broken down and presented through a sequence of filmstrip projections.

The teacher can pause as long as she likes on any one picture.

Many filmstrips are designed to accompany textbooks.

An example of a particularly fine filmstrip in full color is the 37-frame filmstrip on health and nutrition education for primary grades, distributed free by the Cereal Institute, Inc. The titles for each frame are reproduced below.[5] Read them over. Notice how frame No. 26 permits class comment and frame No. 32 calls for oral expression.

Skimpy and a Good Breakfast
1. From: Cereal Institute, Inc. A research and educational endeavor devoted to the betterment of national nutrition.
2. Skimpy and a Good Breakfast.
3. *To the teacher:* The Iowa University Breakfast Studies proved that children have better attitudes and better grades after eating a good breakfast.
4. Here is Bill.
5. He is in a class like ours.
6. Bill is feeling fine.
7. But who is this?
8. His name is Joe. But they call him Skimpy.
9. Skimpy is always last.
10. Skimpy is tired.
11. What do you think is wrong with Skimpy?
12. Skimpy and Bill are friends.
13. The teacher is their friend, too.
14. They say, "Let us have a breakfast party."
15. Everyone helps plan the party.
16. Some children make place mats.
17. Other children make decorations.
18. The party day comes.
19. Some children bring fruit.
20. Some children bring cereal.
21. Some children bring milk.
22. Some children bring bread and butter.
23. They have their breakfast party.
24. Skimpy learns what foods are in a good breakfast.
25. Skimpy begins eating a good breakfast.
26. He follows other ways to Good Health. What are they?
27. Joe and Bill play outdoors in the sunshine.
28. They get plenty of sleep and rest.

---

[5] The Cereal Institute, Inc., 135 S. La Salle Street, Chicago, Illinois, 60603. Used by permission. Two other excellent examples available free from the Institute are *Why Eat a Good Breakfast?* and *Grain from Farm to Table.*

29. They drink plenty of water.
30. They eat the right foods every day.
31. They begin each day with a good breakfast.
32. These foods make a good breakfast. Let us say them together.
33. Remember when Joe used to feel tired?
34. Now Joe feels fine. Do you know why?
35. For health posters and other teaching aids write:

> Cereal Institute, Inc.
> 135 South LaSalle Street
> Chicago, Illinois 60603

36. Puppets are from the film *Bill's Better Breakfast Puppet Show*.
37. The End.

3. Slides. Slides, like filmstrips, are easy to use and relatively inexpensive. One can make a slide or filmstrip from anything that is drawn, written, typewritten, printed, or photographed—and it can be done in full color. Drawings may be made with pencil on etched glass or with special slide ink. It would not be difficult in an intermediate grade class, for example, to sketch the skeleton of the body on glass and project it life-size on a screen. So many slides are readily available today that it often proves more economical in terms of teacher time to purchase ready-made slides.

Most slides are 2 inches × 2 inches; however, the 3½ inch × 4 inch variety are sometimes employed. The latter are more readily used in adapting charts, pictures, tables, and the like from magazines and books since more detail can be shown. Also they can be made by hand more easily. Most slides of a health and biological nature are photographically produced. They may be shown on any one of a number of easy-to-operate projectors. One type of tape recorder is available which will automatically change the slides in a slide projector. This can be a very effective means of putting over a health topic at an exhibit or as part of a display in the main corridor of the school.

4. Opaque Projector. The light from any flat picture may be reflected directly on the screen by means of mirrors and lenses. The opaque projector is flexible enough to handle anything up to six inches square; anything larger can be inserted into it and moved around until the desired part of the picture is on the screen. Its use in the lower grades for showing almost any flat object is great. Although it is heavy to move about, it is inexpensive to use. Small clippings from a newspaper or magazine can be greatly enlarged on a screen. It is a good health motivating device, for children love to see their own health pictures, drawings, charts, and graphs projected on a big screen before the whole class.

In one Wisconsin grade school the opaque projector has been used for years in the food and nutrition area to project proper table settings, color harmony of foods, and food advertisements. A sixth grade studying the content of canned fruits and vegetables found the labels very enlightening. Interest mounted again when poison labels and medical prescription labels were examined. The continued use, therefore, of the opaque projector is limited only by the imagination of the teacher.

5. Overhead Projector. When it comes to a wide variety of uses, the overhead projector reigns supreme. With it, the teacher can stand in front of the semi-darkened room facing the class and project all kinds of transparent materials onto a screen that is behind him and high enough for all students to see without difficulty. For the teacher of health it is a simple matter to sketch, write, or draw on a strip of cellophane with a ceramic or wax pencil, and in color if desired. The chief advantage of this projector is that the teacher can readily project all the details of a lecture while facing the class.

6. Transparencies. With the use of the overhead projector has come an increasing amount of good transparencies. The School Health Education Study materials, distributed by the Minnesota Mining and Manufacturing Company (3M), are supplemented with content-oriented visuals. The teacher is instructed to run these paper visuals and a piece of transparency film through a special device for quickly making tansparencies. Twelve visual packets are available for classroom use and are geared to the health concepts related to consumer health and family living education. Once the transparencies are made and projected, they make the overhead projection of information an effective medium.

Some of the finest prepared transparencies, ready to use and in sharp colors, are distributed free to teachers by the Cereal Institute, Inc. This is a series of 10 inch × 10 inch transparencies pertaining to foods, food selection, and nutritional research findings of interest to primary and intermediate grade pupils. The packet of transparencies is entitled, *Good Health Begins with Good Nutrition* (1968). (See Figure 10–2.)

Overlay transparencies are useful in showing the structure of such items as body organs, cells, muscle tissue, human skin as it would appear under

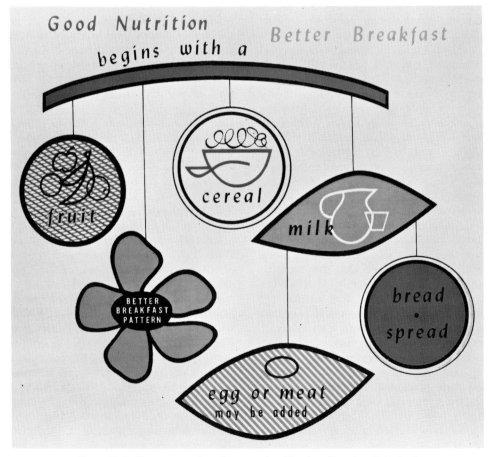

Figure 10–2   Transparency for primary grades. (Courtesy Cereal Institute, Inc.)

the microscope, sense organs, and major areas of the brain. In the text, *The Foundations of Health* (Bucher-Olsen-Willgoose), the overlay transparencies depict the major body organs from superficial structure to internal makeup. The American Dental Association, in its booklet, *How Teeth Grow*, uses overlay transparencies to clearly illustrate the changing pattern of dental development from infancy to the early teens. The booklet is especially practical when children are permitted to look it over and finger the transparencies.

Radio, Television, Record Playing, and Tape Recordings

The Greeks learned chiefly by oral communication, and they discussed what they learned as they learned it. The *Odyssey* and *Iliad* were read in public. Herodotus read his *History* aloud in Athens. Public recital to select audiences by the author himself was the ordinary method of publication.[6]

Learning to listen is something that every child can learn to do fairly well if he is given the opportunity. Today, through the application of electronics, the possibilities for oral communication are virtually limitless.

1. Radio. One teacher has said, "Our boys and girls like to listen to others their own age. It seems to me they learn more from them."

The radio in the classroom is an inexpensive device that is realistic, is authentic, and has emotional impact. It may be used directly by scheduling classes to coincide with some radio programs in order to hear health lectures, interviews, or panel discussions. It may also be used within the classroom as a simulated broadcast with

class members taking part in the production.

From the point of view of health actions, pupils need to be taught how to use the radio and be selective and critical of radio programs. Just as children are taught not to accept everything that appears in print, so they must learn to appraise that which is presented over the radio and television channels.

In New York City radio broadcasts are planned to supplement classroom instruction. The Board of Education's radio station has programs written especially for children in the elementary grades with vocabulary level and attention span correlated with health course study.

Radio offers a real opportunity for children to share health experience with the community and thus accomplish a real service. Actual nutrition activities, for example, may be described. Children talk about what is done to improve school lunches, or the results of a school lunch survey, or how waste was cut down in the lunchroom. In one school a report on physical conditioning exercises was read to the public by a panel of sixth grade pupils. Timely, down-to-earth material is always welcomed by radio station operators.

The number of uses of radio in the health curriculum is almost unlimited. In Montclair, New Jersey, the seventh grade pupils did a broadcast on poliomyelitis over the school radio system and discovered that the broadcast was equally effective whether for radio, a public address system, or a school auditorium program. The preparation and presentation were planned so that they added vividness and meaning to science, English, speech, health, and social studies. In another elementary school a health play was read by several pupils located in the cloakroom and "piped" into the adjoining classroom for general listening. Other topics which lend themselves well to radio are:

---

[6] Toynbee, Arnold J. *Greek Historical Thought from Homer to the Age of Heraclitus.* New York: Dutton Publishing Co., 1924, p. xxv.

An interview with the city health director.

An eyewitness report of a bicycle accident.

A dramatization of a scientific health discovery.

Bringing the health textbook "to life" through lifelike qualities of the broadcaster.

Patent medicine and tobacco advertising—study of truths and half-truths.

Pupil three-minute talk on the value of some food.

A source of radio scripts is the Bureau of Health Education, American Dental Association. A number of short dramas of interest to children are available as 12-inch transcriptions. Examples include: *Tommy Is Three, Linda Gets Ready for School, Sherry and the Apple, The Freckle Faced Rebel.* Sources of additional scripts may be found in *Educator's Guide to Free Transcriptions, Tapes, and Scripts.*

2. Television. A number of schools have access to educational television. Health programs are staged for school audiences. Both professional personnel and schoolchildren may be employed as performers. This can be a fine medium for motivation providing, as, in the case of moving picture films, there is some pertinent discussion prior to and following television presentation. Here sight and sound are combined to teach an entire community. Several intermediate grade school classes, for example, could watch the actual pulling of a bad tooth in a dentist's chair, this to be followed by a special message from the dentist.

Each material aid has its own unique advantages and limitations. Television is a powerful medium, but it is expensive and is often only a one-way communication. Attempting to regiment health classes by means of television would be to violate certain principles regarding pupil interests, needs, and differences. If programs are carefully related to classroom activity, especially following the presentation, it seems logical to expect television to become an effective tool in the promotion of health. However, it must always be evaluated against alternate tools that are available. At the moment, instructional television is an unfinished experiment. It is, in the words of Alvin C. Eurich, standing ". . . at the most significant crossroads in its history. . . . Opportunities have opened . . . to intertwine television fruitfully with other new media."[7]

It is well to keep in mind that research on the successful use of television in the grades indicates that "live" lessons are more warmly received than filmed telecasts. This does not mean that filmed lessons are not worth while; it simply means that the more personal television becomes the more effective it may be.

Home television may be used for pupil assignments somewhat the same way as radio has been used for years, i.e., to appraise "health" commercials and advertising, and to listen to special health talks, demonstrations, news, and plays.

3. Records. Thomas Edison considered the phonograph one of his favorite inventions. Little did he realize that recordings would be successfully used for classroom instruction—a use that is restricted only by the imagination of the teacher.

Records are easy to play, are relatively inexpensive, and are available in many schools today. Disc recordings are owned by children who often enjoy sharing their records with the rest of the group. They give meaning to numerous events, bring authentic sounds into the classroom, and improve the listening habits of boys and

---

[7] Murphy, Judith, and Gross, Ronald. *Learning by Television.* New York: The Fund for the Advancement of Education, August 1966, pp. 6–7.

girls. They constitute two-way communication and can be stopped and discussed with the class.

In the teaching of health, commercial records may be used for health songs and action stories. Other health records may be obtained from the American Medical Association. These are *Health Heroes, Doctors Make History, The Drugs You Use, Slow Poison, Nothing to Fear but Fear,* and several other titles. Still another source of children's health records is Encyclopaedia Britannica Films. Some of the finest 33⅓ rpm transcriptions for classroom use may be obtained from the American Cancer Society, National Interagency Council on Smoking and Health, The National Safety Council, Maryknoll Lending Library, and the United States Rubber Company. By way of example, the United States Rubber Company makes a five minute transcription for school use that encourages the observance of National Fire Prevention Week.

Special recordings for use in sex education classes are distributed by Stanley Bowmar Co., Valhalla, N.Y. 10595. These include *The Story of Growing-Up* (girls) and *What it Means to Grow Up* (boys).

Many state health departments have transcriptions either on records or tapes pertaining to health topics. Also, audio-visual aids services are a source of these teaching aids — particularly the University of Illinois, Indiana University, Syracuse University, and Boston University.

4. Tape Recordings. The tape recorder opens a great many areas to the teacher of health. Tape recorders are not difficult to operate, and the tape is easy to edit and repair. In many respects the tape recorder has more uses in the classroom than the radio or television set. Tape recordings may be purchased. (The periodical, *Tape Recording,* lists most of the tapes available from commercial companies. See also, *Educator's Guide to Free Transcriptions, Tapes, and Scripts,* Educator's Progress Service, Randolph, Wis.)

From the teacher's point of view tape recordings may be used to make permanent behavior patterns and attitudes. From a health instruction viewpoint they make learning more complete by:

a. Bringing health authorities into the classroom. A committee of two or three pupils can visit a busy physician, bakery manager, or water department superintendent and record the answers to pre-arranged classroom questions. Distance is no problem. The world is brought to the classroom.

b. Recording home radio and television commercials, plays, and talks to be used for class discussion and appraisal.

c. Providing a variety of approaches to the same subject. A recording of a health lesson may be reviewed two weeks later with profit. Gives both pupils and teacher an opportunity for self-evaluation.

d. Bringing to the classroom some of the health problems of the community. The teacher's ability to verbalize about a health problem — alcoholism, for example — is at best limited. The tape recorder brings to the students the actual voices of community members who know the problem at first hand. The teacher can use this information, emphasize it, and elaborate upon it; but the raw material of life is here, not lost in abstract verbiage.

One of the most valuable uses of a tape recorder is to play it back to the pupils so that they hear how their own voices sound. Several statements pertaining to a health lesson may actually be read into the machine and played back the next day for class consumption. A "traveling recorder team" may survey the pupils and teachers for their opinions relative to some current health idea, or they may venture into the business area of town to interview the "passing citizen." A sixth grade class in one New York State community questioned quite a number of leading citizens on their opinions relative to fluoridating the city water supply. Another idea often used is to put together a simple story and have it taped exactly as desired for future presentation. A single topic combining humor with good advice is "How to Burn Down Your House."

Textbooks, Periodicals, Pamphlets, and Clippings

The use of the classroom library shelf as well as the school library permits many books, periodicals, pamphlets, and clippings to be helpful in the teaching of a unit of work. Children who like to read stand to gain a great deal from such materials. Other pupils may have to have these items "sugar-coated" in some way in order to profit from them. One method of making a clipping or pamphlet palatable to some students is to project it on a screen by use of the opaque projector. Another way is to have it read aloud by some good reader.

1. Textbooks. In Chapter 9 textbooks were reviewed as a method of teaching. If they are up-to-date and are more than just another reading book, they have value. When the book is accurate in the presentation of facts and illustrations and orderly in the arrangement of materials, it can be used as an effective guide to the health program at a certain grade level. This is particularly true if the pupil is asked to discover things for himself, answer questions, engage in learning activities, and respond to diagrams and situations. Listed below are the publishers of textbooks primarily concerned with health:

American Book Company, New York, N.Y. *The ABC Health Series*, grades 1–8 (1959).

Benefic Press, Chicago, Ill., *The Health Action Series*, grades 1–8 (1955–1961).

The Bobbs-Merrill Co., Inc., Indianapolis, Ind., *Health for Young America Series*, grades 1–8 (1961).

Ginn and Company, Boston, Mass., *New Ginn Elementary Health Series*, grades kindergarten-8 (1969).

Laidlaw Brothers, River Forest, Ill., *Laidlaw Health Series*, grades 1–8 (1966).

Lyons & Carnahan, Chicago, Ill., *Dimensions in Health Series*, grades 1–8 (1965).

Scott, Foresman & Company, Ill., *Curriculum Foundation Series*, *New Basic Health and Safety Program*, grades 1–9 (1964).

The John C. Winston Company, Philadelphia, Pa., *Winston Health Series Revised*, Grades 1–8 (1960).

2. Pamphlets. Probably no other health medium is more wisely used — or mis-used — than the leaflet or pamphlet. Thousands are distributed in school each year, only to end up in wastebaskets. Pamphlets need to be simple and have a definite message. They should be in bold print with lots of color and illustrations and contain some white space so that what is written will stand out. These criteria should also be followed when health leaflets or "handouts" are made in class for home distribution. The accompanying illustration is included in a leaflet which has been widely distributed in Florida. Although limited to black and white, note how attractive it is and the message it has for the parents.[8]

Pamphlets for school use may be obtained from numerous official and nonofficial health agencies. (See Chapter 11.) Most of the large insurance companies, the American Medical Associa-

---

[8] Courtesy Florida State Board of Health, Jacksonville, Fla.

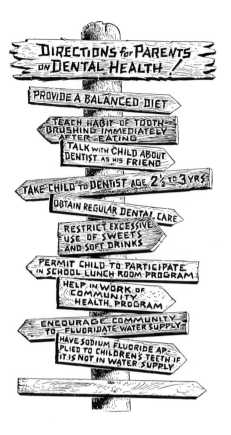

ways; however, a pamphlet cannot be expected to influence attitudes and behavior without being used in conjunction with other methods of health education. They must be informative and motivating, and they must be adapted to each age level. For example, a leaflet such as the one on the basic foods is of little consequence by itself, but when used as a guide for a menu planning project it becomes hard to surpass.

To meet the health and safety needs of pupils, it is recommended that careful consideration be given to the selection of pamphlets, textbooks, and other printed materials. How each applies in a given instance depends upon the specific teaching objectives which have been set up to meet particular needs.

CONTENT

1. Are the facts scientifically accurate?

2. Does the material cover the major health and safety problems of the age group in question?

3. Is all of the information pertinent?

4. Do the selection and arrangement constitute good coverage?

5. Are the ideas essential, significant, and important to clear understanding?

6. Is the content worthy of time and attention in a crowded curriculum?

7. Is the content free of unsound or untrue claims?

PSYCHOLOGICAL VALUES

1. Is the interest appeal strong enough to capture and hold attention?

2. Is the mixture of familiarity and newness such as to foster growth?

3. Is the material suitable for the level of comprehension of the pupils?

4. Does the manner of presentation neither "talk down" to nor "go over the heads" of the intended readers?

5. Is the degree of motivation for action sufficiently potent?

6. Is there educationally objectionable propaganda in the appeal?

tion, the Florida Citrus Commission, and the National Dairy Council represent organizations which distribute particularly well-fashioned leaflets suitable for elementary school classroom use. In recent years there has been a reduction in the number of free materials available for teachers. However, the quality of the inexpensive materials has improved measurably. For years the National Dairy Council has made its wide variety of health leaflets available to teachers, and in sufficient quantity so that each pupil may have his own. *The Story of the Cow* has been written for 12 different grade levels. Third graders are able to use the little 3 inch × 4 inch colored leaflet on the four basic food areas, both in the classroom and at home. Attractive "handouts" such as these may be used in a number of good

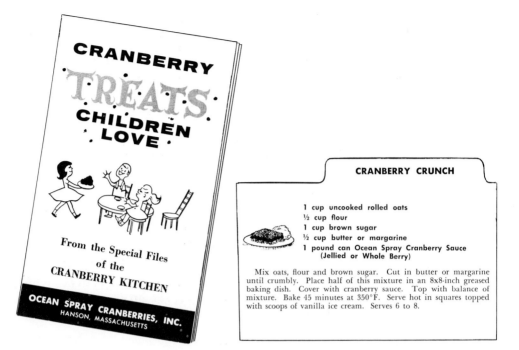

Figure 10–3 Foods to experiment with attract children. (Pamphlet with recipe. Courtesy Ocean Spray Cranberries, Inc., So. Hanson, Mass.)

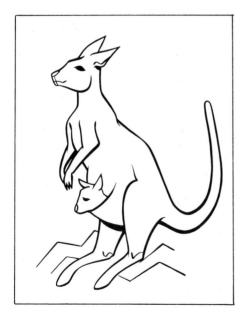

Leave hitch-hiking to the kangeroos. They are built for it, and you and your bike are not. Only one person belongs on your bike . . . and that's YOU. Never hitch rides on cars, trucks or buses. Never follow bikes or cars too closely; allow plenty of room for a safe stop.

Figure 10–4 A page from the attractive pamphlet, *Good Biker Today . . . Good Driver Tomorrow.* (Courtesy Employers Mutuals of Wausau.)

TECHNICAL ATTRIBUTES

1. Are the type size, boldness, and spacing adequate for easy reading?

2. Is the paper stock good from the standpoint of color, contrast, and lack of glare?

3. Is the artistry of design and illustration attractive and effective?[9]

Finally, a word about the use of magazines. The Research Division of the National Education Association has discovered that some of the most imaginative classroom projects are sparked by materials appearing in magazines. Their most common usage is to develop bulletin board displays. They are also employed for useful reference information, for free reading, and for stimulation of student writing. Health articles may be read in class or summarized in understandable language. The most frequently used magazines are *Life, National Geographic, Newsweek, Time, Reader's Digest, Look, Saturday Evening Post, U.S. News and World Report,* and *Holiday.*

3. **Encyclopedias.** Sets of encyclopedias form a wealth of background materials for the classroom. By following the library method of teaching (see Chapter 9) real use may be made of this two-way reference material. Many a statement in an encyclopedia has triggered ideas for pupil activities. Even more important, perhaps, encyclopedias can be used directly by pupils in their search for facts and comments relative to the health unit being studied. It covers all related fields of health, contains bibliographies for the teacher, and provides excellent background material to look over before viewing films, filmstrips, or TV programs. And it often contains a quantity of illustrative diagrams, charts, and maps.

---

[9] Based on Joint Committee on Health Problems in Education of the NEA and AMA, *Health Education,* 5th ed. Washington, D.C.: National Education Association, 1961.

The following sources will be helpful to the teacher in the use of encyclopedias as a teaching aid:

Guide to Britannica Junior. Exercises to to develop basic reference skills. These lessons may be used as a suggestion to the teacher or a class to prepare exercises of their own of similar nature built around the topic of current interest to the group. *Britannica Junior,* Encyclopaedia Britannica, 425 N. Michigan Avenue, Chicago, Ill.

Why an Encyclopedia? A filmstrip for teachers to show how an encyclopedia can broaden and enliven the total school program. (Available on loan. Can be purchased.) Encyclopaedia Britannica.

How to Use the Encyclopedia. Filmstrip showing how to use the modern encyclopedia with an index. *Compton's Pictured Encyclopedia,* F. E. Compton and Co., 1000 N. Dearborn Street, Chicago 10, Ill.

Compton's at Work in the Classroom. A 48-page service book which gives dozens of practical examples of best classroom practice in using an encyclopedia for teaching basic skills in language arts, health, and social studies. Numerous examples are given which show how an encyclopedia can enrich every curriculum area and solve many teaching problems (Free). F. E. Compton and Company.

Look-It-Up-Books, Books I, II, III. Lessons with exercises to introduce the use of encyclopedias to boys and girls, grades three to eight. (Copies upon request, five cents.) *The World Book Encyclopedia, Field Enterprises, Inc.,* Merchandise Mart, Chicago 54, Ill.

4. **Clippings.** One of the finest uses of the health clipping is to tack it to a designated space on a bulletin board where everyone can see it. Clippings from magazines and newspapers include pictures, stories, reports, research, and advertising. Every health topic, particularly in grades four to six, can be bolstered with appropriate clippings. Hardly a week passes by without some of the picture magazines, such as *Life* or *Look,* having an item suited for a health lesson. Pictures of foods, drawings of body parts, and facial expressions may all be

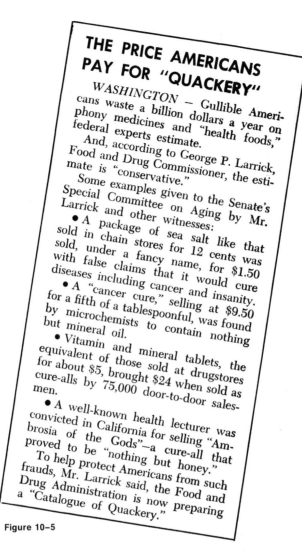

THE PRICE AMERICANS PAY FOR "QUACKERY"

WASHINGTON — Gullible Americans waste a billion dollars a year on phony medicines and "health foods," federal experts estimate.

And, according to George P. Larrick, Food and Drug Commissioner, the estimate is "conservative."

Some examples given to the Senate's Special Committee on Aging by Mr. Larrick and other witnesses:

● A package of sea salt like that sold in chain stores for 12 cents was sold, under a fancy name, for $1.50 with false claims that it would cure diseases including cancer and insanity.

● A "cancer cure," selling at $9.50 for a fifth of a tablespoonful, was found by microchemists to contain nothing but mineral oil.

● Vitamin and mineral tablets, the equivalent of those sold at drugstores for about $5, brought $24 when sold as cure-alls by 75,000 door-to-door salesmen.

● A well-known health lecturer was convicted in California for selling "Ambrosia of the Gods"—a cure-all that proved to be "nothing but honey."

To help protect Americans from such frauds, Mr. Larrick said, the Food and Drug Administration is now preparing a "Catalogue of Quackery."

Figure 10–5

posted on a bulletin board or projected on a large screen.

Study Guides and Workbooks

There is some use in health teaching for these aids providing they encourage students to be active—to try something out, to experiment, to listen, to observe, or to discuss. Their use, therefore, is strictly related to how practical they can make such topics as dental health, communicable disease, sleep, and exercise. If they contain a profusion of outlines, charts, or lists and appear to be a substitute for such approved methods as the discussion, demonstration, and lecture, their use should be limited.

A good elementary school workbook is attractive. It has directions for study, self-instructive techniques, and self-corrective exercises. It contains pictures, practice exercises, and testing material. Provision is made for individual differences and for developing initiative and independence.

In many of the elementary school

health readers there is a teacher's edition or guidebook section which provides the teacher with a number of proven ideas for classroom use. Good examples may be found in these guides that help in lesson planning— discussion topics, games, experiments, songs, and poems. The guides give teachers a wealth of ideas because they often contain stories, posters, and drawings which may be used to make the teaching of health more rewarding.

Pictures, Photographs, Posters, and Mobiles

A collection of pictorial materials, illustrating as far as possible every health topic which the teacher expects to cover during the school year, is one of the best stock in trade items any teacher can possess.

1. Pictures and Photographs. Pictures crystallize ideas and form much of the basis for thinking. Industry and business spend a fortune each year on pictures to put their story across. Pictures are everywhere today in magazines, folders, and booklets. Good photographs are also available or may be made through a school project. Once used, the outstanding pictures and photographs should be filed in an accessible folder for future use.

Suitable health instruction pictures should include such items as groups of healthy children with smiling faces; pictures of pets and other animals eating the same foods as children (pigs drinking milk, rabbits eating green vegetables, chickens picking up grain in the barnyard); the fire engine en route to a fire, the policeman directing traffic, and the like.

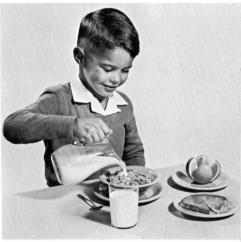

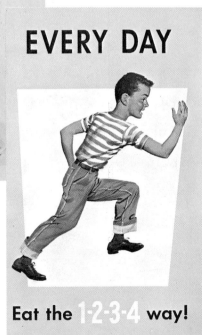

Figure 10–6 An action photograph displayed with an action pamphlet. (Pamphlet from the Food Chart for Children, courtesy National Dairy Council.)

In posture instruction in the upper grades, the ordinary flat photograph may serve as a superior teaching aid. "Before" and "after" posture photographs are helpful in teaching the benefits of good posture, especially from the point of view of appearance. The Polaroid Land Camera has been successfully employed to show boys and girls how they look as they stand at ease. Since there is no waiting for the picture to be developed, one can "witness the anxiety, then the reaction of subjects when they see their picture a minute after the shutter is clicked." This is without doubt the psychological moment for optimum health teaching.

A multitude of heterogeneous pictures will only confuse a student. To obtain the best results with pictures use only a few well chosen ones for a pertinent illustration. Pictorial materials may be mounted and passed around for individual inspection or exhibited on a board. They may also be projected by the opaque projector.

2. Posters. The thousands of billboards spread across the land have only one purpose: to put over an idea in one fleeting glance. Posters accomplish the same purpose.

Posters have become an expressive form of American art. Their chief purpose is stimulation. Thus they may be used to introduce a unit or call attention to some facts in a phase of instruction. A good poster should be simple, large (28 inches × 22 inches), have bold and colored lettering that is easily read and understood. If it can be interesting enough to cause a chuckle, adroit enough to promote discussion, and clever enough to haunt the mem-

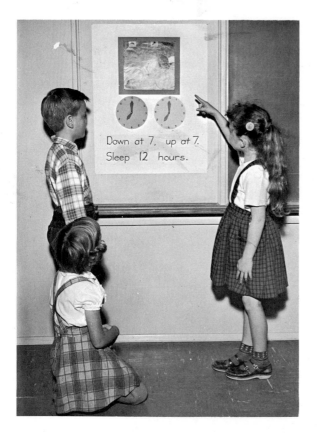

Figure 10-7 What can a photograph do?

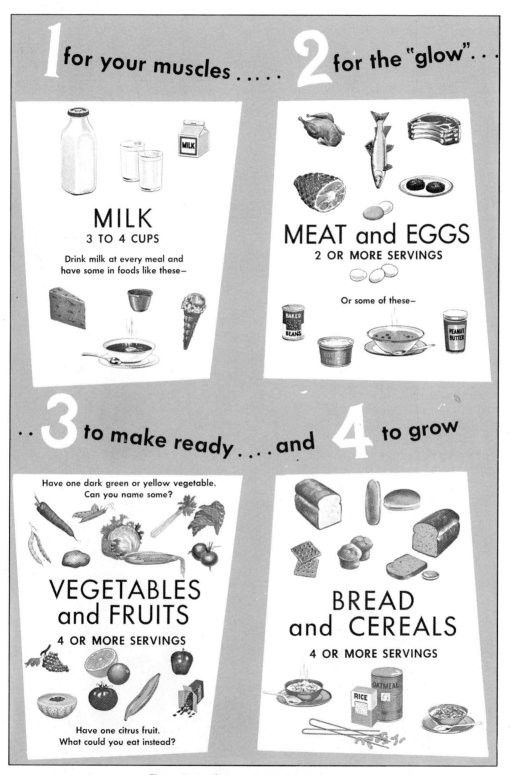

Figure 10–8   (Courtesy National Dairy Council.)

ory, it has just about everything that is needed to make it a useful teaching aid. If, however, it functions only as another implement, requiring the support of more basic teaching aids, then it is of limited value. Too often posters have been used solely as a wall decoration, having been left on display far beyond the point of attracting notice. They are effective only when they are *frequently changed.*

Numerous manufacturers of foods, toothpastes, school furniture, and dairy products are excellent sources of poster materials. Practically all of the large insurance companies distribute, free of charge, colorful wall posters relating to health and safety practices. Some examples of the more effective free posters for primary and intermediate grade use may be obtained from:

American Cancer Society
American Dental Association
Elementary school (large) posters (set of four)
Elementary school (miniature) posters (25 sets)
Toothbrushing chart
Bicycle Institute of America

Educators Mutual Life Insurance Co.:
Many posters, especially relating to posture and body mechanics.
Employers Mutual of Wausau:
Be a Better Biker
Sound Suggestions for Swimmers and Splashers
Mouth-to-Mouth Artificial Respiration
Every Day Seat Belts Prevent Injury and Death
Equitable Life Assurance Society:
Pets—Choosing, Keeping Pets for Healthier and Safe Companions.
The Day Begins with Breakfast
The Rest Is up to You—Does Your Sleep Really Rest You?
Good Posture Pays Off
Take Stock of Your Health
Florida Citrus Commission:
Several large, colorful posters relative to oranges and vitamin C.
The National Dairy Council:
Numerous posters depicting appetizing dairy products which are immediately related to efficiency of children.
National Livestock and Meat Board:
Food nutrition posters. Colorful, clear, 19 inches × 28½ inches printed, adapted from booklet, *You and Your Engine.* Part of elementary school nutrition unit.
The Foods You Need Every Day
The Foods I Eat

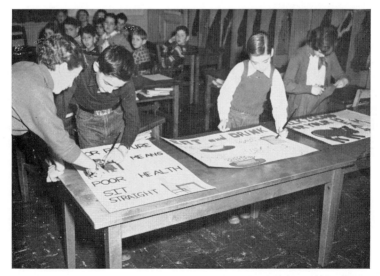

Figure 10–9   Poster drawing is fun. (Courtesy Campus School, State University of New York, Oswego, N.Y.)

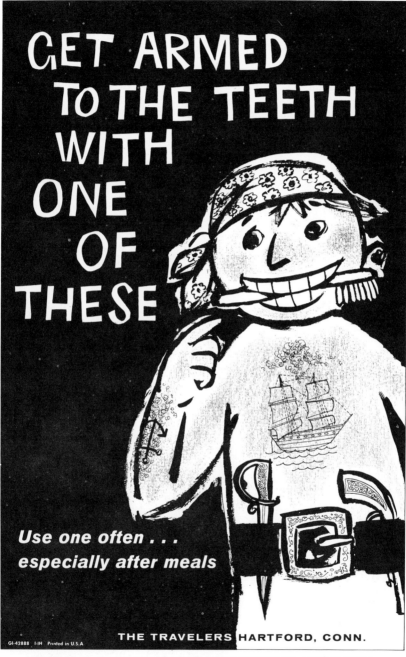

Figure 10–10   Poster. (Courtesy The Travelers Insurance Co., Hartford, Conn.)

Also separate posters on proteins, calories, vitamins, calcium, phosphorus, and iron.

Pepsodent:
Honor roll chart for "Clean Teeth Club"

National Commission on Safety Education:
A number of posters from the Classroom Series Program
Playground Safety
Special Activities Are Fun
Let's Be Safe Passengers

The National Safety Council:
Colorful, eye-catching safety posters, 8½ inches × 11½ inches for elementary school use

Travelers Insurance Co.:
Several colorful 12 inch × 24 inch health posters for primary grades

In working with posters the best learning probably takes place when children make their own. This is especially true when the poster making is directly related to the particular

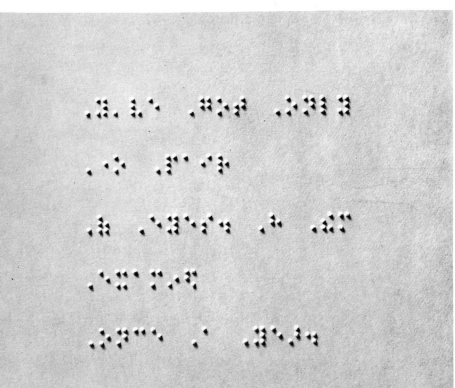

This is Braille. It says:

"You've got only one pair of eyes. Have them examined once a year."

Better Vision Institute.

Figure 10–11   Poster. (Courtesy The Better Vision Institute.)

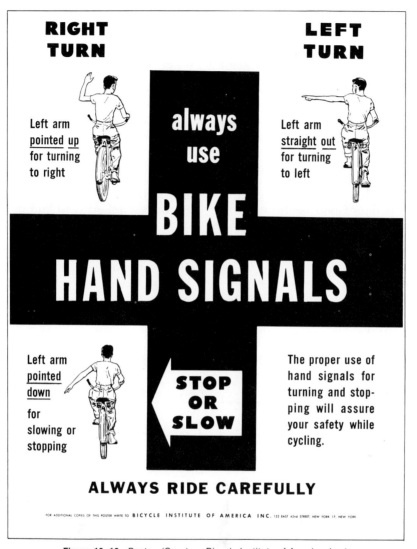

Figure 10–12   Poster. (Courtesy Bicycle Institute of America, Inc.)

health topic, is clear and forceful, is well designed, is colorful, and has easily understood titles with brief captions. An example of a poster that meets these qualifications and would be attractive on a fifth-grade bulletin board is on page 338.[10]

Artistic posters may be fashioned

from wrapping paper, scrap tin, tinfoil, box tops, magazine pictures, wallpaper, and the usual art supplies. Even comic book clippings and newspaper cartoons may be used in making the poster. These sometimes serve to make the poster more attractive and humorous.

Once health posters are discussed in class they may be hung about the room for a short period. The better ones may be selected for a main corridor bulletin

---

[10] Prepared by the State of New York, Division of Safety, Albany, N.Y. Current poster material is available on request.

board, the lunchroom, or the physical education locker room.

It is possible to purchase excellent 24 inch × 36 inch wall charts for keeping records of pupil achievements: physical fitness records, growth records, activities calendars, and colorful bulletin board-type materials which may be erased and used again and again.

A positive slogan displayed in a good place can be very effective in the elementary school. Such slogans as "Good Food for Good Teeth" or "Your Carriage, Madam" are far more effective than the negative type of slogan which begins with "Don't" do this or that.

More and more posters are employing cut-out figures and superimposed materials over the foundation surface. Items are readily tacked, stapled, or glued to the surface and provide another dimension for observation. A "Susie Goodtooth" may be made in poster form for a bulletin board. She is made of foods which build healthy teeth. A milk carton is used for the body, an orange for the head, small leaves of spinach or chard for the hair, carrots for the feet and legs (small end fitted into the bottom of the carton), and celery stalks for her arms. An alternate method is to find pictures of these foods and paste them on a large piece of poster paper.

Simple line expressions can tell more sometimes than fancy drawings. Mental health is well depicted this way:

JANUARY 1969

SUN	MON	TUE	WED	THU	FRI	SAT
			1	2	3	4
5	6	7	8	9	10	11
12	13	14	15	16	17	18
19						25
26						

AN ACCIDENT-FREE YEAR depends on you

SIMPLE LINE EXPRESSIONS

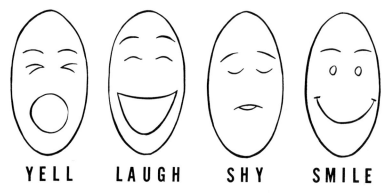

YELL   LAUGH   SHY   SMILE

3. The Health Mobile. Under the direction of the clever teacher a rather stimulating health "mobile" may be constructed. This may consist of wooden signs, printed on both sides, a wire frame, and string. To learn about food values a fourth grade class might build and hang a mobile such as the following:

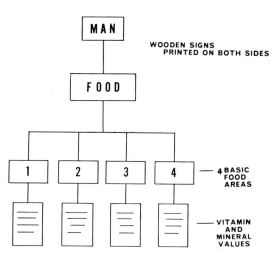

This mobile is different enough from the usual display that the pupils can learn the four basic food groups more easily. Here they also see the values inherent in each group. The wooden signs may be made in class or in the elementary industrial arts laboratory.

These are superior to cardboard signs. Also, as an alternative to using signs for vitamin and mineral values, the class might cut out and hang pictures of the various human organs affected. Example, the eyeball for vitamin A, or the skeleton for calcium.

Cartoons, Sketches, Stick Drawings, Strip Drawings, and Writing Pads

This is a materials area that is closely related to the one on pictures and posters. It covers everything from a sketch or diagram of an object or process to the more elaborate cartoons, strip drawings, and stick men drawings. Such items as these are excellent for presenting abstract ideas in visual form, summarizing, informing, showing relationships, demonstrating positions and operations and the development of structures.

1. Cartoons. The perfect cartoon needs no caption. The symbolism conveys the message, for the best cartoons make their point immediately.

If the teacher will watch carefully for cartoons having to do with health, she will find a number of excellent ones appearing each week in popular magazines and newspapers.

In some respects cartoons work bet-

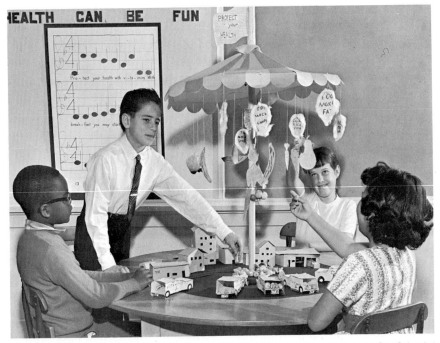

Figure 10–13   A variety of mobile. (Courtesy *Health Education Journal,* Los Angeles City Schools.)

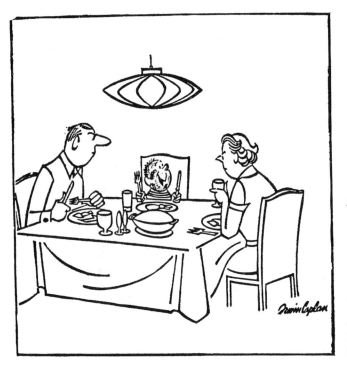

"Why should I wash—I'm inoculated against everything, ain't I?"[11]

<hr />

[11] Reproduced through courtesy of Irwin Caplan, McNaught Syndicate, Inc., and the *American Legion Magazine.*

ter with intermediate grade children, probably because a first-rate cartoon has emotional impact. This is arranged by the clever cartoonist who is able to play with humor, mockery, satire — qualities that are generally appreciated more by older children.

In using such a medium in health teaching, one must be careful that pupils do not accept the message of the cartoon uncritically. Cartoons are very often all "black" or "white," or they oversimplify without qualification. Moreover, they cannot be used repeatedly as can pictures and photographs. They become outdated rapidly. They must be considered because surveys indicate that they are among the most popular aids used by teachers. And where they are not obtained from initial sources they may be made in the classroom. In fact, original health cartoons frequently help students think for themselves and apply what they know about health to the cartoon.

2. Sketches and Drawings. A pencil sketch or drawing made with a pen, pencil, or special crayon may make health facts more vivid. A class studying posture, for example, may see what is involved in a straight line type of posture when a simple sketch is drawn of building blocks.

Where a drawing of the heart might appear too complicated to arouse interest, a simple sketch would serve the purpose. It helps, of course, if the teacher has skill in this area. If not, it would be better to try some other means of audio-visual enlightenment.

Drawings and diagrams are valuable at all age levels. Primary grade children seem to appreciate the line drawing that outlines a process. In a study of foods, an outline of how the grain passes from the farmer's field to the bakery and ultimately to the bread on the table is of real interest. The diagram of a water supply from the original source to the clean glass or the story of milk from the cow to the table are other examples that may be nicely diagrammed. Some of these items may be put on transparencies by pupils themselves.

Drawings, sketches, and diagrams may also be put together by the teacher or the class using magazine prints, newsprint, wrapping paper, window shades, or anything else that can be brought to class to work with. These materials may be large sheets of paper, chart cloth, old bedsheets, large paper panels, or classroom chalkboards.

3. Strip Drawings ("Comics"). Here a story is told through a series of drawings, frequently called "comics."

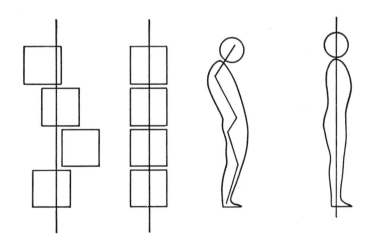

A large per cent of the fourth, fifth, and sixth graders in this country are avid readers, reading several comic books each week. And, significantly, they tend to remember fairly well what they read. This has implications for health teaching, for if pupils will read and enjoy drawings because they are clear, are easy reading, and are "personal," then health strips may be developed which will do the same thing.

A number of health comic strips have successfully used for several years. The principal ones were developed and are distributed by the American Dental Association. They are colorful, full size, and may be obtained free of charge.

A number of free health comic books are available from the Food and Drug Administration, U.S. Public Health Service. The comic *Dennis the Menace Takes a Poke at Poison* is especially well written. So are the several "Sparky" fire stories distributed by the National Fire Protection Association: *Early Man and Fire, Man Learns More about Fire, Hello, I Am Fire, Is This Your Home?* Employers Insurance of Wausau has a comic-style booklet, *A Tale of Two Bike Riders,* and the Public Health Committee of the Paper Cup and Container Institute has a large number of food and sanitation comic cartoons available for general use.

4. Writing Pads. These pads of paper may be as big as or bigger than 2 feet × 3 feet. They are usually supported on an easel and used very much the same as a chalkboard. They have a distinct advantage over the chalkboard in that sketches, diagrams, and notes may be prepared well in advance of the class period. This is especially helpful in the crowded school with inadequate blackboard space. To many children it is simply a different medium—a fact to keep in mind when new sources of motivation are sought.

Charts, Tables, Graphs, and Maps

Whereas posters are centered on one idea, most charts, tables, graphs, and maps carry more explanatory information. By way of example, a teaching chart or table may contain a grouping of certain vitamins in one area and minerals in another, together with a number of details about each. This makes it a self-contained instructional unit which requires class study to make it completely useful.

1. Charts and Tables. Information is arranged in lists. Facts, figures, and even pictures are organized in some way so that the visible parts are related to the whole. The ramifications of a whole concept or idea are presented at once. The danger here is that the table or chart may include too much detail or too many words.

A proper chart should have a title large enough to be seen across an ordinary classroom. Lettering should be clear with strong colors on a neutral or light background. It may be several square feet in size and hung from the ceiling, or small enough to be duplicated and distributed to each pupil. It may be mounted on heavy paper, a bulletin board, or ordinary flannel. In any case it should not remain on display beyond its period of usefulness.

It is not difficult to make an elaborate table or chart when it comes to depicting health and disease statistics, the nutritional breakdown of food into calories, or something similar. Care must be taken, however, to limit the detail to the primary and intermediate grade level of comprehension.

Health charts with the most instructional value are those which the pupils make themselves, and are based on data which they have assembled. In one Southern school the primary grade boys and girls put together a chart which they called *A Trip Through*

A TRIP   THROUGH HEALTHLAND

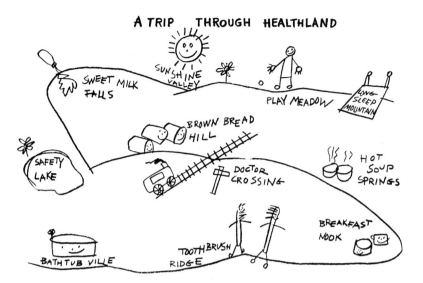

Healthland.[12] It was constructed with felt mounted on heavy paper. The medium of light colors was also applied to make it attractive.

At each "stop" on the "trip through healthland" the importance of that area was discussed and personal problems were raised and talked about.

Every elementary teacher should have a chance to look over the *Good Health Record* charts distributed by the Kellogg Company, Battle Creek, Michigan. The students keep these current on a day-to-day basis, recording habits of cleanliness, eating, sleeping, and helping at home and at school. Other chart materials are available free from Proctor & Gamble, *The Ivory Inspection Patrol*—wall charts which may be taken home by pupils for personal inspection—and from the American Dental Association.

Most children enjoy charting their progress and keeping their own records. This becomes a kind of self-testing activity—a means of comparing oneself today with what one did yesterday or with someone else in the

12 Originated and reported by Mary Charles Garrett of Gainesville, Fla.

class. The *Good Health Record,* made available (free) to teachers by the Kellogg Company, is an example of a chart useful over a four week period.

Another attractive chart used especially in health teaching is one for measuring pupil height in the ordinary classroom. The *How Tall Chart* of the Travelers Insurance Company, Hartford, Connecticut, fits inconspicuously on a closet door or wall. It hangs so that the bottom of the chart is $2\frac{1}{2}$ feet above the floor. Height may be measured to the nearest quarter inch.

Tables are usually more complete than charts. They afford the viewer detail. They are often referred to as table-charts because they are set up in chart form with straight columns. Consider the usefulness of such a table as the accompanying one to a sixth grade studying the topic of wholesome meats.

2. Graphs and Maps. A graph diagrams quantity, development, function, or relationship of factors. There are graphs that are horizontal or bar, line, pictorial, and circular or pie. All may be effectively used in health teaching. Excellent multi-colored bar graphs for health teaching may be ob-

Some Household Tests for Food Wholesomeness

Food	Indications of Spoilage or Contamination	Comments
CANNED FOOD	Swelled top and bottom. Dented areas along the side seam. Abnormal odor of contents. Indications of foaming. Milkiness of liquor above food.	These indications of spoilage apply to canned vegetables, meats, fish and poultry. Home-canned meats and vegetables should be cooked thoroughly before being served.
FISH	Gills gray or greenish. Eyes sunken. Flesh is easily pulled away from bones. Fingernail indentation persists in flesh Rigidity not present.	Off-odor can be detected quite frequently in spoiled fish.
SHRIMP	A pink color develops on upper fins and near the tail. Off-odor similar to ammonia is often detectable.	Some types of shrimp are naturally pink. Cooked shrimp also develops a pink or salmon color. Both of these are wholesome if the odor is not abnormal.
MEAT	Off-odor is detectable. Slimy to touch.	Beef usually spoils first on the surface. Pork usually spoils at the juncture of bone and meat in the inner portions. To test for spoiled pork it may be necessary to use a pointed knife to reach the interior of the meat. An off-odor on the knife is an indication of spoilage.
DRESSED POULTRY	Stickiness appears first under the wing. At the juncture of legs and body and on the upper surface of the tail end. Darkening of the tips of the wings sometimes indicates spoilage.	Dressed poultry should be washed thoroughly before cooking and the hands likewise should be washed after handling the poultry.

tained from the Evaporated Milk Association.

The graph on page 345 has a message for upper grade children. It clearly illustrates how well cereal and milk "go together" to furnish a breakfast meal.[13] It may be seen that cereal contributes most of the nutrients supplied less generously by milk and vice versa.

A map is something more than a dia-

gram or line drawing. It generally starts somewhere and goes somewhere. It may be like an automobile road map or a sketch of the terrain made by a Boy Scout.

A map may be made on any health subject. It is different from the physical, economic, and political maps made available by a supplier and used in geography and social studies; it is generally made by the students. Primary graders, for example, may derive considerable benefit from mapping the route from home to school. In one school, as a part of a lesson on safety, all pupils drew a picture map showing

---

[13] Adapted from the graph in the booklet, *The "Cream of Wheat" Story,* distributed free by the Cream of Wheat Corp., Box M, Minneapolis, Minn., 55413. (Used by permission.)

Cereal and Milk—Nutritional "Go-Togethers"

Enriched Quick "Cream of Wheat" with fresh whole milk and sugar is a perfect breakfast combination. This chart shows you how these nutritious foods complement each other. For example, when you eat 1 ounce (dry weight) of Enriched Quick "Cream of Wheat" along with 4 ounces of fresh whole milk and a teaspoon of sugar, about 99% of the Iron comes from the cereal and the remaining 1% from the milk. But then, from this same combination you will get about 71% of the Riboflavin from the milk. The cereal contributes most of the nutrients supplied less generously by the milk and vice versa.

Nutritionists recommend a "Basic Breakfast Pattern" which supplies about 600 calories and makes a good contribution of almost every essential nutrient. Enriched Quick "Cream of Wheat" with milk plus a serving of citrus fruit fills the bill!

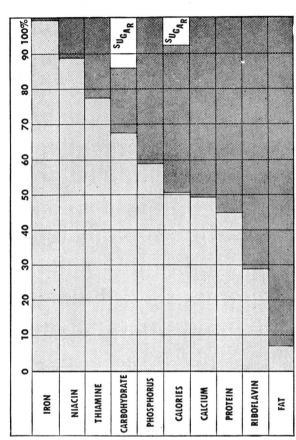

  MILK

  CEREAL

the route from home to school. They were encouraged to make them complete, even to including such hazards as water holes, angry dogs, inviting junkyards, houses under construction, a pile of dirt, and the like. When the maps were completed they were studied by the class so that the hazardous places could be discussed. Some new routes were created to avoid the hazards. The routes were further appraised from the point of view of the bicycle rider. The maps were so revealing that the pupils carried the discussion beyond walking and bicycling to automobile and bus safety.

Another map particularly suited to health teaching in the elementary school is the spot map. It may be a map of the community or an ordinary road map. It could be stuck with a small colored-head pin to show the exact spot where an automobile accident occurred during the preceding month. In one school the pupils marked the spots on the map of the school grounds where accidents occurred. They counted everything from cut elbows, scraped knees, and blisters, to serious falls and minor emergencies. Once the map was well covered with pins, the class stopped to analyze the situation in an attempt to do something about it.

Flash Cards and Flip Charts

Flash cards have titles printed on each side for use in flashing certain information before the pupils. An idea is brought home on a small card. These cards may be in the form of charts, such as the food value charts of the National Dairy Council, and they may be mounted on hinged display panels and flipped one at a time by the teacher.

Flash cards and flip charts may be used to train pupils for quick reaction and correct responses. To many pupils they are a novelty, and, as such, command attention. A series of questions

and answers on school safety may be displayed before the class on 13 inch × 22 inch panels, or the logical progress of a certain food may be followed through the processes of assimilation, digestion, and elimination.

A series of 36 large flip charts, expressly created for kindergarten or grade one pupils, are the *How About You?* health charts published by Ginn and Company. These 17 inch × 20 inch full color charts were described on p. 143, Chapter 7.

Teaching with flash cards permits the teacher to put over a concept that is brief and to the point. The word *Stop* or *Go* or *Caution* has a message all by itself. A series of words arranged to cover health instruction in one class period might read (1) Health, (2) Food, (3) Music, (4) Rest, and (5) Happiness. As the essential ingredients of a healthy person are mentioned, the particular key word on the chart or card is flipped for the class to see. Finally, if the flip chart is helpful in keeping the pipils' minds on the speaker's track, it is equally helpful in keeping the speaker's mind on it.

Bulletin Boards, Chalkboards, Flannel Boards, Felt Boards, and Magnetic Boards

All of these boards are essentially teaching tools to motivate and inform students through the display of photographic, graphic, and other study materials. It is the base of each of these that is different.

1. The Bulletin Board. Practically every classroom has some kind of bulletin board which is used from time to time to display health materials. The materials displayed should have a unifying theme. They should be authentic and easy to read. Simplicity should be the rule in organizing material for elementary schoolchildren. One should ask these questions:

Is there a center of interest?

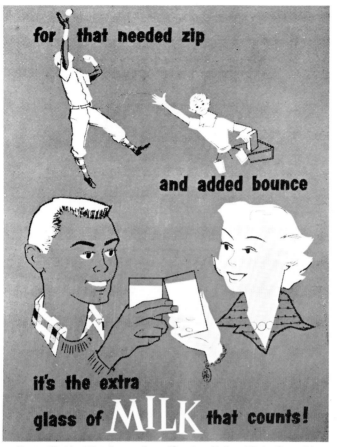

Figure 10–14   Attractive captions. (Courtesy National Dairy Council.)

Is there beauty of line and form?

Do the materials go well together?

Is the total arrangement well-balanced?

Is there repetition of color?

Is a feeling of unity created?

Does the arrangement tell a story?

Captions for bulletin boards have great value. A challenging question or statement accompanying the material may have much to do with the value derived from the display. Captions which tell little, such as *Foods for Health,* or *This Is Posture Week,* can be improved by making them read *Eat Your Way to Good Health* and *How Do You Look to Your Friends?* Other captions which relate to health clip-pings or the health topic being studied might read: *Have You Seen These? Do You Know? Stop—Look—Read.*

Notice that in arranging the pictures or other materials the teacher places the largest number of pictures in the bottom row to give strength to the arrangement. The same procedure is followed when color is used—the darkest colors are concentrated near the bottom of the display.

The bulletin board, when used in health teaching, can arouse interest in many things such as special health week (safety, posture), seasonal wearing apparel, current discussion topics, or local health events. If bulletin

HAVE YOU SEEN THESE?

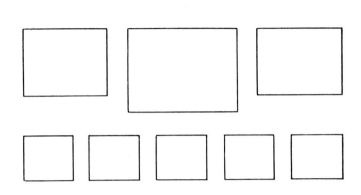

boards are especially colorful and make a good first impression early in September, there is a fairly good chance they will be purposely seen by pupils whenever they pass by them. Needless to say, the materials must be changed frequently.

Three-dimensional display can enhance the appearance of the bulletin board. Real objects brought from home may be hung or tacked to the board with particular attention given to space, color, and shape. In fact, when children help plan and organize the bulletin board display, it is more apt to be read than otherwise. The pupils may print their own captions, mount their materials, and take care to label each item with the name of the child who made it or brought it to school. An odorless and stainless bulletin board wax may be used in place of thumbtacks to hold three-dimensional as well as flat objects.

At Chautauqua Central School, Chautauqua, N.Y., what started as a health project of one class became the interest of the entire school. The project was a *Health Bulletin Board* that was extremely colorful and was changed weekly. Students gathered regularly to review it, and parents even visited the school each week to see what was new. Here short interest-

ing items were posted. Here is an example of a notice to all sixth grade athletes:

−NOTICE−

100 words —

Best advice for amateur and professional athlete alike, say Dr. Jean Mayer and Beverly Bullen: Eat a variety of foods daily—Enriched or whole grain bread and cereal, milk or cheese, meat or an alternate, fruits and vegetables.

Special Pre-Event Meal Instructions for Strenuous Contests:

- Avoid a heavy meal within three to four hours before the game.
- For endurance events, concentrate on foods high in carbohydrate, low in fat. Include generous amounts of cereal, bread, jam, honey.
- To prevent disabling discomfort during the game, avoid high protein and bulky foods.
- Omit coffee, tea, alcohol to avoid a depressing effect later.

---

2. Chalkboard. This is well known to classroom teachers, yet it is often used in such a way that it is not very effective. The work should be clear, legible, and highlighted with colored chalk. The chalkboard is sometimes suitable for projected items such as a sketch of the body or a diagram of an infected tooth. Chalk markings and erasures are then made without disturbing the outline of the picture.

3. Flannel Boards and Felt Boards. Flannel or felt is unique in that once the background is constructed it may be developed into any type of diagram, graph, chart, or bulletin board. Moreover, this may be done while the class watches, and, like a blackboard or chalk talk, the teacher can add portions of the chart or diagram as the lesson unfolds until the story is complete.

The flannel or felt is stretched over a 2 foot × 3 foot stiff board, usually on an easel. Velvet, velveteen, suede cloth, or flocking may also be used. Material which will cling to this includes coarse sandpaper, flannel, felt, terry cloth, or Floktite. All titles, captions, letters, and models are pasted to one of these adhering substances. It is a simple matter after this to arrange and rearrange the board materials. In one school a pie graph of the four basic food groups was put together piece by piece in four operations while the teacher told the class about each category of food. By the time she added piece Number 4 the class was well on the way to visualizing how the parts make up the whole — the balanced diet. Here, the pie graph and the felt board techniques were effectively employed to give meaning to a health lesson which would be difficult to duplicate through some other medium.

In a second grade class in Garden City, New York, the children made up a large number of food items which were attached to the board. They were then asked to select from the board those foods that would make a good breakfast, lunch, and dinner. With practice the pupils were able to do a reasonably good job in planning a full day's diet. Such a technique in learning is another worthy way to help boys and girls of varying abilities engage in a stimulating learning experience.

4. Magnetic Boards. Closely associated with the flannel board is the magnetic board. This is essentially a metal sheet upon which magnets may be attached for a number of purposes of representation. The board may be covered with a thin layer of cardboard or oilcloth or some other material which will not hinder the action of the magnet. One form of this board is truly flexible in all situations. Not only is it permanently magnetized, but it has a chalk writing surface and is available with brightly colored plastic symbols and indicators enabling the teacher to plan and illustrate almost anything. In terms of health instruction, this aid may be used to teach such things as fire routes for fire drills or air raids, moving foods from one plate to another, showing the spread of cold germs, illustrating the hands of the clock at bedtime, placing children and equipment on the school playground, and as many others as the teacher's imagination will permit.

Collections, Specimens, Models, and Mirrors

Children of elementary school age seem to enjoy collecting all kinds of things. Research studies have indicated that one may tell the chronological age of a child by the items found in his pocket. It is not difficult, therefore, to interest boys and girls in collecting health specimens of one kind or another.

1. Collections and Specimens. Newspaper clippings, magazine articles, and cartoons ·may be collected for bulletin board display. Other items such as eight or ten animal teeth for a dental health lesson present a challenge to the average nine or ten year old which he generally meets directly. In one fourth grade class the boys and girls made a collection of empty cereal boxes. Every known cooked and dry cereal was represented and displayed. This was done to initiate a unit on breakfasts. It promoted much interest, especially after the boxes were examined to see what food values the cereals contained. In a fourth grade class that was talking about food spoilage, several persons were asked to bring a good item and a spoiled one to class, for example, a good grapefruit and a bad one, a sound potato and an unsound one, a fresh stalk of celery and a withered one. There was as much interest created by the bad specimen as by almost anything else brought to class that school year.

Other ideas for collections of health-centered articles include:

Canned food labels	Candy bar wrappers
Foods that clean teeth (apples, celery)	Samples of good and poor sneakers
Household cleaning agents	Varieties of apples
Animals and human teeth (also bones and hair)	Drinking utensils used over the years
Potentially dangerous implements (knives, axes, sharp pencils, chisels)	Pressed leaves and stalks of eatable plants (wild)

2. **Models** The true value of a model lies in its degree of accuracy. It helps also if it has several characteristics to attract the eye.

A number of biological supply houses sell excellent models of the various body parts. Merely demonstrating or exhibiting these, however, does not necessarily promote understandings and appreciations. Associating a model of the digestive system with a machine that processes foods, or a model of the heart with a mechanical instrument is not enough. The teacher must project the idea that the digestive tract or heart or anything else is merely a part of the whole man, that man is not a machine —for no machine repairs itself or reproduces itself. In other words, a model is, at best, only a poor copy of the real thing, but it may be quite helpful in creating favorable concepts. A model of the human ear, for instance, may help teach the fact that careless blowing of the nose can be dangerous. This is more important to understand than learning all of the names of the parts of the inner ear. An exploratory examination of the mechanics of the inner ear, however, may be the item that impresses the children the most. The way the model is used is probably more important than the model itself. If somehow the student can get the idea that the human body is the greatest of wonders, a real appreciation will be born. Man wonders over many things, said St. Augustine, but "man himself is the most wonderful."

The use of models in the field of safety has been quite effective. They have been fashioned out of cardboard, wood, clay, plastics, and similar materials. A simple extension ladder built to scale may be leaned against a model of a house with a caption over it that reads: ANCHOR A LADDER FIRMLY IN THIS MANNER. The building of health models lends itself well to the construction method of teaching. Other models more elaborate in nature may be obtained through advance planning.

The inner workings of the human body are strikingly revealed in a life-size transparent model woman which the American Medical Association is sending around the country as part of its health education program. Formed from a sheet of lustrous Tenite butyrate plastic, the model shows with

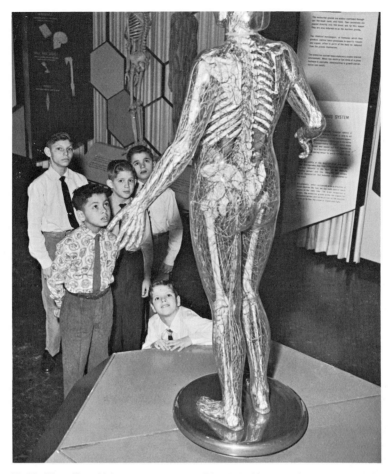

Figure 10-15 "Juno," world-famous transparent talking lady. (Courtesy Cleveland Health Museum.)

remarkable clarity the structure of 25 organs and the blood circulation system.

Five layers of the optically clear plastic are used from front to back to provide realism to the depth and location of organs lying deep within the body. Butyrate was chosen for the model not only because of its ease and detail of forming but because of its exceptional resistance to impact and breakage and ability to withstand the rigors of shipment. Traveling companion of the figure of the AMA tour is a sister model showing the body's 200-bone skeleton and its network of nerves.

A unique feature of the models is an electronic device which progressively lights up the various organs and systems as a tape recording describes and discusses their functions.

3. **Mirrors.** A large share of health teaching is concerned with personal appearance. The use of a single full length mirror can do much to impress growing boys and girls. Children may look at themselves in terms of cleanliness and neatness. Many children have never seen themselves in a full length mirror. Also, when it comes to posture improvement, there is no finer medium than the mirror. Full length mirrors hinged together are the most desirable for they allow several viewing angles. Successful posture work

is done when children not only hear about how they should stand, but also "see how they feel" in front of the mirror.

Exhibits and Museums

The educational exhibit, whether a simple affair in the corner of a classroom or an elaborate museum layout, has considerable value in the health instruction area. It tends to have its greatest value when it is a product of the pupils who help to design and develop it.

The properly conceived health exhibit tells something. It is the "unified dramatization of a single idea. . . . The singleness of the theme is the essence of the exhibit."[14] Unfortunately too many exhibits try to tell everything but end up filling the mind of the viewer with a disconnected assortment of facts and figures. One sometimes forgets that the human brain can absorb only so much.

A good health exhibit takes careful planning and time to prepare. Here are some useful standards to follow for making school exhibits:

Use only one central idea in the exhibit.

Place the exhibit where it is certain to be seen.

The exhibit is something to look at, not to read.

Make all labels short and simple, uniform and legible.

Motion attracts attention.

See that the exhibit is well lighted.

Use color to add interest and attractiveness.

Employ sound and various mechanisms to add charm to the exhibit.

If the classroom teacher will follow this list of standards when an exhibit is being prepared, success of this teaching technique will be assured.

---

[14] Patterson, Raymond S., and Roberts, Beryl J. *Community Health Education in Action.* St. Louis: C. V. Mosby Co., 1951, p. 212.

Too often a room is filled with pictures, diagrams, models, charts, objects, and other symbols, yet they do not represent an interest-compelling presentation. In short, equally as important as the aid itself is an understanding of the teaching methods through the exhibit medium.

The construction method of teaching is applicable to the building of displays for exhibits and museums. Children have excellent ideas when it comes to presenting these materials. In just two items — color and motion — imagination can be boundless. The exhibits that stand out in almost any room are those which employ color and motion. Colored posters, colored paper, paint, or cloth add spice to the display. A simple battery-driven device or a turntable from a discarded phonograph puts motion into the exhibit. Music and other sounds may be supplied by automatic record players. Questions may be asked and answers given over a simple telephone circuit. Most local telephone companies are happy to cooperate in such a project by lending the necessary equipment to the teacher. In fact, there are many people in every community who willingly go out of their way to help the classroom teacher. An orthodontist, for example, will lend plaster casts of teeth, which may be displayed along with the teeth of horses and cows and the jawbones of other animals. A taxidermist in Florida will lend alligator teeth, while his contemporary in Wyoming will lend one of the elk.

At almost any time of the year displays may be obtained for exhibit purposes from official and non-official health agencies. Most state health departments have such displays. In New York State two of the most popular have dealt with tuberculosis and fluoridation. Other displays may be obtained from the local heart or mental hygiene association, the county health association, the National Foundation, the American Red Cross, the American

Dental Association, the National Tuberculosis Association, the National Safety Council, and many other health organizations. Safety displays are often prepared by traffic safety personnel in industry and business. And, of course, one should not overlook the local police department and its safety efforts.

The way an exhibit is used is the key to whether or not pupil behavior is changed in any appreciable way. Generally, there is an intrinsic interest in pupil-built exhibits—an interest that may accompany a particular display *if the teacher requires the pupils to use the materials.* Children should be permitted to touch, feel, and otherwise examine much of the exhibit. There should be answers to their questions. Even a formal listing of questions on a sheet of paper may help to guide some students in securing answers from the exhibit. More than one teacher has employed a simple version of the true-false questionnaire for the pupil to complete as he studies the exhibit.

Additional activity may be involved when electric buttons are pressed or little doors are opened. In the Cleveland Health Museum there is a food facts and fallacies exhibit which employs the "lift-up door" technique.[15]

_____

[15] The Cleveland Health Museum, Cleveland, Ohio, has a long history of experimenting with the more effective ways of visualizing health concepts. Among its most successful attempts has been the production of a series of suitcase exhibits created for classroom use.

Here, a question is asked, such as "Are celery and fish special brain foods?" After the pupil ponders the answer for a few seconds he simply lifts the hinged door and finds the answer. "No. There are no such things as brain foods." Other examples from this excellent display which support this method of teaching include the following:

Q. "Are raw eggs more digestible than cooked eggs?"
A. "No. Soft or hard cooked eggs are more digestible."
Q. "Is Vitamin A margarine as good as butter?"
A. "Yes. Vitamin A margarine contains the same amount of vitamin A as butter."
Q. "Is it safe to leave food standing in open tin cans?"
A. "Yes, if food is properly refrigerated."

True-false questions may also be used with this "lift-up door" technique. Following are two examples used for sixth graders in the Cleveland Health Museum:

Q. "Potatoes have more minerals and vitamins than a head of lettuce. True or false."
A. "True. Lettuce has few minerals and vitamins while potatoes contain iron, vitamins B and C."
Q. "Calcium pills are a good substitute for milk. True or False."
A. "False. Milk contains valuable minerals, vitamins, and proteins in addition to calcium."

The elementary school health museum may be built in a spare room or in the corner of a large classroom, but

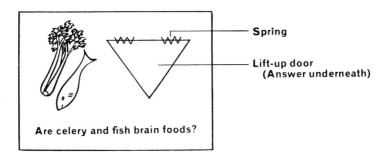

Spring

Lift-up door
(Answer underneath)

Are celery and fish brain foods?

this is not easy to accomplish. A museum differs from the usual exhibit in that it is permanent. For this reason very few schools have a museum. Space is at a premium in most buildings, and unless the whole school has easy access to the museum, it will soon lose its usefulness. The short-term exhibit, therefore, will be more practical for elementary school use, and the museum will be more practical if set up as a resource area in the community.

Permanent museums have been gaining in popularity since the Century of Progress World's Fair in Chicago (1933–1934). One of the first to be established was the Mayo Foundation Museum of Hygiene and Medicine in Rochester, Minnesota, opened in 1935. A year later the Cleveland Health Museum was incorporated. The Dallas (Texas) Health Museum was organized in 1946, and in 1952 the now famous Lankenau Hospital Health Museum opened in a suburb of Philadelphia. This was followed by the establishment of the Hinsdale Health Museum in a Chicago suburb in 1959, and by 1963 the Reading (Pennsylvania) Hospital had its health museum in operation. People of all ages are discovering that the value of a permanent health museum is great indeed; it is an educational institution, alive and vital—not a static, smelly mausoleum.

There is little doubt that the community health museum is a real force in the area of public health and school health education. The constantly replaced and modernized exhibits of the Dallas Health and Science Museum make it one of the outstanding educa-

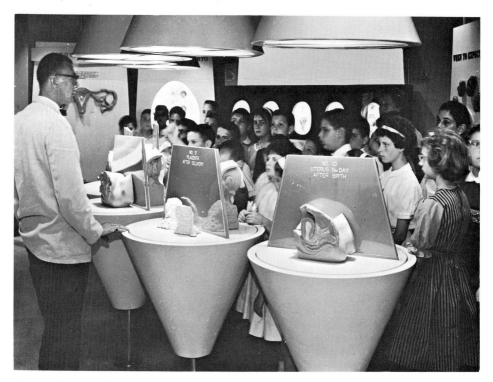

Figure 10–16 Class of schoolchildren hear a museum staff instructor talk on "Wonder of Life" display. (Courtesy Cleveland Health Museum.)

tional forces in that section of the United States. The Cleveland Health Museum is without doubt the finest example of a museum set up to educate in matters of health. For almost three decades thousands of schoolchildren and adults have visited this institution to see such superb exhibits as: Human Genetics; the Hall of Health, which shows how the body is put together and how it works; the plastic engravings, "From Egg to Embryo"; the transparent talking woman; the transparent tooth; the famous Dickinson sculptured models showing human birth and growth; the sound of the beating heart; truths and misconceptions relative to food and nutrition; and many more. The educational department of this one museum supplies hundreds of schools annually with materials for use in various phases of health and human biology.

One of the most successful projects originated by the Cleveland Health Museum is that of the portable exhibits for health teaching in the classroom. These suitcase exhibits have traveled widely, and teachers and nurses have been instructed in teaching from the materials presented. To facilitate this, a seven-minute magnetic tape recording was made for each exhibit, describing in detail and giving teachers pointers on what to stress at different grade levels as well as suggestions for class projects. A mimeographed teacher's manual was also developed.

"A health museum's visitors," says Bruno Gebhard, "are motivated, not by a love of aesthetics as in an art museum, or a curiosity about nature as in a natural history museum, but by a strong interest in their own physical and mental well-being. This appeal is a powerful magnet and enables the health museum to educate its visitors, once attracted to its doors, in personal health as well as in public health."[16] Finally, and perhaps more important than anything else, the modern health museum is a place where one goes to look at something that is available without obvious propaganda, "and where one is saved from any kind of commercialism."[17]

THE MATERIALS CENTER

One of the problems confronting teachers is the storage of materials and equipment. For the teacher of several decades ago who was concerned primarily with one textbook for each subject, the problem of selection, handling, and storage of these materials was relatively simple. However, with the increase in variety and quantity of instructional aids came the problem of their management. This has been resolved in some of the larger elementary schools by the organization of a resource or materials center.

A materials center is a vital force in the health instruction program, especially if one person is given the responsibility for its direction. Regardless of size, a few of the services which the center can offer classroom teachers and pupils are:

Make available a central source for all types of teaching materials.

Assist in locating and obtaining needed teaching aids.

Assist with the production of classroom materials.

Organize and keep current a file of all health instructional materials and equipment in the school building and a file of community resources.

---

[16] Gebhard, Bruno, and Doyle, Winfield G. "Health Museum at Work," from a paper read at the 85th Annual Meeting of the American Public Health Association, Cleveland, November 11, 1957.

[17] Gebhard, Bruno. "Development of Health Museums in the U.S.A.," *Health Education Journal* (London), 20:87–96, May 1962.

Maintain equipment and materials in a good state of repair.

Inform teachers of new materials.

Organize in-service training in the use of equipment for pupils and teachers.

Questions for Discussion

1. Prepare a checklist of material aids for teaching, and survey one or two elementary schools to see how many of these aids are in use. Are they being employed in any unique way for health instruction?

2. Do you remember ever building an exhibit or creating a health model for class use? If so, do you think your participation changed you in any way?

3. Prepare a brief chart in two parts: (1) "Ways in Which TV Can Help Health Instruction," and (2) "Ways in Which TV May Interfere with Health Instruction."

4. In your opinion, what is the difference between seeing a good film dealing with the work of the heart or some other organ, and hearing an interesting broadcast on this function?

5. Do you see the health museum as influential in helping students form concepts of healthful living? Does it have more or less to offer than a well-run classroom program in school?

6. As a classroom teacher interested in health instruction, what value would there seem to be in coordinating the activities and materials of the community health agencies with those of the school?

Suggested Activities

1. Visit a curriculum library and look over several brands of health textbooks suitable for primary or intermediate grade pupils. Generally, the level of word difficulty and the pictures will approximate the age level of the pupils for which the text is intended. However, the content may vary considerably between brand books for a particular grade level. What are some of your specific observations? The School Health Education Study research report (pp. 129–140) should be helpful. (See *Selected References.*)

2. Formulate a list of health and safety misconceptions. What kinds of teaching aids and materials of instruction might seem appropriate for helping pupils overcome these inadequacies? Opposite the list of misconceptions, write down your suggestions.

3. Seek out and read research data having to do with the effective use of health materials. Do you find evidence to suggest that media such as instructional television or tape recordings are more effective than the more traditional media?

4. Visit a materials center that has been established to serve the many and varied needs of teachers in a school system. Find out how it functions and how regularly it is used by the elementary classroom teachers.

5. Examine the educational program of some health museum. If possible, do this through a personal visit (Cleveland, Dallas, Chicago, Philadelphia). If a visit is not possible, write to a museum director for this kind of information. Finally, make comments on the "uniqueness" or "sameness" of the program as compared with what the schools are doing in your area.

Selected References

Cox, Helen M. "Sex Education Via Instructional Television." *Journal of Health, Physical Education, and Recreation*, 37:71–72, April 1966.

Educators Guide to Free Science Materials, Mary S. Saterstrom (ed.). Randolph, Wisconsin: Educator's Progress Service, annual.

Fox, Willard. "Care and Feeding of Bulletin Boards." *Education*, 83:362–363, February 1963.

Gary, Ralph. "Television for Children." *Journal of Education, 144*:1–27, February 1962.

Gillespie, D. K. "Differential Unit Assignment." *Journal of School Health*, 36:80–86, February 1966.

Haag, Jessie Helen. *School Health Program*. New York: Holt, Rinehart and Winston, Inc., revised 1965.

Hainfield, Harold. "Home-made Mannequin for First Aid Classes." *Journal of Health, Physical Education, and Recreation*, 37:65–67, February 1966.

Harris, William H. "Suggested Criteria for Evaluating Health and Safety Materials." *Journal of Health, Physical Education, and Recreation*, 35:26–27, February 1964.

Kinder, James S. *Using Audio-Visual Materials in Education*. New York: American Book Co., 1965.

Mayshark, Cyrus, and Foster, Roy A. *Methods in Health Instruction: a Workbook Using the Critical Incident Technique*. St. Louis: C. V. Mosby Co., 1966.

McTaggart, Aubrey C. "The Readability of Health Textbooks." *Synthesis of Research in Selected Areas of Health Instruction*. The School Health Education Study, National Education Association, 1963, pp. 129–140.

Schneider, Robert E. *Methods and Materials of Health Education*, 2nd ed. Philadelphia: W. B. Saunders Co., 1964.

School Health Education Study. *Synthesis of Research in Selected Areas of Health Instruction*. Washington, D.C.: National Education Association, 1963.

Smolensky, Jack, and Bonvechio, L. Richard. *Principles of School Health*. Boston: D. C. Heath and Co., 1966.

Tuck, Miriam L. "Experimental Demonstration as a Method of Stimulating Learning." *Journal of School Health*, 35:172–175, April 1965.

Turner, C. E., Sellery, C. Morley, and Smith, Sara Louise. *School Health and Health Education*, 5th ed. St. Louis: C. V. Mosby Co., 1966, Part 5.

Yost, Charles P. *Teaching Safety in the Elementary School*. Washington D.C.: American Association for Health, Physical Education, and Recreation, 1962.

Sources of Free and Inexpensive Teaching Aids

CHAPTER 11

The teacher who puts to use some of the great variety of free and inexpensive teaching aids stands a better chance of doing an effective job of teaching health than the one who still clings to the textbook method. It is not that textbooks have a lower value; it is that they simply are not adequate by themselves. Today boys and girls develop the habit at an early age of keeping up with what is happening in the world by seeing and hearing contemporary material – pamphlets, films, filmstrips, recordings, and exhibits. And in the field of health a vast amount of good material is available. One of the reasons for this is that many organizations are interested in child health.

The health curriculum, having lost its old-fashioned rigidity, now employs a variety of health materials to supplement books and teacher lectures; this is a more practical means of recording and reporting the current scene. But it réquires considerable work on the part of the teacher to locate and select these materials for classroom use. Even when there is a materials center in the

358

school, it is still helpful to have some knowledge of what is available and from what official, non-official, or commercial agency it may be obtained.

A number of organizations and agencies have educational consultants who are of real help to teachers, providing they have sufficient information to work with. When ordering materials, it is well to mention the age group to be served, the number of children in the class, the type of materials desired, and the special area of interest. Some companies or agencies will then go out of their way to supply useful aids to learning. In fact, in several instances they will develop new materials if the teacher can show that there is a need for them.

The Reliability of Health Information

Teachers are becoming more and more aware of health materials and sources of health information. They are being exposed from all sides to a variety of pamphlets, booklets, and products designed to overcome health problems or, at least, to bear on mental and physical well-being. How reliable is this material? Is it loaded with advertising in order to sell a product?

Health information must be evaluated before it is used in the classroom. Ordinarily there is little reason to question the materials and aids of a well-known organization such as the American Red Cross or the American Medical Association. And there are numerous commercial organizations that conscientiously promote health as their primary purpose, followed by the promotion of their own product. This is well demonstrated by the fact that it is sometimes difficult to find the name of the commercial organization or its product on the school health literature.

The evaluation of health information, whether it is read, heard, or seen, may be determined in part by appraising the publisher, association, or agency. One might ask the following questions:

Is the agency recognized as having a good reputation in the field of health?

Why has the health information been presented?

Is the purpose of the communication to give facts on which to base personal opinion and beliefs? To improve living?

Is the purpose to sell specific products or ideas without reference to the scientific value of the product?

Is the purpose simply to entertain?

What are the qualifications of the specific author or speaker?

Is the material up to date?

What is the opinion of others, such as medical experts, public or private agencies, and reliable friends familiar with the topic?

OFFICIAL HEALTH AGENCIES

Organizations that have been established by law to accomplish specific health maintenance, promotion, and control are generally designated as official health agencies. These include city, county, state, and Federal government organizations. Very often a wealth of free teaching aids is available from these groups:

City and County Health Departments — Child health material in the form of pamphlets for teacher use. Films and certain poster material may also be on hand.

State Health Departments — In almost every state there is much in the way of child and teacher health pamphlets, monthly magazines or bulletins, films, special health exhibits, and speakers available for school use. In addition to this, several states publish catalogs dealing specifically with health education sources of materials and other audio-visual aids.

State Universities — In many states the unit of the state university having to do with public health or school health provides pamphlets, bulletins, and special charts for school use within the state. Other institutions, such as Indiana University, Syracuse University, or Boston University, have an extensive division which supplies a wide variety of audio-visual aids. Sample materials are generally available for out-of-state use.

Federal Government —

Department of Health, Education, and Welfare Office of Education Washington, D.C., 20025	Special booklets, primarily for teacher use, on food, community, grooming, prevention and control of illness. Lists of materials are available with no charge for single copies.
Superintendent of Documents U.S. Government Printing Office Washington, D.C., 20025	Considerable health information for teacher use which may be adapted to healthful school living and health teaching. A catalog should be secured before materials are ordered.

U.S. Public Health Service Washington, D.C., 20201	This organization has many health interests including the National Institutes of Health, health research, statistics, and promotion.
U.S. Children's Bureau Division of Reports Washington, D.C., 20025	Numerous catalogs, child health pamphlets, and lists.
The United Nations World Health Organization Geneva, Switzerland (or New York, N.Y., 20006)	A large number of picture booklets dealing with world health conditions. Useful in studying community health and social studies.

NON-OFFICIAL HEALTH AGENCIES

In almost every American community there are groups of citizens banded together for the express purpose of promoting health. Generally their interest is centered on some special disease or abnormality such as poliomyelitis, tuberculosis, mental illness, heart disease, or crippled children. These groups are, without a doubt, in a position to be of immense service to the schoolteacher if the teacher will call upon them.

Non-official agencies generally include *voluntary health agencies, commercial organizations*, and *professional associations*. Their scope of influence is great and includes health education services for the entire community, its industries, and its schools. If the agency is a state or national one, its sphere of influence is almost unlimited.

With the tremendous growth in the number of charitable institutions and foundations in this country over the last quarter century, it is becoming increasingly difficult to differentiate between a purely voluntary health organization and a professional association. Many voluntary health organizations began at the local level with a handful of volunteers and blossomed through the years into full-fledged national groups with considerable professional zeal. In any case, both categories of organization exist to help in any way they can.

The staff and members of these citizen and professional worker groups help the schools enrich curricula, add resources, carry on research, and improve the school health programs. The schools in turn offer to these agencies an excellent channel for working towards personal and community health. Certainly there are common goals; "child health is everybody's business." Moreover, there are common activities involving the home and the school. Some of the agency activities include:

Making available to school personnel the latest health information.

Providing teaching aids.

Helping in the preparation of resource units.

Helping with special short-term projects.

Helping with in-service education of teachers.

Providing the means for demonstrations and studies.

Enriching the curriculum.

Interpreting the school health program and needs of the community.

Helping in interpretation to the parents.

Voluntary and Professional Health Agencies

A selected number of the more productive voluntary and professional health agencies that have proven to be of immeasurable service to elementary teachers are as follows:

Alcoholics Anonymous, 305 E. 45th Street, New York, N.Y., 10017.

American Academy of Pediatrics, 1801 Hinmon Avenue, Box 1034, Evanston, Ill., 60204.

American Association for Health, Physical Education, and Recreation, Department of the National Education Association, 1201 16th Street, N.W., Washington, D. C., 20036.

American Cancer Society, 219 E. 42nd Street, New York, N.Y., 10017.

American Dental Association, 211 E. Chicago Avenue, Chicago, Ill., 60611.

American Foundation for the Blind, 15 W. 16th Street, New York, N.Y., 10011.

American Hearing Society, 919 18th Street, N.W., Washington, D.C., 20006.

American Heart Association, 44 E. 23rd Street, New York, N.Y., 10010.

American Hospital Association, 840 N. Lake Shore Drive, Chicago, Ill., 60611.

American Institute of Family Relations, 5287 Sunset Boulevard, Los Angeles, Calif., 90027.

American Medical Association, 535 N. Dearborn Street, Chicago, Ill., 60610.

American Optometric Association, Department of Public Affairs, 700 Chippewa Street, St. Louis, Mo., 63119.

American Public Health Association, 1790 Broadway, New York, N.Y., 10019.

American National Red Cross, 17th and D Streets, N.W., Washington, D.C., 20006. (Contact local chapters for materials.)

American School Health Association, 515 E. Main Street, Kent, Ohio, 44241.

American Social Hygiene Association, 1740 Broadway, New York, N.Y., 10019.

Arthritis Foundation, 10 Columbus Circle, New York, N.Y., 10019.

Better Vision Institute, 630 Fifth Avenue, New York, N.Y., 10020.

Child Study Association of America, 132 E. 74th Street, New York, N.Y., 10021.

Cleveland Health Museum, 8911 Euclid Avenue, Cleveland, Ohio, 44106.

Health Information Foundation, 420 Lexington Avenue, New York, N.Y., 10017.

Hogg Foundation for Mental Health, University of Texas, Austin, Tex., 78712.

Muscular Dystrophy Associations of America, 1790 Broadway, New York, N.Y., 10019.

National Association of Hearing and Speech Agencies, 919 18th Street, N.W., Washington, D.C., 20006.

National Association for Mental Health, 10 Columbus Circle, New York, N.Y., 10010.

National Commission on Safety Education, 1201 16th Street, N.W., Washington, D.C., 20036.

National Congress of Parents and Teachers, 700 N. Rush Street, Chicago, Ill., 60637.

National Council on Alcoholism, 2 E. 103rd Street, New York, N.Y., 10029.

National Education Association, Division of Elementary Education, 1201 16th Street, N.W., Washington, D.C., 20036.

National Foundation, 800 Second Avenue, New York, N.Y., 10017.

National Interagency Council on Smoking and Health, P.O. Box 3654, Central Station, Arlington, Va., 22203.

National Multiple Sclerosis Society, 257 Park Avenue South, New York, N.Y., 10010.

National Publicity Council for Health and Welfare, Inc., Park Avenue South, New York, N.Y., 10010.

National Recreation Association, 8 W. 8th Street, New York, N.Y., 10011.

National Safety Council, 425 N. Michigan Avenue, Chicago, Ill., 60611.

National Society for Crippled Children and Adults, Inc., 2023 W. Ogden Avenue, Chicago, Ill., 60603.

National Society for the Prevention of Blindness, Inc., 79 Madison Avenue, New York, N.Y., 10016.

National Tuberculosis Association, 1790 Broadway, New York, N.Y., 10019.

Nutrition Foundation, Inc., 99 Park Avenue, New York, N.Y., 10016.

Planned Parenthood Federation of America, Inc., 515 Madison Avenue, New York, N.Y., 10022.

Public Affairs Committee, 381 Park Avenue South, New York, N.Y., 10016.

Rutgers Center for Alcohol Studies, The State University, Rutgers, New Brunswick, N.J.

Sex Education and Information Council of U.S. (SEICUS), 1855 Broadway, New York, N.Y., 10023.

United Cerebral Palsy Associations, Inc., 321 W. 44th Street, New York, N.Y., 10017.

Commercial Organizations and Associations of Industry

There are many business and commercial agencies which publish materials especially fitted for elementary school use. The list of individual industries that offer printed matter is a long one. It is customary today for practically every commercial organization to promote its product through bulletins, brochures, posters, and other advertising media. Many of these companies have suitable products that are legitimate in terms of health promotion. In the area of foods there are a number of firms that sell a healthful product and employ sound health teaching techniques to promote it. There are also a large number of companies which promote a valid health concept as a public service item. For instance, a company promoting dental health through charts, leaflets, and films puts over a basic idea. This in turn is good business for it sells more dental products. When people buy more dental products, this is an indication that their health behavior has been favorably changed. In view of this, a number of commercial firms in several areas have formed their own associations. These associations of industry make available, often in unlimited quantity, a number of health items for the classroom teacher to use with her pupils.

There follows a partial list of national sources of especially reliable and generous companies and associations of industry. No attempt is made here to list specific materials offered by these sources, but in many cases catalogs are available, and in most cases the name of the agency will indicate to some extent the subject matter and scope of its material.

Aetna Life Affiliated Companies, Education Department, 151 Farmington Avenue, Hartford, Conn., 10015. Leaflets and motion pictures on safety for teachers and pupils, special tests.

American Automobile Association, Traffic Safety Department, 1712 G. Street, N.W., Washington, D.C., 20036. Pamphlets and films on traffic safety; also safety project materials.

American Bakers Association, Public Relations Department, 1700 Pennsylvania Avenue, N.W., Washington, D.C., 20036. Booklets on bread for intermediate grades. Contact state bakers associations for additional materials.

American Institute of Baking, Consumer Service Department, 400 E. Ontario Street, Chicago, Ill., 60611. Pamphlets, posters, self-testing charts, colorful guides to eating, record forms.

American Insurance Association, Safety Department, 85 John Street, New York, N.Y., 10038.

Armour and Company, Public Relations Department, 401 N. Wabash Street, Chicago, Ill., 60690. Maps, charts on foods.

Association of American Soap and Glycerine Products, Inc., Cleanliness Bureau, 295 Madison Avenue, New York, N.Y. Pamphlets, posters, radio and TV scripts.

Athletic Institute, 805 Merchandise Mart, Chicago, Ill., 60650.

Behavioral Research Laboratories, Box 577, Palo Alto, Calif., 94300.

Bicycle Institute of America, 122 E. 42nd Street, New York, N.Y., 10017.

The Borden Company, The Borden Building, 350 Madison Avenue, New York, N.Y., 10017. Pamphlets on milk values and uses.

Cereal Institute, Inc., Educational Director, 135 S. LaSalle Street, Chicago, Ill., 60603. Classroom teaching units, food charts, and graphs.

Church and Dwight Company, Inc., 70 Pine Street, New York, N.Y. 10005. Charts, comics, and pamphlets on dental health.

Colorado Wheat Administrative Commission, Mr. Dwayne E. Williams, Administrator, 1636 Welton Street, Denver, Colorado, 80202.

Connecticut Bakers Association, Mrs. Lee Silva, Secretary, 85 Belcher Road, Wethersfield, Connecticut, 06109. (Honors requests from Connecticut only.)

Cream of Wheat Corporation, Box M, Minneapolis, Minn., 55413. Educational Activities Inc., Box 392, Freeport, N.Y., 11520. Action records for physical fitness and rhythmics.

Educators Mutual Life Insurance Company, Lancaster, Pa. Pamphlets and posters on safety.

Eli Lilly Company, 740 S. Alabama Street, Indianapolis, Ind., 46206.

Employers Mutuals of Wausau, 407 Grant Street, Wausau, Wisc., 55402.

Encyclopaedia Britannica Films, Inc., Britannica Building, 425 N. Michigan Avenue, Wilmette, Ill., 60611. Filmstrips, slide films, movies, cartoons, and records. (Rentals only.)

Equitable Life Assurance Society of the United States, 1285 Avenue of the Americas, New York, N.Y. Posters, booklets for intermediate grades and up.

Evaporated Milk Association, 910 17th Street, N.W., Washington, D.C., 20036. Flash cards, graphs, and leaflets on milk equivalent values.

Films Incorporated, Public Relations Department, 1150 Wilmette Avenue, Wilmette, Ill. Cartoons and catalogs for all age levels.

Florida Citrus Commission, P.O. Box 148, Lakeland, Fla., 33802. Posters, pamphlets, movies on citrus fruits.

Ford Motor Company, Information Department, Dearborn, Mich., 48127. Traffic safety materials.

General Mills, Inc., Education Section, 9200 Wayzata Boulevard, Minneapolis, Minn., 55426. Nutrition education teaching aids.

Gerber Baby Foods, Fremont, Michigan. Nutrition pamphlets.

Hartford Fire Insurance Company, Hartford, Conn. Fire prevention activities and songs; teacher booklets.

H. J. Heinz Company, P.O. Box 57, Pittsburgh, Pa., 15230. Food charts and stories of origin of various foods.

Indiana Bakers Association, Mr. Ferd A. Doll, Secretary, 1941 E. 30th Street, Indianapolis, Indiana, 46218. (Honors requests from Indiana only.)

International Harvester Company, 180 N. Michigan Avenue, Chicago, Ill. 60601. Pamphlets and posters relative to personal safety.

John Hancock Mutual Life Insurance Company, Health Education Service, P.O. Box 111, Boston, Mass. Catalogs, teacher material on food, illness, safety, first aid, and community health.

Johnson & Johnson, Educational Division, New Brunswick, N.J., 08903. Charts, pamphlets, films on first aid and safety, and programmed instruction first aid for grade six.

Kansas Wheat Commission, Mr. G. C. Fowler, Administrator, 1021 N. Main Street, Hutchinson, Kansas, 67501.

Kellogg Company, Department of Home Economics Services, Battle Creek, Mich., 49016. Breakfast food pamphlets and charts.

Kimberly-Clark Corporation, Educational Department, Neenah, Wis., 54947. Menstrual physiology chart and films; pamphlets, guides on common cold.

Kraft Cheese Company, 500 Peshtigo Court, Chicago, Ill., 60690. Nutrition.

Lederle Laboratories Division, American Cyanamid Co., Pearl River, N.Y., 10965. Child health and nutrition.

Lever Brothers Company, Public Relations Division, 390 Park Avenue, New York, N.Y., 10022. Cleanliness charts for primary grade teachers.

Licenced Beverage Industries, Inc., 155 E. 44th Street, New York, N.Y., 10017.

Maltex Company, Burlington, Vt. Food charts, posters, and leaflets on breakfast foods.

Metropolitan Life Insurance Company, Health and Welfare Division, 1 Madison Avenue, New York, N.Y., 10010. Catalogs, exhibits, films, filmstrips, booklets for teachers on all diseases and the school health instruction program; health bulletin for teachers.

Missouri Bakers Association, Mr. Louis F. O'Konski, Jr., Secretary, 1016 Central Street, Kansas City, Missouri, 64105. (Honors requests from Missouri only.)

Money Management Institute, Prudential Plaza, Chicago, Ill., 60601. Consumer health materials.

National Board of Fire Underwriters, 85 John Street, New York, N.Y., 10038.

National Dairy Council, Program Service Department, 111 N. Canal Street, Chicago, Ill., 60606. Health education materials, exhibits, films, filmstrips, displays, animals for feeding experiments. Local chapters are rich in materials especially suited for primary and intermediate grades; health bulletins for teachers.

National Fire Protection Association, Public Relations Department, 60 Batterymarch Street, Boston, Mass. 02110. Posters, pamphlets, safety lists, comics, fire inspection blanks, charts, quizzes.

National Foot Health Council, 272 Union Street, Rockland, Mass., 02370. Posters, radio scripts, cartoons, pamphlets, and children's foot size charts.

National Livestock and Meat Board, 36 S. Wabash Avenue, Chicago, Ill., 60603. Self-testing charts, food graphs, colored posters of the various cuts of meat, pamphlets on food values of meat.

National Social Welfare Assembly, Inc., 345 E. 46th Street, New York, N.Y., 10017. Health comic books.

North Dakota State Wheat Commission, Mr. Paul E. R. Abrahamson, Adminstrator, 316 N. Fifth Street, Bismarck, North Dakota, 58501.

Ocean Spray Cranberries, Inc., Executive Offices, Hanson, Mass., 02341. Pamphlets, films, food recipes, and food record charts.

Paper Cup and Container Institute, Public Health Committee, 250 Park Avenue, New York, N.Y., 10017. Periodicals on food handling, food service sanitation, films, and health reprints.

Pennsylvania Bakers Association, Mr. Robert H. Maurer, Secretary, 407 N. Front Street, Harrisburg, Pa., 17101. (Honors requests from Pennsylvania only.)

Personal Products Company, Milltown, N.J., 08850. Charts, posters, leaflets regarding menstruation.

Pet Milk Co., 1406 Arcade Building, St. Louis, Mo., 63101. Nutrition pamphlets and charts.

Pharmaceutical Manufacturers Association, 1155 15th Street, N.W., Washington, D.C., 20005. Films and booklets on general health topics.

The Procter and Gamble Company, P.O. Box 171, Cincinnati, Ohio, 45201. Booklets and materials for dental health. Several excellent posters in color.

The Prudential Insurance Company of America, Advertising and Sales Promotion, Prudential Plaza, Newark, N.J., 07101. General school health pamphlets for teachers.

Scott Paper Company, Home Service Center, Philadelphia, Pa., 19113. Menstral health pamphlets.

Sealtest Foods Consumer Service, 605 3rd Avenue, New York, N.Y., 10016. Food charts and graphs.

Smith, Kline, and French Laboratories, Philadelphia, Pa., 19101. Posters, exhibits, leaflets, and films on mental health.

South Dakota Wheat Commission, Mr. August Snyder, Executive Director, P.O. Box 549, Pierre, South Dakota, 57501.

Stanley Bowmar Company, Inc., Valhalla, N.Y., 10595. Records for creative activities and rhythmics.

Sunkist Growers, Box 2706, Sunkist Building, Los Angeles, Calif., 90054. Teaching units on nutrition, posters, pamphlets.

Swift and Co., Union Stockyards, Chicago, Ill., 60609.

Tampax, Incorporated, Educational Director, 161 E. 42nd Street, New York, N.Y., 10017. Anatomical charts, student pamphlets, and special instruction materials for teachers on the subject of menstruation.

Tennessee Bakers Association, Mr. R. L. Pettigrew, Secretary, P.O. Box 266, Nashville, Tennessee, 37202. (Honors requests from Tennessee only.)

Texas Gulf Bakers Council, Mr. Robert H. Ruhe, Exec. Dir., P.O. Box 11125, Houston, Texas, 77016. (Honors requests from Texas only.)

The Travelers Insurance Company, Hartford, Conn., 06115. Charts on growth, height-weight, and posture, and several colorful posters.

United Fresh Fruit and Vegetable Association, 777 14th Street, N.W., Washington, D.C., 20005. Leaflets on foods for elementary level.

United States Beet Sugar Association, Tower Building, Washington, D.C. Teaching kits and charts.

Washington Wheat Commission, Mr. Wayne B. Gentry, Administrator, 409 Great Western Building, Spokane, Washington, 99201.

Wheat Flour Institute, Supervisor of Distribution, 14 E. Jackson Boulevard, Chicago, Ill., 60604. Posters, filmstrips, pamphlets, and catalogs pertaining to nutritious breakfast foods.

SOURCES OF AIDS FOR HEALTH TEACHING UNITS

A list of sources of health teaching materials for a major area of study cannot contain every known aid, nor would one want it to, because some sources are better than others for teaching a certain health topic. The teacher's time is at a premium, and following up several leads to sources takes time. It is the purpose of the author, therefore, to limit the following list to those sources of *teaching* aids which have proved to be especially valuable in the health instruction program in the elementary schools.[1] All sources listed are for the students to read or see themselves. They have been carefully selected with this in mind.

The sources are set up by health topics which are in keeping with the major activity areas referred to in Chapter 8. The type of teaching aid (i.e., film, pamphlet, poster), the specific name of the aid, and the name of the agency supplying it are listed.

1. Personal Cleanliness and Appearance*

a. Pamphlets or Leaflets

Cups Through the Centuries, Paper Cup and Container Institute.

Everybody Smile, American Dental Association.

Eyes That See and Ears That Hear, John Hancock Mutual Life Insurance Company.

Facts about Vision, American Optometric Association.

Hearing Is Priceless — Protect It, American Hearing Society.

It's Smart to Protect your Sight, U.S. Public Health Service.

Professor Ludwig Von Drake's IQ, National Society for the Prevention of Blindness.

On Every Lip, Paper Cup and Container Institute.

Only One Pair of Ears for Life, American Hearing Society.

Signs of Eye Trouble in Children, National Society for the Prevention of Blindness.

Sunglasses, National Society for the Prevention of Blindness.

Take Care of Your Eyes, National Society for the Prevention of Blindness.

Teachers Tell, Paper Cup and Container Institute.

The Eye in Sight, American Optometric Association.

The Language of Light, National Society for the Prevention of Blindness.

The Little Seeing Book, Pharmaceutical Manufacturers Association.

The Story of Soap, Procter and Gamble Company.

---

[1] For additional sources see *Educator's Guide to Free Films, Filmstrips, Transcriptions, Tapes and Scripts,* Educators Progress Services, Randolph, Wis. (annual).

*Includes the care of the special senses.

b. Films*

A More Attractive You, Modern Talking Picture Service.
Body Care and Grooming, McGraw-Hill Book Company.
Care of the Hair and Nails, Encyclopaedia Britannica Films, Inc.
Care of the Skin, Encyclopaedia Britannica, Films, Inc.
Choosing Clothes for Health, Coronet Instructional Films.
Cleanliness and Health, Coronet Instructional Films.
Eyes and Their Care, Encyclopaedia Britannica Films, Inc.
Hear Better: Healthy Ears, Coronet Instructional Films.
How Billy Keeps Clean, Coronet Instructional Films.
How the Ear Functions, Knowledge Builders.
Joan Avoids a Cold, Coronet Instructional Films.
Johnny's New World, National Society for the Prevention of Blindness.
Kitty Keeps Clean, Young America Films.
Let's be Clean and Neat, Coronet Instructional Films.
Platform Posture, Young America Films.
Running for Sheriff, Charles Cahill and Associates.
See Better: Healthy Eyes, Coronet Instructional Films.
The Doctor Is Your Friend, National Tuberculosis Association.
Ways to Good Habits, Coronet Instructional Films.
Your Cleanliness, Young America Films.
Your Ears, Young America Films.
Your Eyes, Young America Films.
Your Friend the Doctor, Coronet Instructional Films.
Your Health at School, Coronet Instructional Films.
Your Teeth, Young America Films.

c. Filmstrips

Care of the Hair and Nails (Health story), Encyclopaedia Britannica Films, Inc.
Care of the Skin (Health story), Encyclopaedia Britannica Films, Inc.
Checking Your Health, Educational Record Sales.
Health Habits (Health story), Encyclopaedia Britannica Films, Inc.
Healthy, Happy, and Wise, Popular Science.
How We See and Hear, Moody Institute of Science.
How Your Ears Work, Popular Science.

---

*The addresses of film and filmstrip sources may be found on page 385.

Keeping Clean, McGraw-Hill Book Company.
Keeping Neat and Clean, Educational Record Sales.
Keeping Well and Happy, National Tuberculosis Association.
Let's Stand Tall, Society for Visual Education.
Protecting Our Eyes and Ears, McGraw-Hill Book Company.
Special Senses, Keystone View Co.
The Ears, Young America Films.
The Eyes, Young America Films.
The Science of Personal Appearance, McGraw-Hill Book Company.
This Is You, Encyclopaedia Britannica Films, Inc.
You and Your Clothes, Young America Films.
You and Your Ears, Encyclopaedia Britannica Films, Inc.
Your Eyes at Work, Popular Science.
Your Skin and Its Care, Popular Science.

d. Posters

Be Fair—Cover Your Coughs and Sneezes, National Tuberculosis Association.
Common Cold, John Hancock Mutual Life Insurance Company.
How to Catch a Cold, Kimberly-Clark Corporation.
Only One Pair of Ears for Life, American Hearing Society.
Physical Fitness Posters, National Dairy Council.
Reading Takes Seeing, American Optometric Association.
School Time, Vision Exam Time, American Optometric Association.
Seeing and Hearing, American Medical Association.
To Fight Germs—Wash Your Hands, National Tuberculosis Association.

e. Charts

Cross Section of the Eye, National Society, for the Prevention of Blindness.
One Out of Four Children Need Eye Care, National Society for the Prevention of Blindness.
Snellen, Symbol E Charts, National Society for the Prevention of Blindness.
The Ivory Inspection Patrol, Procter and Gamble.

f. Radio Scripts

(From University of Texas, Bureau of Research in Education by Radio)
Care of the Skin
Cleanliness
Importance of Good Vision
We Wash Our Hands Before We Eat

g. Tape Recordings

Health Is Wealth (HC15), New York State University College of Agriculture, Cornell University, Ithaca, N.Y.

Are We Responsible for Our Own Good Health? Audio-Visual Aids Service, University of Illinois.

h. Selected Stories for Children

(P) Primary Level, (I) Intermediate Level

About Glasses for Gladys (I), Mary K. Erickson (Melmont).

All Ready for Winter (P), Leone Adelson (McKay).

Health Can Be Fun (P), Munro Leaf (Lippincott).

Lesson in Loveliness (I), J. W. Scott (Macrae, Smith).

Look at Your Eyes (I), Paul Showers (Crowell).

Manners Can Be Fun (P), Munro Leaf (Lippincott).

Nothing to Wear but Clothes (I), F. K. Jupo (Aladdin).

Our Insect Friends and Foes (I), W. A. Dupuy (Winston).

Our Wonderful Eyes (P), J. Perry (McGraw-Hill).

Our Senses and How They Work (I), H. Zimm (Morrow).

Somebody Called Boo (P), L. Gardner (Watts).

Story of Your Coat (P,I), Clara Hollos (International Publishing Co.)

The Clean Pig (P), Leonard Weisgard (Scribner).

Tim and His Hearing Aid (I), E. C. Ronnei and Joan and Max Porter (Dodd).

Time Out for Living (P), D. E. Patridge and C. Mooney (American Book).

True Book of Health (P), O. U. Haynes (Children's Press).

World of Invisible Life (I), Mary Stephenson (Wilcox and Follet).

You and Your Senses (I), L. Schneider (Harcourt).

Your Ears (I), Irving and Ruth Adler (John Day).

Your Eyes, (I), Irving and Ruth Adler (John Day).

Your Manners Are Showing (I), B. Betz (Grossett).

2. Activity, Sleep, Rest, and Relaxation

a. Pamphlets or Leaflets

A Boy and His Physique, National Dairy Council.

A Girl and Her Figure, National Dairy Council.

A Girl and Her Figure and You, National Dairy Council.

Eat and Grow, Evaporated Milk Association.

Johnny Makes the Team, American Medical Association.

Letters to Tony, Evaporated Milk Association.

Physical Fitness, U.S. Government Printing Office.

Relax! You're a Bundle of Nerves, The Borden Company.

Seven Paths to Fitness, American Medical Association.

Sleep, the Restorer, John Hancock Mutual Life Insurance Company.

What the Classroom Teacher Should Know and Do about Children with Heart Disease, American Heart Association.

Working and Playing, Evaporated Milk Association.

b. Films

American Square Dance, Coronet Instructional Films.

Day at the Fair, Coronet Instructional Films.

Dress for Health, Encyclopaedia Britannica Films, Inc.

Exercise and Health, Coronet Instructional Films.

Fun That Builds Good Health, Coronet Instructional Films.

How the Body Uses Energy, McGraw-Hill Book Company.

Human Machine, Moody Institute of Science.

Improving Your Posture, Coronet Instructional Films.

Play in the Snow, Encyclopaedia Britannica Films, Inc.

Playtown U.S.A., The Athletic Institute.

Safety on the Playground, Encyclopaedia Britannica Films, Inc.

Sleep for Health, Encyclopaedia Britannica Films, Inc.

Water Safety, Young America Films.

You and Your Helpers, Coronet Instructional Films.

Your Child's Health and Fitness, AAHPER, Washington, D.C., 20036.

c. Filmstrips

At Home in the Evening, Popular Science.

Checking Your Health, Encyclopaedia Britannica Films, Inc.

Exercise for Happy Living, Encyclopaedia Britannica Films, Inc.

Getting Ready for Bed, Popular Science.

Posture and Exercise, Encyclopaedia Britannica Films, Inc.

Rest and Sleep, McGraw-Hill Book Company.

Rest and Sleep, Young America Films.

Sleep and Rest, Popular Science.

Sleep for Health, Encyclopaedia Britannica Films, Inc.

Working and Playing Together, McGraw-Hill Book Company.

d. Posters

A Day with the Wide Awakes, General Mills, Inc.

Change of Pace, Equitable Life Assurance Society of United States.

Health Is Not Just Luck, General Mills, Inc.

Lift with Your Legs, Not Your Back, American Medical Association.

Physical Fitness, American Medical Association.

Physical Fitness (4), Educational Activities, Inc.

Physical Fitness (9 posters), National Dairy Council.

Sleep Tonight for Pep Tomorrow, National Tuberculosis Association.

The Rest Is Up to You, Equitable Life Assurance Society of United States.

e. Charts

Day to Day Good Health Records, Kellogg Company.

Eyes That See, John Hancock Mutual Life Insurance Company.

Your Heart and How It Works, American Heart Association.

f. Radio Scripts

Batter Up, National Safety Council.

Fresh Air and Sunshine, Bureau of Research in Education by Radio, University of Texas.

Sleep and Rest, Bureau of Research in Education by Radio, University of Texas.

Swimming Is Fun, National Safety Council.

Vacation Daze, National Safety Council.

g. Comics

The Adventures of Eva, Pora, and Ted, Evaporated Milk Association.

h. Records

Basic Rhythms, BR1 (Ruth Evans), Stanley Bowmar Co.

Honor Your Partner Records, Educational Activities, Inc.

Lullabies for Sleepy Heads, Dorothy Olsen, RCA Victor.

Music for Relaxation, Melochrino Strings, RCA Victor.

Physical Fitness Activities, Album 14, Primary Grades (Durlacher), Stanley Bowmar Co.

Rhythmic Play Series (K-3), Educational Record Sales.

The Sleepy Family (A35), Children's Record Center, 2858 W. Pico Boulevard, Los Angeles, Calif.

Toy Shop Album (A4—Grades 1—6), Activity Records.

Why Do I Have to Go to Sleep? (P156), Children's Record Center.

i. Tape Recordings

Health at Summer Camps (AC19), New York State University College of Agriculture, Cornell University, Ithaca, N.Y.

j. Selected Stories for Children

(P) Primary Level, (I) Intermediate Level

Bedtime for Frances (P), H. Hoban (Harper and Bros.).

Boo, Who Used to Be Scared of the Dark (P), Munro Leaf (Random House).

Child's Good Night Book (P), Margaret Wise Brown (W. R. Scott).

Child's Treasury of Things to Do (P), Caroline Horowitz (Hart).

Forty Rainy Day Games and Play Alone Fun (P), Caroline Horowitz (Hart).

Going to Camp (P,I), Helen Beck (Daye).

Health Can Be Fun (P), Munro Leaf (Lippincott).

Hustle and Bustle (P), Louis Slobodkin (Macmillan).

Jimmy's Own Basketball (I), M. B. Renick (Scribner).

Joey Gets the Golf Bug (I), J. Sherman (Little, Brown).

Lifeline (I), L. Schneider (Harcourt).

Sleepy ABC (P), Margaret Wise Brown (Lothrop).

Switch on the Night (P), R. Bradbury (Pantheon).

The Dream Book (P), Margaret Wise Brown (Random House).

Time for Sleep (I), Millicent Selsam (W. R. Scott).

Touchdown for Tommy (I), M. Christopher (Little, Brown).

While Susie Sleeps (P), Nina Scheider (W. R. Scott).

Who's Afraid of Thunder? (I), H. E. Sandman (Sterling).

3. Nutrition and Growth

a. Pamphlets or Leaflets

A Guide to Better Nutrition, H. J. Heinz Company.

A Nutrition Guide, General Mills, Inc.

Animals That Give People Milk, National Dairy Council.

Bananas for Us, United Fruit Company.

Better Breakfast Activities, Cereal Institute, Inc.

Citrus as Aid to Health and Beauty, Florida Citrus Commission.

Citrus Industry Story, Sunkist Growers.

Classroom Food Facts and Fun, Wheat Flour Institute.

Cooking Is Fun, National Dairy Council.

Eat a Good Breakfast, Kellogg Company.

Eat a Good Breakfast to Start a Good Day, Cereal Institute, Inc.

Eat and Grow, General Mills, Inc.

Eat to Live, Wheat Flour Institute.

Elementary School Nutrition, National Livestock and Meat Board.

Enriched Bread, American Institute of Baking.

Evaporated Milk Drinks, Evaporated Milk Association.

Facts about Evaporated Milk, Evaporated Milk Association.

Facts about Nutrition (PHSP-917), U.S. Public Health Service.

Foods for Growing Boys and Girls, Kellogg Company.

Foodway to Follow, American Institute of Baking.

Fresh Citrus for Vitamin C, Sunkist Growers.

From Flour to Bread, Wheat Flour Institute.

Fruit and Vegetable Facts and Pointers on Nutrition, United Fresh Fruit and Vegetable Association.

Functions of Food in Nutrition, National Livestock and Meat Board.

Hello U.S.A., National Dairy Council

How to Conduct a Rat Feeding Experiment, Wheat Flour Institute.

How Your Body Uses Food, National Dairy Council.

Ice Cream Is Good, National Dairy Council.

It's Smart to Eat Breakfast, Kellogg Company.

Jane and Jimmy Learn about Fresh Fruits and Vegetables, United Fresh Fruit and Vegetable Association.

Letters to Tony, General Mills, Inc.

Maybe I'll Be a Milkman, National Dairy Council.

Meat Builds Better Breakfasts, National Livestock and Meat Board.

Meat Snacks for Better Health, National Livestock and Meat Board.

My Friend the Cow, National Dairy Council.

Nutrition Aids Grade One Through Eight, Kellogg Company.

Nutrition Information Test (Grade 3), General Mills, Inc.

Nutrition Information Test (Grades 4, 5, 6), General Mills, Inc.

Our Bread and Butter, in Pioneer Days and Today, National Dairy Council.

Our Food—Where It Comes From, National Dairy Council.

School Lunch, National Dairy Council.

The Banana Story, United Fruit Company.

The Grains Are Great Foods, Kellogg Company.

The Nutrition Ladder, Florida Citrus Commission.

The School That Learned to Eat, General Mills, Inc.

The Story of the Cereal Grains, General Mills, Inc.

The Story of Food Preservation, H. J. Heinz Company.

Uncle Jim's Dairy Farm, National Dairy Council.

What Did You Have for Breakfast This Morning?, National Dairy Council.

What to Eat and Why, John Hancock Mutual Insurance Company.

What Will I Be from A to Z?, National Dairy Council.

What's on Your Table?, Aetna Life Affiliated Companies.

Wild Bill Hickock Breakfast Games, Kellogg Company.

You and Your Engine, National Livestock and Meat Board.

Your Daily Bread, American Bakers Association.

b. Films

Better Breakfasts, U.S.A., Cereal Institutes, Inc.

Dairy—Farm to Door, Charles Cahill and Associates.

Digestion of Foods, Encyclopaedia Britannica Films, Inc.

Eat for Health, Encyclopaedia Britannica Films, Inc.

Food and Growth, Encyclopaedia Britannica Films, Inc.

Food Stores, Encyclopaedia Britannica Films, Inc.

Food, the Color of Life, National Dairy Council.

Foods That Build Good Health, Coronet Instructional Films.

Foundation Foods, Avis Films, Inc.

Fundamentals of Diet, Encyclopaedia Britannica Films, Inc.

Good Eating Habits, Coronet Instructional Films.

Good Table Manners, Coronet Instructional Films.

Growing Up Day by Day, Encyclopaedia Britannica Films, Inc.

Journey to Bananaland, United Fruit Company.

Judy Learns About Milk, Young America Films.

Health—You and Your Helpers, Charles Cahill and Associates.

Milk, Encyclopaedia Britannica Films, Inc.

Save Those Teeth, Encyclopaedia Britannica Films, Inc.

Something You Didn't Eat, Association Films.

Something You Didn't Eat, U.S. Department of Agriculture.

The Best Way to Eat, Florida Citrus Commission.

The King Who Came to Breakfast, Association Films.

The Wheat Farmer, Encyclopaedia Britannica Films, Inc.

Two Little Rats, National Dairy Council.

Uncle Jim's Dairy Farm, National Dairy Council.

Understanding Vitamins, Encyclopaedia Britannica Films, Inc.

Visit to Dairyland U.S.A., National Dairy Council.

Water We Drink, Coronet Instructional Films.

Whenever You Eat, Association Films.

You and Your Food, National Dairy Council.

Your Food, McGraw-Hill Book Company.

Your Food, Young America Films.

c. Filmstrips

A Right Breakfast, Society for Visual Education.

Beef—From Store to Table, National Livestock and Meat Board.

Bill's Better Breakfast Puppet Show, Cereal Institute, Inc.

Digestive System, Young America Films.

Eat Well: Live Well, McGraw-Hill Book Company.

Food Around the World, National Dairy Council.

Foods for Health, Young America Films.

Grain from Farm to Table, Cereal Institute, Inc.

Guide to Breakfast, Kraft Foods.

Guide to Cheesemaking, Kraft Foods.

How Food Becomes You, National Dairy Council.

How Food Is Digested, McGraw-Hill Book Company.

How We Get Our Foods, Society for Visual Education.

Proper Food, Encyclopaedia Britannica Films, Inc.

Skimpy and a Good Breakfast, Cereal Institute, Inc.

Story of Wheat, Wheat Flour Institute.

The Essentials of Diet, McGraw-Hill Book Company.

The Power of Food, National Livestock and Meat Board.

We Grow, National Dairy Council.

Why Does Food Spoil? McGraw-Hill Book Company.

Why Eat a Good Breakfast?, Cereal Institute, Inc.

You and Your Food, Young America Films.

d. Posters

A Day with the Wide Awakes, General Mills, Inc.

A Guide to Good Eating, National Dairy Council.

Child Feeding Posters (3 posters), National Dairy Council.

Food Nutrient Posters (6), National Livestock and Meat Board.

Foods, United Fresh Fruit and Vegetable Association.

Foods You Need Every Day, National Livestock and Meat Board.

Foodway to Follow, American Institute of Baking.

Good Foods Help You Grow, National Tuberculosis Association.

Let's Make Butter, National Dairy Council.

Make Lunch Count, National Dairy Council.

Milk from Farm to Family (6 posters), National Dairy Council.

More Milk Please, National Dairy Council.

My Growth Record, National Dairy Council.

Ready for Breakfast, National Dairy Council.

School Lunch, National Dairy Council.

Series of Posters about Citrus Fruits (8), Florida Citrus Commission.

Start a Better Day with a Better Breakfast, National Livestock and Meat Board.

Surprise for Mother Pictures, National Dairy Council.

The Day Begins with Breakfast, Equitable Life Assurance Society of the United States.

The Four Food Groups, Florida Citrus Commission.

The Wheel of Good Eating, American Institute of Baking.

What Did You Have for Breakfast This Morning? National Dairy Council.

Which Are You? General Mills, Inc.

e. Charts

A Basic Breakfast Pattern, Cereal Institute, Inc.

A Guide to Good Eating, National Dairy Council.

Availability Guide for Fruits and Vegetables, United Fresh Fruit and Vegetable Association.

Bananaland, United Fruit Company.

Better Breakfast for Primary Children, Florida Citrus Commission.

Colored Food Value Charts, National Livestock and Meat Board.

Conserving Minerals and Vitamins, General Mills, Inc.

Day to Day Good Health Record, Kellogg Company.

Facts About Foods, H. J. Heinz Company.

Food Chart, General Foods Corporation.

Food Mobile, American Institute of Baking.

Foods for Growing Boys and Girls, Kellogg Company.

For the Calcium You Need, Evaporated Milk Association.

Grains—Origin of Cereal Breakfasts, Cereal Institute, Inc.

Its Always Breakfast Time Somewhere, National Dairy Council.

Kernel of Wheat, Wheat Flour Institute.

Milk from Farm to Family, National Dairy Council.

Mother Hubbard's Cupboard, General Mills, Inc.

My Daily Food Record, National Livestock and Meat Board.

My Growth Record, National Dairy Council.

Nutritive Values of Fruits and Vegetables, United Fresh Fruit and Vegetable Association.

Potato Calorie Bar Charts, United Fresh Fruit and Vegetable Association.

Safari Breakfast Game, Kellogg Company.

School Lunch Evaluation Charts, General Mills, Inc.

School Lunch Record, National Dairy Council.

School Teaching Charts on Beet Sugar, United States Beet Sugar Association.

Shield of Good Health, Wheat Flour Institute.

Vitamin Food Chart, The "Cream of Wheat" Corporation.

Wall Meat Charts, National Livestock and Meat Board.

We Work Together, Wheat Flour Institute.

f. Maps

Armour Food Source Map, Armour and Company.

g. Radio Scripts

Better Breakfast, Cereal Institute, Inc.
The School Lunch, Bureau of Research in Education by Radio, University of Texas.
We Need a Balanced Diet, Bureau of Research in Education by Radio, University of Texas.

h. Models

Better Breakfast Cut-outs, Florida Citrus Commission.
Dairy Farm, National Dairy Council.
Food Model, National Dairy Council.
It's Always Breakfast Time Somewhere, National Dairy Council.
Story Display Banners, United Fresh Fruit and Vegetable Association.
Urban Panorama, National Dairy Council.

i. Transparencies

Good Health Begins with Good Nutrition (6), Cereal Institute, Inc.

j. Selected Stories for Children (P) Primary Level, (I) Intermediate Level

About Food and Where It Comes From, (I), T. Shannon (Melmont).
Around the World in Eighty Dishes (I), L. Blanche (Harper).
At the Bakery (P), L. Colonius and G. Schroeder (Melmont).
Baker Bill (P), Jean Barr (Whitman).
Basketful, the Story of Our Foods (I), J. Eberle (Crowell).
Brazil, Giant to the South (I), Alice Hagar (Macmillan).
Chickens and How to Raise Them (I), L. Darling (Morrow).
Chocolate Touch (P,I), P. S. Cathing (Morrow).
Cook-A-Meal Cookbook (I), G. Clark (W. R. Scott).
Everybody Eats (P), M. M. Green (W. R. Scott).
Farmer and His Cows (P), L. Floethe (Scribner).
Fish (I), R. Fawcett (Gawthorne).
Fun with Cooking (I), Mae Freeman (Random House).
Great Nutrition Puzzles (I), D. Callahan (Scribner).
It's Always Breakfast Time Somewhere (I), M. C. Letton (National Dairy Council).
Jimmy, the Groceryman (P), Jane Miller (Houghton).
Krista and the Frosty Foods (P,I), H. Olds (Messner).
Let's Take a Trip to a Fishery (P), S. Riedman (Abelard).

Milk for You (P), W. G. Schloat (Scribner).
Milk Production (P), J. Perry and C. Slauson (Longmans).
Milkman Freddy (I), Elizabeth Halfman (Messner).
Miss B's First Cook Book (I), Percy Hoffman (Bobbs).
Nothing to Eat but Food (I), Frank Jupo (Aladdin).
Plants That Feed Us (I), C. Fenton (Day).
Story Book of Foods (P,I), M. Petersham (Winston).
Story Book of Wheat (P), M. Petersham (Winston).
Stories from the Americas (I), F. Henuis (Scribner).
Sugar (I), R. Fawcett (Gawthorne).
The Apple That Jack Ate (P), William R. Scott (W. R. Scott).
The Lunchbox Story (P), M. Goldberg (Holiday House).
The Milk That Jack Drank (P), W. R. Scott (Cadmus).
The Wonderful Egg (I), W. G. Schloat (Scribner).
This Is the Bread That Betsy Ate (P), Irma Black (W. R. Scott).
To Market We Go (P), Jane Miller (Houghton).
Walkabout Down Under (I), K. S. Foote (Scribner).
What the World Eats (I), H. H. Webster (Houghton).
Where's the Bunny? (P), Ruth Carroll (Oxford University Press).
Who Dreams of Cheese? (P), Leonard Weisgard (Scribner).
Wonderful Baker (I), M. L. Hunt (Lippincott).
Your Food and You (I), H. S. Zim (Morrow).

4. Dental Health

a. Pamphlets or Leaflets

A Drop in the Bucket, U.S. Public Health Service.
A Visit to the Dentist, American Dental Association.
Betty and Bobby, the Baker Twins, Lambert Pharmacal Company.
Dental Health Education, American Dental Association.
Even Dragons Have Teeth, American Dental Association.
Food and Care for Dental Health, National Dairy Council.
Food and Care for Good Dental Health, National Dairy Council.
For Good Teeth and a Healthy Mouth, Church and Dwight Company.
Frank Visits the Dentist, American Dental Association.
Fresh Oranges, Important for Sound Teeth, Sunkist Growers.
Good Teeth, Government Printing Office.

How Bright the Smile, Florida Citrus Commission.

How to Take Care of Your Teeth, Procter and Gamble Company.

How Teeth Grow, National Dairy Council.

I'm Going to the Dentist, American Dental Association.

Kit Goes to the Dentist, Health Education Service.

Little Red Sky, Church and Dwight Company.

My Friend Nick, Church and Dwight Company.

Teeth and How to Care for Them, Pepsodent Division, Lever Brothers Company.

Teeth Talk, Travelers Insurance Company.

The Way to a Smile, Procter and Gamble Company.

They Are Your Teeth, National Dairy Council.

Tom Visits the Dentist, Procter and Gamble Company.

Tommy's First Visit to the Dentist, American Dental Association.

Toothbrushing, American Dental Association.

Toothbrushing, Church and Dwight Company.

When I Grow Up, National Dairy Council.

Your Guide to Dental Health, American Dental Association.

b. Films

Billy Meets Tommy Tooth, American Dental Association.

Case of the Missing Tooth, American Dental Association.

Gateway to Health, National Apple Institute.

How Teeth Grow, Encyclopaedia Britannica Films, Inc.

It Doesn't Hurt, Coronet Instructional Films.

Learning to Brush, American Dental Association.

Our Teeth, Knowledge Builders.

Project Teeth, American Dental Association.

Save Those Teeth, Encyclopaedia Britannica Films, Inc.

Sights and Sounds Around the Dental Chair, American Dental Association.

Teeth Are to Keep, Encyclopaedia Britannica Films, Inc.

The Beaver's Tale, American Dental Association.

The Teeth, Encyclopaedia Britannica Films, Inc.

Tommy's Day, Young America Films.

Tommy's Healthy Teeth, National Dairy Council.

What Do You Know about Teeth? American Dental Association.

Your Teeth, Young America Films.

c. Filmstrips

Billy Meets Tommy Tooth, American Dental Association.

Brush Up on Your Teeth, Canadian National Film Board.

Johnny's Magic Toothbrush, American Dental Association.

Let's Visit the Dentist, National Dairy Council.

Primary Grade Health Series, National Dairy Council.

Save Those Teeth, Encyclopedia Britannica Films, Inc.

Strong Teeth, McGraw-Hill Book Company.

Tale of a Toothache, Society for Visual Education.

Ten Little People and Their Teeth, Canadian National Film Board.

The Teeth, Encyclopaedia Britannica Films, Inc.

The Teeth, Young America Films.

Your Teeth and Their Care, Popular Science.

You're on Parade, Society for Visual Education.

d. Posters

Armed to the Teeth, Florida Citrus Commission.

Begin Early, National Dairy Council.

Big Pains, Travelers Insurance Company.

Brush Your Teeth, Eat Good Foods, Visit Your Dentist, National Dairy Council.

Elementary School Posters (set of 4), American Dental Association.

How We Take Care of the Teeth, National Dairy Council.

Teeth, American Dental Association.

They're Your Teeth, National Dairy Council.

e. Charts

Elementary School Posters (4 each) American Dental Association.

Four Food Groups, National Dairy Council.

Honor Roll – Clean Teeth Club, Pepsodent.

How to Brush the Teeth (21″ × 25½″), American Dental Association.

Ivory Inspection Patrol Chart, Procter and Gamble Company.

Toothbrushing Chart, American Dental Association.

f. Records

Friendly Doctor Drillum Fillum, J-209 Columbia Records.

Willie and a Little Tooth, J-184 Columbia Records.

g. Toothbrushing Kits

American Dental Association (M10 kit), Procter and Gamble Company.

h. Models

Look at Your Teeth – Everyone Else Does, American Dental Association.

Tooth Model, Association of Casualty and Surety Companies.

Toothbrushing Model (M13 new), American Dental Association.

i. Radio Scripts

Care of the Teeth, Bureau of Research in Education by Radio, University of Texas.
Terry's Trip to the Moon, American Dental Association.
The Freckle Faced Rebel, American Dental Association.

j. Selected Stories for Children (P) Primary Level, (I) Intermediate Level

Child's Book of Teeth (I), H. W. Ferguson (World Book).
Let's Be Healthy (P), W. W. Charters (Macmillan).
Let's Go to a Dentist (P), N. Buckheimer (Putnam).
Milk for You (P), W. G. Schloat (Scribner).
Milkman Freddy (I), Elizabeth Hoffman (Messner).
One Morning in Maine (P), R. McClusky (Viking).
Your Wonderful Teeth (P,I), W. G. Schloat (Scribner).

5. Body Structure and Operation

a. Pamphlets or Leaflets

Blood's Magic for All, American Red Cross.
Foot Health Exercises, National Foot Health Council.
Good Posture in the Little Child, U.S. Children's Bureau.
Heart Disease, U.S. Public Health Service.
It's a Breeze, American Red Cross.
Pounds and Inches, Metropolitan Life Insurance Company.
The Breath of Life. Aetna Life Insurance Company.
The Heart and Circulation, American Heart Association.
The Wonder of You, American Institute of Baking.
These Sitting Americans, American Seating Company.
When I Grow Up, National Dairy Council.
Wonder Stories of the Human Machine (7 stories), American Medical Association.
Your Children's Feet and Their Care, National Foot Health Council.
Your Heart, Metropolitan Life Insurance Company.

b. Films

Back on the Job, American Heart Association.
Breathing, Encyclopaedia Britannica Films, Inc.
Circulation, United World Films.

Digestion in Our Bodies, Coronet Instructional Films.
Endocrine Glands, Encyclopaedia Britannica Films, Inc.
Functions of the Nervous System, Knowledge Builders.
Healthy Lungs, Coronet Instructional Films.
Heart, Lungs, and Circulation, Coronet Instructional Films.
I Never Catch a Cold, Coronet Instructional Films.
Mechanisms of Breathing, Encyclopaedia Britannica Films, Inc.
Muscles and Bones of the Body, Coronet Instructional Films.
Obesity, National Dairy Council.
Posture Habits, Coronet Instructional Films.
Rest That Builds Good Health, Coronet Instructional Films.
Sitting Right, Association Films.
Sleep for Health, Encyclopaedia Britannica Films, Inc.
The Huffless, Puffless Dragon, American Cancer Society.
The Human Body, National Dairy Council.
Wonder Engine of the Body, American Heart Association.
Wonder of Our Body, Moody Institute of Science.
Work of the Kidneys, Encyclopaedia Britannica Films, Inc.
Your Nervous System, Coronet Instructional Films.

c. Filmstrips

Harvey and Blood Circulation, International Film Bureau.
How the Heart Works, Popular Science.
How to Grow Well and Strong, McGraw-Hill Book Company.
How to Grow Well and Strong, Popular Science.
Human Respiration, Popular Science.
Nervous System, Young America Films.
Respiratory System, Young America Films.
Skin, Hair, and Nails, McGraw-Hill Book Company.
Straight and Tall, Young America Films.
Systems of the Body, Educational Activities, Inc.
The Heart — How It Works, McGraw-Hill Book Company.
The Human Cell, American Cancer Society.
Use of Artificial Respiration, McGraw-Hill Book Company.
We Grow, National Dairy Council.
You the Living Machine, Encyclopaedia Britannica Films, Inc.
Your Blood System, Curriculum Films.
Your Bones and Muscles, Popular Science.
Your Heart and Lungs, Popular Science.
Your Posture — Good or Bad, Young America Films.

d. Posters

ACS Bulletin Board Posters (7 each), American Cancer Society.

Foot Health Exercises (several posters), National Foot Health Council.

Good Posture Pays Off, Equitable Life Assurance Society of United States.

Mouth to Mouth Artificial Respiration, Employers Mutuals of Wausau.

Posture on Parade (for girls), National Dairy Council.

The Breath of Life, Aetna Life Insurance Company.

Walk and Be Healthy, National Foot Health Council.

Which One Is a Fake?, American Cancer Society.

e. Charts

Bone Structure, National Livestock and Meat Board.

Heart Charts (12), American Heart Association.

He Needs Your Blood, American Red Cross.

How Tall, The Travelers Insurance Company.

Human Body (kit), Owen Publishing Company, Danville, N.Y.

My Growth Record, National Dairy Council.

Physical Growth Record for Boys, American Medical Association.

Physical Growth Record for Girls, American Medical Association.

Your Heart and How It Works, American Heart Association.

f. Radio Scripts

Good Posture, Bureau of Research in Education by Radio, University of Texas.

g. Records

Childhood Rhythms for Intermediate Grades (Evans CHR-3), Stanley Bowmar Company

Childhood Rhythms for Lower Grades (Evans CHR-1), Stanley Bowmar Company, Valhalla, N.Y.

Creative Rhythm Album (Burns-Wheeler), Stanley Bowmar Company.

My Heart and I, American Heart Association.

h. Models

The Heart and Circulation, American Heart Association.

i. Selected Stories for Children (P) Primary

Level, (I) Intermediate Level

A Baby Is Born (P), L. I. Mitton and J. N. Seligmann (Simon & Schuster).

All About Eggs (P), Selsan Millicent (W. R. Scott).

All About the Human Body (I), B. Glemser (Random).

All About Us (I), Eva Evans (Capital).

All Kinds of Babies and How They Grow (P), Selsan Millicent (W. R. Scott).

Brave Gives Blood (I), Philip and Mirina Eisenburg (Messner).

Growing Story (P), Ruth Krauss (Harper).

Growing Up (P), Karl DeSchweintz (Macmillan).

How We Grow (I), P. O'Keefe and C. H. Maxwell (Winston).

How Your Body Works (I), H. Schneider (W. R. Scott).

Linda Goes to the Hospital (I), Nancy Dudley (Coward-McCann).

Push and Pull (I), P. Blackwood (McGraw-Hill).

The Smallest Boy in the Class (I), J. Beim (William Morrow).

What's Inside of Me? (I), Herbert S. Zim (Morrow).

What's Inside of Me? (P), Herbert S. Zim (Morrow).

When I Am Big (P), R. P. Smith (Harper).

Wonders Inside You (P), L. Cosgrove (Dodd).

Wonders of the Human Body (I), A. Ranelli (Viking).

Your Body and How It Works (I), P. Lauber (Random House).

Your Heart and How It Works (I), H. Zim (Morrow).

6. Prevention and Control of Disease

a. Pamphlets or Leaflets

Acne—What You Can Do about It, Health Education Service.

A Hot War Against the Common Cold, Kimberly-Clark Corporation.

Colds and Other Respiratory Diseases, Travelers Insurance Company.

Common Cold, U.S. Public Health Service.

Common Sense about Common Diseases, Equitable Life Assurance Society.

Cups Through the Centuries, Paper Cup and Container Institute.

Health Heroes Series, Metropolitan Life Insurance Company.

I Promise Common Sense, Kimberly-Clark Corporation.

Men Against Disease, American Red Cross.

Old King Cold, American Medical Association.

On Every Lap, Paper Cup and Container Institute.

Poliomyelitis—Teacher's Guide, National Foundation.

Sickness at Home, Equitable Life Assurance Society.

The Common Cold, Equitable Life Assurance Society.

The Truth about Cancer, Health Education Service.

b. Films

Avoiding Infections, Encyclopaedia Brittannica Films, Inc.

Cleanliness and Health, Coronet Instructional Films.

Common Cold, Encyclopaedia Britannica Films, Inc.

Goodbye, Mr. Germ, National Tuberculosis Association.

Health Heroes: the Battle Against Disease, Metropolitan Life Insurance Co.

House Fly, Encyclopaedia Britannica Films, Inc.

How to Catch a Cold, Kimberly-Clark Corporation.

I Never Catch a Cold, Coronet Instructional Films.

Immunization, Encyclopaedia Britannica Films, Inc.

Joan Avoids a Cold, Coronet Instructional Films.

Let's Have Fewer Colds, Coronet Instructional Films.

Life in a Drop of Water, Coronet Instructional Films.

Spot Prevention, U.S. Public Health Service.

Story of Dr. Jenner, Teaching Film Custodians.

Story of Louis Pasteur, Teaching Film Custodians.

The Body Fights Bacteria, McGraw-Hill Book Company.

The Fight Against Microbes, International Film Bureau.

The Inside Story, National Tuberculosis Association.

Tiny Water Animals, Encyclopaedia Britannica Films, Inc.

Unmasking the Germ Assassins, International Film Bureau.

Water We Drink, Coronet Instructional Films.

Your Health, Disease and Its Control, Coronet Instructional Films.

c. Filmstrips

Avoiding Infections (Treating a Cold), Encyclopaedia Britannica Films, Inc.

Cancer, the Challenge to Youth, American Cancer Society.

Checking Your Health, Encyclopaedia Britannica Films, Inc.

Common Cold, Encyclopaedia Britannica Films, Inc.

Communicable Diseases, Young America Films.

Controlling Germs, Curriculum Films.

Florence Nightingale, Metropolitan Life Insurance Company.

Germ Invaders, McGraw-Hill Book Company.

Health Heroes, Metropolitan Life Insurance Company.

Helping the Body Defenses Against Disease, McGraw-Hill Book Company.

Keeping Ourselves Healthy, Curriculum Films.

Keeping Sickness Away, McGraw-Hill Book Company.

Keeping Well, Young America Films.

Madame Curie, Metropolitan Life Insurance Company.

Making Water Safe to Drink, McGraw-Hill Book Company.

The Little Pink Bottle, National Foundation.

The Water We Drink, Young America Films.

Walter Reed and the Conquest of Yellow Fever (with transcription), Metropolitan Life Insurance Company.

We Have You Covered, Society for Visual Education.

d. Posters

How to Catch a Cold, Kimberly-Clark Corporation.

How to Cure a Cold, Kimberly-Clark Corporation.

How to Spread a Cold, Kimberly-Clark Corporation.

Protect Them with Shots. National Tuberculosis Association.

Remember the Fundamentals (Sanitation), Paper Cup and Container Institute.

Soap Before Soup, Travelers Insurance Company.

We Had Polio Vaccine, National Foundation.

e. Records

Chest X-ray Song, National Tuberculosis Association.

Doctors Make History, American Medical Association.

Health Heroes, American Medical Association.

Rainy Days, National Safety Council.

The Constant Invader (15 each), Wisconsin Anti-Tuberculosis Association.

f. Charts

I Promise Common Sense, Kimberly-Clark Corporation.

g. Radio Scripts From Bureau of Research in Education by Radio, University of Texas)

Fly Control

Health Living Radio Broadcast (kit of 30 scripts)

Keep Your Cold at Home

Mosquito Control

Safe Water Supply

We Wash Our Hands Before We Eat

h. Selected Stories for Children (P) Primary Level, (I) Intermediate Level

Conquest of Disease (I), L. Martin (Coward).

Doctors and Nurses; What They Do (I), C. Greene (Harper & Row).

Doctors and What They Do (I), H. Coy (G. P. Putnam's Sons).

Dr. Trotter and His Big Gold Watch (P), H. Gilbert (Abingdon).

Have a Happy Measle, a Merry Mumps and a Cheery Chickenpox (I), J. Bendick (Whittlesey House).

Health Can Be Fun (P), Munro Leaf (Lippincott).

Johnny Goes to the Hospital (P), J. Sener (Houghton).

Linda Goes to the Hospital (P), N. Dudley (Coward).

Modern Medical Discoveries (I), E. Bigland (Criterion).

Moptop (P), D. Freeman (Viking).

Our Insect Friends and Foes (I), W. A. DuPuy (Winston).

The Clean Pig (P), Leonard Weisgard (Scribner).

The First Book of Microbes (I), L. Lewis (Watts).

The Water That Jack Drank (P), William R. Scott (W. R. Scott).

True Book of Health (P), Mary Brockman (Scribner).

What's Inside of Me? (P), Herbert S. Zim (Morrow).

7. Safety and First Aid

a. Pamphlets or Leaflets

About Electricity, National Fire Protection Association.

Artificial Respiration, American Medical Association.

Bicycle Riding Clubs, Bicycle Institute of America.

Bicycle Safety in Action, National Commission on Safety Education.

Bicycle Safety Information Test, National Safety Council.

Bicycle Safety Test, Bicycle Institute of America.

Bicyclists' Safety Rules, Bicycle Institute of America.

Bike Regulations in the Community, Bicycle Institute of America.

Bike Safety Program, Bicycle Institute of America.

Children and Matches, National Fire Protection Association.

Falling, Falling, Falling, Employers Mutuals of Wausau.

Fatal Fallacies, The Travelers Insurance Company.

Fire Prevention Guide, Intermediate, American Red Cross.

Fire Prevention Guide, Primary, American Red Cross.

First Aid Now! Pharmaceutical Manufacturers Association.

First Aid (Programmed instruction), Behavioral Research Laboratories.

First Aid Facts, Johnson & Johnson.

Good Biker Today—Good Driver Tomorrow, Employers Mutuals of Wausau.

Helpful Hints on Bicycle Care for Safe Riding, American Red Cross.

Home Sweet (non-poisonous) Home, Employers Mutuals of Wausau.

In Case of Fire, National Fire Protection Association.

Junior Bicycle Courts, Bicycle Institute of America.

Read the Label, National Fire Protection Association.

Safe at Home and in the Community, John Hancock Mutual Life Insurance Company.

Safe Play to Save Sight, National Society for the Prevention of Blindness.

Seat Belts Save, American Medical Association.

Standard Rules for School Safety Patrols, National Safety Council.

Ten Little Tasters, U.S. Public Health Service (Food and Drug Administration).

The Safest Route to School, American Automobile Association.

Units in Safety Education for Grades 5 and 6, National Commission on Safety Education.

When the Unexpected Happens, John Hancock Mutual Life Insurance Company.

You and Your Bicycle, American Red Cross.

Your Clothing Can Burn, National Fire Protection Association.

b. Films

A Monkey Tale (Bicycle Safety), Encyclopaedia Britannica Films, Inc.

Bicycle Rules of the Road, Employers Mutuals of Wausau.

Bicycle Safety Skills, Coronet Instructional Films.

Children at Play with Poison, U.S. Public Health Service (Food and Drug Administration).

Emergency 77, Metropolitan Life Insurance Company.

Fifty Thousand Lives, Johnson & Johnson.

Fire Exit Drill at Our School, Coronet Instructional Films.

Fireman, Encyclopaedia Britannica Films, Inc.

First Aid Now, Pharmaceutical Manufacturers Association.

Help Wanted, Johnson & Johnson.

I'm No Fool as a Pedestrian, American Automobile Association.

I'm No Fool with a Bicycle, American Automobile Association.

Playground Safety (2nd ed.), Coronet Instructional Films.

Primary Safety: In the School Building, Coronet Instructional Films.

Safe Living at Home, Coronet Instructional Films.

Safe Living at School, Coronet Instructional Films.

Safe Living in Your Community, Coronet Instructional Films.

Safe Through Seat Belts, International Film Bureau, Inc.

Safe Use of Tools, Coronet Instructional Films.

Safest Way, American Automobile Association.

Safety Begins at Home, Young America Films.

Safety Belts for Susie, Charles Cahill and Associates.

Safety in Winter, Coronet Instructional Films.

Safety on the Playground, Encyclopaedia Britannica Films, Inc.

Safety on the Streets, Encyclopaedia Britannica Films, Inc.

Safety on the Way, Coronet Instructional Films.

Safety with Fire, Coronet Instructional Films.

School Bus and You, Progressive Films.

School Bus Safety with Strings Attached, Employers Mutuals of Wausau.

School Rules—How They Help Us, Coronet Instructional Films.

Special Delivery, Employers Mutuals of Wausau.

Stop, Look, and Think, Charles Cahill and Associates.

Water Safety, Young America Films.

You and Your Bicycle, Progressive Films and Employers Mutuals of Wausau.

c. Filmstrips

Be a Better Pedal Pusher, Society for Visual Education.

Bicycle Safety, Curriculum Films.

Controlling Fire, McGraw-Hill Book Company.

Electrical Hazard, Stanley Bowmar Company.

Happy Hollow Makes the Honor Roll, Society for Visual Education.

Home Safety, Encyclopaedia Britannica Films, Inc.

I'm No Fool Having Fun, McGraw-Hill Book Company.

I'm No Fool with a Bicycle, McGraw-Hill Book Company.

I'm No Fool with Fire, McGraw-Hill Book Company.

Keeping Food Safe to Eat, McGraw-Hill Book Company.

Play Safety, Encyclopaedia Britannica Films, Inc.

Playing in City Streets, Curriculum Films.

Safe and Sure with Electricity, McGraw-Hill Book Company.

Safety at School, Curriculum Films.

Safety Helpers, Encyclopaedia Britannica Films, Inc.

Safety in the Summer, Curriculum Films.

School Safety, Encyclopaedia Britannica Films, Inc.

Street Safety, Encyclopaedia Britannica Films, Inc.

Vacation Safety, Encyclopaedia Britannica Films, Inc.

Wintertime Safety, McGraw-Hill Book Company.

d. Posters

A Clean House Seldom Burns, National Fire Protection Association.

Always Use Bike Hand Signals, Bicycle Institute of America.

Be a Better Biker, Employers Mutuals of Wausau.

Be Sure Your Bike Is Ready to Go, Bicycle Institute of America.

Bike Safety Aids, Bicycle Institute of America.

Ducks Can't Sink, National Commission on Safety Education.

First Aid, Ross Laboratories.

In and Out of Traffic, National Commission on Safety Education.

Let's Be Safe Passengers, National Commission on Safety Education.

Playground Safety, National Commission on Safety Education.

Prevent Fire, National Fire Protection Association.

Safe Steps Through School, National Commission on Safety Education.

Seat Belts, American Medical Association.

Special Days Are Fun, National Commission on Safety Education.

Sports Accidents, American Medical Association.

Stop Carelessness—Prevent Accidents, International Harvester Company.

Stop Fires, Save Lives, American Insurance Association.

Wait on the Curb for Your Go Signal, American Automobile Association.

e. Charts

Check List for Child Safety, American Red Cross.

Child Poisoning, Health Education Service.

First Aid, Metropolitan Life Insurance Company.

Home Fire Safety Check List, National Fire Protection Association.

Special Days Are Fun, National Commission on Safety Education.

Summertime Safety, National Commission on Safety Education.

f. Records

Fire on Thunder Hill, American Forest Products Industries, Inc.

Safety Through Music, Educational Activities, Inc.

g. Comics

A Tale of Two Bike Riders, Employers Mutuals of Wausau.

Dennis the Menace Takes a Poke at Poison, U.S. Public Health Service.

Early Man and Fire, National Fire Protection Association.

Hello. I Am Fire! National Fire Protection Association.

Man Learns More about Fire, National Fire Protection Association.

Sparky, National Fire Protection Association.

Sparky Makes a Home Fire Inspection, National Fire Protection Association.

h. Radio Scripts

Benny, the Matchstick, National Safety Council.

Bobby Grows Up, National Safety Council.

Carl, the Bear Cub, National Safety Council.

Child Safety Stories, National Safety Council.

Danger, Children at Play, National Safety Council.

Fire Prevention, Bureau of Research in Education by Radio, University of Texas.

Fire Safety, National Safety Council.

Happy and Safe Thinking, National Safety Council.

Lady from Safety Land, National Safety Council.

Let's Play Safe, Bureau of Research in Education by Radio, University of Texas.

Louis Agazzi Fuertes, National Safety Council.

Make Your City Safer, National Safety Council.

Mary and the Broken Glass, National Safety Council.

Needles and Pins, National Safety Council.

On a Bicycle Not Built for Two, National Safety Council.

Our Animal Show, National Safety Council.

Out of the Night, National Safety Council.

Safe Water Supply, Bureau of Research in Education by Radio, University of Texas.

The Bat Blinky, National Safety Council.

The Safety Elf, National Safety Council.

The Twins Have Safety Trouble, National Safety Council.

To Walk in the Night, National Safety Council.

Worrying Bike, National Safety Council.

i. Selected Stories for Children (P) Primary Level, (I) Intermediate Level

Andy and the School Bus (P), J. Beim (Morrow).

Big Fire (P), E. Olds (Houghton).

Binkey's Fire (P), Sally Scott (Harcourt).

Country Fireman (P), J. Beim (Morrow).

Dr. Squash, the Doll Doctor (P), Margaret Wise Brown (Simon & Schuster).

Fireman for a Day (I), Z. K. McDonald (Messner).

Fireman Fred (P), Jean Barry (Whitman).

First Book of Firemen (I), Mary Elting (Watts).

Forest Fireman (P, I), Bill and Rosalie Brown (Coward).

Going to Blazes (I), R. V. Masters (Sterling).

Hercules, Story of an Old Fashioned Fire Engine (P), Hardie Gramatsky (Putnam).

I Want to Be a Policeman (P), C. Greene (Children's Press).

Johnnie Wants to Be a Policeman (I), W. J. Granberg (Aladdin).

Let's Find Out about Safety (I), M. Shapp (Watts).

Mountain Courage (I), D. Hawkins (Doubleday).

Pat and Her Policeman (I), F. Friedman (Morrow).

Rags, the Firehouse Dog (P), E. Morton (Winston).

Red Light, Green Light (P), Margaret Wise Brown (Doubleday).

Safety Can Be Fun (P), Munro Leaf (Lippincott).

The Bike Lesson (P), S. and J. Berenstain (Random House).

The Firefighter (I), H. B. Lent (Macmillan).

The Little Igloo (P), L. Beim (Harcourt Brace).

The New Fire Engine (P), Jay Barnum (Morrow).

Time and the Brass Buttons (P, I), Ruth Tooze (Messner).

Walkabout Down Under (I), K. S. Foote (Scribner).

Watch Out (I), Norah Smaridge (Abington).

8. Mental Health

a. Pamphlets or Leaflets

A Happy Day, National Dairy Council.

All Around Me, Continental Can Company.

Children of the Evening, Hogg Foundation for Mental Health.

Emotional Health in Work and Play, American Medical Association.

Getting Along with Brothers and Sisters, Child Study Association of America.

Habits, Habits, Habits, Equitable Life Assurance Society.

How Teachers Can Build Mental Health, American Medical Association.

Mental Hygiene in the Classroom, American Medical Association.

Six to Twelve, John Hancock Mutual Life Insurance Company.

Teachers Listen, the Children Speak, U.S. Children's Bureau.

The Teacher's Role in Mental Hygiene, American Medical Association.

Three Cheers for a Big Smile, National Dairy Council.

What Is Mental Illness? U.S. Public Health Service.

b. Films

Act Your Age, Coronet Instructional Films.

Adventuring Pups, Young America Films.

Are You Popular? Coronet Instructional Films.

Attitudes and Health, Coronet Instructional Films.

Case 258, National Council on Alcoholism.

Don't Be Afraid, Encyclopaedia Britannica Films, Inc.

Feeling Left Out, Coronet Instructional Films.

Good Sportsmanship, Coronet Instructional Films.

Growing Up, Coronet Instructional Films.

How Do You Do, Young America Films.

How Friendly Are You? Coronet Instructional Films.

How Honest Are You? Coronet Instructional Films.

If These Were Your Children (Adult), Metropolitan Life Insurance Company.

Jimmy Rabbitt, Bailey Films.

Let's Play Fair, Coronet Instructional Films.

Making Life Adjustments, McGraw-Hill Book Company.

Mental Health, Encyclopaedia Britannica Films, Inc.

Other Fellow's Feelings, Young America Films.

Out of Orbit, National Council on Alcoholism.

Overcoming Worry, Coronet Instructional Films.

Planning for Success, Coronet Instructional Films.

Sky Guy, Coronet Instructional Films.

The Outsider, Young America Films.

The Ugly Duckling, Coronet Instructional Films.

To Your Health, World Health Organization.

Ways to Good Habits, Coronet Instructional Films.

You and Your Family, Association Films, Inc.

You and Your Friends, Association Films, Inc.

You and Your Time, Association Films, Inc.

c. Filmstrips

Getting Acquainted, McGraw-Hill Book Company.

Health Helpers, Encyclopaedia Britannica Films, Inc.

Keeping Children Happy, McGraw-Hill Book Company.

Let's Have a Party, Society for Visual Education.

Manners at Home, Educational Record Sales.

Manners at School, Educational Record Sales.

Mike Finds out about Friendship, Society for Visual Education.

Orphan Willie, Canadian National Film Board.

Promises Are Made to Keep, Encyclopaedia Britannica Films, Inc.

Sense and Nonsense, Popular Science.

Share the Sandpile, Society for Visual Education.

Sharing with Neighbors, Encyclopaedia Britannica Films, Inc.

The Little Cloud, Society for Visual Education.

The Raggedy Elf, Society for Visual Education.

We Play Together, Stanley Bowman Co.

We Work Together, Stanley Bowman Co.

Working and Playing Together, McGraw-Hill Book Company.

d. Posters

Change of Pace, Equitable Life Assurance Society of United States.

e. Plays (From Mental Health Materials Center)

The Daily Special

What Did I Do?

f. Radio Scripts

Are You Afraid? National Safety Council.

Mental Health, Bureau of Research in Education by Radio, University of Texas.

Mind Alone (No. 7), American Medical Association.

Trouble Comes in Threes, National Dairy Council.

g. Selected Stories for Children (P) Primary Level, (I) Intermediate Level

A Friend Is Someone Who Likes You (P), J. Walsh (Harcourt Brace).

A Name for Obed (P), E. C. Phillips (Houghton).

A Race for Bill (I), M. N. Wallace (Nelson).

Ann and the Sand Dobbies (I), John Colburn (Seabury Press).

"B" Is for Betsy (P), Carolyn Haywood (Harcourt).

Child of the Silent Night (I), Edith Hunter (Houghton Mifflin).

David's Bad Day (P), Ellen McKean (Vanguard).

Even Steven (P), W. Lipkind (Harcourt).

Fair Play (P), Munro Leaf (Lippincott).

Finders Keepers (P), W. Lipkind (Harcourt).

Granite Harbor (I), D. Bud (Macmillan).

Growing Story (P), Ruth Krauss (Harper).

Growing Up (P), Karl DeSchweintz (Macmillan).

Here's a Penny (P), Carolyn Haywood (Harcourt).

How to Behave and Why (I), Munro Leaf (Lippincott).

Jerry at School (P), Kathryn Jackson (Simon & Schuster).

Judy's Journey (I), Lois Lenski (Lippincott).

Let's Do Better (P, I), Munro Leaf (Lippincott).

Love Is a Special Way of Feeling (P), J. Walsh (Harcourt Brace).

Manners to Grow on (P), T. Lee (Doubleday).

Mine for Keeps (P), Jean Little (Little, Brown).

My Friend Johnny (P), Vane Earle (Lothrop).

Noise in the Night (I), A. Alexander (Rand).

North Fork (I), Doris Gates (Viking).

Old Can and Patrick (I), Ruth Sawyer (Viking).

Out to Win (I-Boys), M. G. Bonner (Knopf).

Peter's Treasure (I), C. I. Judson (Houghton).

Petunia (P), Roger Duvoisin (Knopf).

Play Fair (P, I), Munro Leaf (Lippincott).

Sad Day—Glad Day (P), Vivian Thompson (Holiday House).

Shaken Days (I), Doris Gates (Viking).

Something to Live By (I), Dorothea Kopplin (Doubleday).

Switch on the Night (P), R. Bradbury (Pantheon).

The Night the Storm Came (P), G. Relyea (Aladdin).

The Smallest Boy in the Class (I), M. Wohlberg (Morrow).

The Ugly Duckling (I), Hans C. Anderson (Harcourt).

The Very Little Girl (P), P. Krasilovsky (Doubleday).

The Wonderful Year (I), Nancy Barnes (Messner).

Timid Timothy (P), G. Williams (W. R. Scott).

Understood Betsy (I), C. L. Judson (Houghton).

What Do They Say? (P), Ellen McKean (Vanguard).

What Is She Like? (I), Mary Brockman (Scribner).

What's That Noise? (I), L. Kauffman (Lothrup).

9. Sex and Family Living Education

a. Pamphlets or Leaflets

A Baby Is Born (Teacher), American Social Health Association.

A Story about You, American Medical Association.

Accent on You, Tampax Incorporated.

Are You in the Know? Kimberly-Clark Corporation.

At What Age Should a Girl Be Told about Menstruation? Kimberly-Clark Corporation.

Boy and His Physique, National Dairy Council.

Boys Want to Know, American Social Hygiene Association.

From Fiction to Facts, Tampax Incorporated.

Girl and Her Figure, National Dairy Council.

Growing Up and Liking It, Personal Products Corporation.

How Shall I Tell My Daughter? Personal Products Corporation.

In the Good Old Summertime, American Red Cross.

It's Time You Knew. Tampax Incorporated.

Life with Brothers and Sisters, American Social Hygiene Association.

Off to a Beautiful Start, Scott Paper Company.

Play Time Is Happy Time, American Red Cross.

Put Our Toys Away, American Red Cross.

Safe Living in the Home, American Red Cross.

Safety at Christmas, American Red Cross.

Sex Education for the Ten Year Old, American Medical Association.

Some Questions and Answers about V.D., American Social Hygiene Association.

Summer Is Here, American Red Cross.

The Doctor Answers Some Practical Questions on Menstruation, American Association For Health, Physical Education and Recreation.

The Gift of Life, American Social Hygiene Association.

The Heart of the Home, American Heart Association.

The Human Story, Scott, Foreman, and Co.

The Story of Life, American Medical Association.

The World of a Girl, Scott Paper Company.

Very Personally Yours, Kimberly-Clark Corporation.

What to Tell Your Children about Sex, Child Study Association of America.

Why Girls Menstruate, American Medical Association.

Your Own Story, American Social Hygiene Association.

You're a Young Lady Now, Kimberly-Clark Corporation.

b. Films (P) Primary Level, (I) Intermediate Level

A Happy Family (P), Classroom Film Distributors. Family relations between a seven year old girl, her younger brother, older sister, and their parents. Depicts how members of the family have learned to live together.

Baby Animals (P), McGraw-Hill Book Company. Elementary.

Farm Babies and Their Mothers (P), Film Associates.

Friendship Begins at Home (P), Coronet Instructional Films.

Growing Up (P), Coronet Instructional Films. Elementary material.

Growing Up Day by Day (P), Encyclopaedia Britannica Films, Inc. Explains the principles of physical, mental, social, and emotional growth to children by comparing members of a group of eight year olds at a birthday party. Explains that actions should vary at different ages and that, as a child grows older, he should learn to do more for himself and others.

Human and Animal Beginnings (P), E. C. Brown Trust. 22 minutes in color. Young children express their beliefs about origin of human life in drawings. Starts with newborn baby and compares with animal babies. Reviews egg development (human and animal) at one month, four months, six months, and nine months.

Kittens—Birth and Growth (P), Bailey Films. Robin and Billy are present when their cat "Millie" gives birth to four kittens. Shows the kittens nursing, crawling, playing, and being weaned. Emphasizes the care the children give to the kittens.

Mike Finds out about Growing (P), Society for Visual Education. Elementary.

Mother Hen's Family (The Wonders of Birth) (P), Coronet Instructional Films. 10 minutes. Depicts how eggs are hatched by hens. Shows a small boy, with the help of his father, following the process from the laying of the eggs to the hatching of the chicks. The boy charts on a calendar the time of setting to the day of the hatching.

Tabby's Kittens (P), Kindergarten.

What Do Fathers Do? (P), Churchill Films. Develops father's image of providing for family's needs. Tells of importance of being on time to work, of cooperation with others, and how happy people are who like their work and perform it well. (Fourth grade.)

Your Family (P), Coronet Instructional Films.

Boy to Man (I), Churchill Films. 16 minutes in color. Depicts the physical changes of the adolescent as well as complete glandular development. For boys 11–14; may also be used with girls. (Excellent for sixth or seventh grade.)

Everyday Courtesy (I), Churchill Films. Pupils arrange and present an exhibit on courtesy. Invitations are written by children to their parents and guests. Regards courtesy in connection with invitations, telephone conversations, introductions, and entertaining guests.

Growing Girls (I), Encyclopaedia Britannica Films, Inc.

Growing Up (Preadolescence) (I), McGraw-Hill Book Company. 10 minutes in color. Silhouette and animal photography regarding the development of twins. Discusses irregular growth, glands involved in growth, sex differences in growth. Emphasizes diet, relaxation, recreation, and rest.

Human Growth (I), Wexler Film Productions. 20 minutes, 16 mm., color. Shows a seventh grade class viewing and discussing animated film that traces human growth from conception to adulthood. Differences in male and female structural development are emphasized. (Revised.)

Human Reproduction (I), McGraw-Hill Book Company. 22 minutes, 16 mm. Stresses the biological normalcy of human reproduction. Models and animated drawings depict the anatomy and physiology of the male and female reproductive organs.

It's Wonderful Being a Girl (I), Personal Products. 20 minutes in color. This is an excellent film on menstruation. It presents a fine philosophy of being a girl.

Molly Grows Up (I), Personal Products. Upper elementary—junior high.

Story of Menstruation (I), Kimberly-Clark Corporation. 10 minutes in color. Animated drawings and diagrams present, in a direct and scientific way, the story of this natural phenomenon.

The Day Life Begins (I), Carousel Films. 23 minutes.

The Endocrine System (I), Encyclopaedia Britannica Films, Inc.

The Story of Menstruation (I), Walt Disney Productions.

You and Your Five Senses (I), Walt Disney Productions. Jiminy Cricket develops theme "All your pets are smart, but the only thinking animal is you. You use thought and reason with your five senses. Animals use their senses entirely by instinct."

You and Your Parents (I), Coronet Instructional Films.

Your Body During Adolescence (I), McGraw-Hill Book Company. Shows the seven glands that regulate human life and growth with emphasis on the pituitary and sex glands. Outlines changes that take place in the bodies of boys and girls.

c. Filmstrips

About Your Life, Denver Public Schools, Denver, Col. (Grade 5).

After School Hours, Popular Science.

Confidence Because ... You Understand Menstruation, Personal Products Corporation.

Families Around the World, Encyclopaedia Britannica Films, Inc.

Family Fun, Encyclopaedia Britannica Films, Inc.

Finding Out How Animals Grow, Society for Visual Education.

Fun at the Beach, McGraw-Hill Book Company.

Fun on a Picnic, Curriculum Films.

Getting Ready for School, Popular Science.

How Babies Are Made, Creative Scope Inc. (Grades K–3).

Janet Helps Mother, Curriculum Films.

Let's Visit Our Friends, Society for Visual Education.

Miss Brown's Class Goes to the Zoo, Eye Gate House (Grades 2–3).

Reproduction in Flowers, Eye Gate House (Grades 4–6).

d. Posters

What Happens During Menstruation? Personal Products Corporation.

e. Charts

Beginning the Human Story: A New Baby in the Family, Scott, Foresman and Co.

Female Anatomical Charts, Tampax, Incorporated.

Keeping our Home Free from Fire, National Commission on Safety Education.

What Happens During Menstruation? Personal Products Corporation.

f. Records

Family Recreation (H29), New York State

University College of Agriculture, Cornell University, Ithaca, N.Y.

g. Slides

How Babies Are Made, Creative Scope, Inc., 509 5th Avenue, New York, N.Y., 10017.

Happy Vacation (H56), New York State University College of Agriculture, Cornell University.

House of Darkness, National Safety Council.

Stop–Look–Listen (H70), New York State University College of Agriculture, Cornell University.

The Story of Growing Up (Girls), Stanley Bowmar Co.

What It Means to Grow Up (Boys), Stanley Bowmar Co.

h. Selected Stories for Children (P) Primary Level, (I) Intermediate Level

A Baby Is Born (P), M. I. Levine and J. H. Seligmann (Golden Press).

A Chimp in the Family (P), Charlotte Beeker (Messner).

A Doctor Talks to 5 to 8 Year Olds (P), D. Z. Meilach (Budlong Press).

A Doctor Talks to 9 to 12 Year Olds (I), M. U. Lerrigo and M. Cassidy (Budlong Press).

A Story about You (I), M. O. Lerrigo and M. J. Senn (American National Association).

About Eggs and Creatures That Hatch from Them (I), M. Uhl (Melmont).

All Kinds of Babies and How They Grow (P), S. E. Millicent (W. R. Scott).

Animal Babies (P), Ylla (Harper).

Animals As Parents (P), M. Selsam (Morrow).

Baby Sister for Francis (P), R. Hoban (Harper & Row).

Big Lion, Little Lion (P), M. Schlein (Albert Whitman & Co.).

Birthday of Obash (P), A. Chalmers (Viking).

Boo, Who Used to Be Scared of the Dark (P), Munro Lead (Random House).

Daddies (P), L. Carton (Random House).

Daddy and Me (P), Monte Stein Jonathan (Scribner).

Daddy Is Home (P), D. Blomquist (Holt, Rhinehart, Winston).

Exploring Home and Family Life (I), H. Fleck (Prentice-Hall).

Facts of Life for Children (I), (Child Study Association).

Finding Yourself (I), M. O. Lerrigo (American Medical Association).

Fine Eggs and Fancy Chicks (P), M. Marks (Dial).

Growing Up (I), K. De Schweitz (Macmillan).

Happy Little Family (P), R. Candill (Winston).

Holiday on Wheels (I), C. Wooley (Morrow).

How Animals Live Together (I), M. Selsam (Morrow).

How Life Is Handed on (I), C. Beck (Harcourt Brace).

Kid Brother (P), J. Beim (Morrow).

Laurie's New Brother (P), M. Schlein (Abelard-Schuman, Ltd.).

Manners Can Be Fun (P), Munro Leaf (Lippincott).

Mommies (P), L. Carton (Random House).

Mommies Are for Loving (P), R. Penn (Putnam's Sons).

Peter and Caroline (P), S. Hegeler (Abelard-Schuman Ltd.).

Possum (P), R. McClung (Morrow).

Red Bantam (P), L. Fatio (McGraw-Hill Book Company).

Seeds Are Wonderful (I), W. Foster and P. Queree (Melmont).

Sigurd and His Brave Companions (I), S. Undset (Knopf).

Sky Bed, a Norwegian Christmas (I), T. T. Grundrun (Scribner).

Squirrels in the Garden (P), O. Earle (Morrow).

Stepsister Sally (P), H. F. Daringer (Harcourt).

The Chosen Baby (P), V. P. Wasson (Lippincott).

The Human Story (I), S. Hoftein (Scott-Foresman).

The People Upstairs (I), Phyllis Cote (Doubleday).

The Story of Life (I), M. O. Lerrigo and M. J. Senn (American National Association).

The Wonder of Life (I), M. I. Levine and J. H. Seligmann (Simon & Schuster).

The Wonderful Story of How You Were Born (P), J. Gruenberg (American Social Hygiene Association).

The Wonderful Year (I), Nancy Barnes (Messner).

True Book of Health (P), O. V. Haynes (Children's Press).

Two Little Birds and Three (P), J. Kepes (Houghton).

Wait and See (P), C. Georgion (Harvey House).

What Makes Me Tick? (I), H. Ruchlis (Harvey House).

What's Inside of Animals? (P), H. S. Zim (Morrow).

When Boy Likes Girl (I), A. Stowe (Random House).

Whitefoot—the Story of a Wood Mouse (I), R. McClung (Morrow).

You and the World Around You (P), M. Selsam (Doubleday).

Young Man of the House (P), Mabel L. Hunt (Lippincott).

10. Community Health

a. Pamphlets or Leaflets

Bicycle Riding Clubs, Bicycle Institute of America.

Bike Regulations in the Community, Bicycle Institute of America.
Clean Water, U.S. Public Health Service.
Crusade of the Christmas Seal, National Tuberculosis Association.
Fire Prevention Guide (Primary), American Red Cross.
Fire Prevention Guide (Intermediate), American Red Cross.
Hot Tips on Food Protection, U.S. Public Health Service.
Medical Uses of Blood, American Red Cross.
Some Facts . . . Why Blood Is Needed, American Red Cross.
Something in the Air, Employers Mutual of Wausaw.
Suggestions on What to Teach about Cancer, American Cancer Society.
The Doctor Is Your Friend, National Tuberculosis Association.
The Long Adventure, National Tuberculosis Association.
Your Friend the Doctor, American Medical Association.

b. Films

Choosing a Doctor, McGraw-Hill Book Company.
Community Health Is Up to You, McGraw-Hill Book Company.
Defending the City's Health, Encyclopaedia Britannica Films, Inc.
Disaster and You, American Red Cross.
Farm Animals, National Dairy Council.
From the Heart of Town, American Red Cross.
Fun on the Playground, Encyclopaedia Britannica Films, Inc.
Mosquito, Encyclopaedia Britannica Films, Inc.
Policemen—Day and Night, Charles Cahill and Associates.
The Doctor, Encyclopaedia Britannica Films, Inc.
The Fireman, Encyclopaedia Britannica Films, Inc.
The Water We Drink, Coronet Instructional Films.
Uncle Jim's Dairy Farm, National Dairy Council.
Your Friend the Doctor, Coronet Instructional Films.
Your Health in the Community, Coronet Instructional Films.

c. Filmstrips

Community Sanitation, Young America Films.
Fun at the Beach, McGraw-Hill Book Company.
Health Heroes (with transcription), Metropolitan Life Insurance Company.
Keeping Sickness Away. McGraw-Hill Book Company.
Maintaining Community Health, Young America Films.

Making Water Safe to Drink, Popular Science.
On the Road to the Country, Curriculum Films.
Our Health Department, Encyclopaedia Britannica Films, Inc.
Safeguarding Our Food, Young America Films.
Safety in the Community, Young America Films.
Sewage Disposal, McGraw-Hill Book Company.
The School That Learned to Eat, General Mills, Inc.
The Water We Drink, Young America Films.
Tommy and His Health Department, Educational Activities, Inc.
Vacation in the City, Curriculum Films.
Walter Reed and the Conquest of Yellow Fever (with transcription), Metropolitan Life Insurance Company.
Waste Disposal for the Community, Encyclopaedia Britannica Films, Inc.
Water for the Community, Encyclopaedia Britannica Films, Inc.

d. Charts

He Needs Your Blood, American Red Cross.
I Promise Common Sense, Kimberly-Clark Corporation.
Keeping Your Home Free from Fire, National Commission on Safety Education.

e. Records

Fire on Thunder Hill, American Forest Products Industries, Inc.
The Constant Invaders, Wisconsin Anti-Tuberculosis Association.
Tommy and His Health Department, Educational Activities, Inc.

f. Radio Scripts

Danger, Children at Play, National Safety Council.
Fly Control, Bureau of Research in Education by Radio, University of Texas.
Home Safety, National Safety Council.
Keep Your Cold at Home, Bureau of Research in Education by Radio, University of Texas.
Know Your Traffic Laws, National Safety Council.
Make Your City Safer, National Safety Council.
Out of the Night, National Safety Council.
Safe Water Supply, Bureau of Research in Education by Radio, University of Texas.
Swimming and Water Safety, Bureau of Research in Education by Radio, University of Texas.
To Walk in the Night, National Safety Council.

g. Selected Stories for Children

(P) Primary Level, (I) Intermediate Level
A Chimp in the Family (P), Charlotte Becker (Messner).

A Walk in the City (P), Rosemary Dawson (Viking).

Boating Is Fun (I), R. Brindze (Dodd).

Brave Gives Blood (I), Philip and Mirina Eisenburg (Messner).

Camp-in-the-Yard (P), V. Thompson (Holiday).

Come to the City (P), Ruth Tensen (Pertly & Lee).

Fireman for a Day (I), Z. K. MacDonald (Messner).

First Book of Nurses (I), M. Etting (Watts).

Johnny Goes to the Hospital (P), J. Sever (Houghton).

Johnny Wants to Be a Policeman (P,I), W. J. Granberg (Aladdin).

Let's Go Fishing (I), Lee Wulff (Lippincott).

Little Town (P), Bertrand Elmer Hader (Macmillan).

Our Insect Friends (I), W. A. DuPuy (Winston).

Pat and Her Policeman (I), F. Friedman (Morrow).

Su-Mei's Golden Year (I), M. H. Bro (Doubleday).

The Discontented Village (I), Rose Dobbs (Coward-McCann).

The Fight to Save America's Water (I), U.S. Public Health Service.

The Water That Jack Drank (P), William R. Scott (W. R. Scott).

The Wonderful Farm (P), M. Ayme (Harper).

Tim and the Brass Buttons (P), Ruth Tooze (Messner).

True Book of Policemen and Firemen (P), I. Miner (Children's Press).

While Susie Sleeps (P), N. Schneider (W. R. Scott).

11. Tobacco, Alcohol, and Drugs

a. Pamphlets or Leaflets

A Light on the Subject of Smoking, U.S. Children's Bureau.

About Alcohol and Narcotics, Licenced Beverage Industries, Inc.

Alcohol, Science and Society, Center for Alcohol Studies, Yale University.

Alcoholics Anonymous — 44 Questions, Alcoholics Anonymous.

Charlie's Party, Connecticut State Department of Mental Health, Hartford, Conn.

Cigarette Smoking and Cancer, American Cancer Society.

Drugs and Driving, U.S. Food and Drug Administration.

Facts about Alcohol, Connecticut State Department of Mental Health, Hartford, Conn.

Facts on Alcoholism, National Council on Alcoholism.

How Alcohol Affects the Body, Connecticut State Department of Mental Health, Hartford, Conn.

I'll Choose the High Road, American Cancer Society.

My Dear, This'll Kill You! National Tuberculosis Association.

No. 4 Knocks on Every Door, National Council on Alcoholism.

Of Cats and People, National Council on Alcoholism.

Smoking — It's up to You, Health Education Service.

Smoking and Illness, National Clearinghouse for Smoking and Health.

Thirteen Steps to Alcoholism, National Council on Alcoholism.

To Your Health, American Medical Association.

What to Tell Your Parents about Smoking, American Heart Association.

Why Nick the Cigarette Is Nobody's Friend, U.S. Children's Bureau.

b. Films

Alcohol in the Human Body, Indiana State Board of Health.

Alcoholism, Encyclopaedia Britannica Films, Inc.

Alcoholism, the Hidden Disease, National Council on Alcoholism.

Barney Butt, American Heart Association.

Breaking the Habit, American Cancer Society.

Drug Addiction, Encyclopaedia Britannica Films, Inc.

Drunk Driving, Teaching Film Custodians.

Flagged for Actions, National Film Board of Canada.

From One Cell, American Cancer Society.

Huffless, Puffless Dragon, American Cancer Society.

Is Smoking Worth It? American Cancer Society.

Narcotics — Why Not? Charles Cahill and Associates.

One Day's Poison, National Film Board of Canada.

Out of Orbit, National Council on Alcoholism.

Should You Drink? McGraw-Hill Book Company.

Smoking and You, American Heart Association.

Tobacco and the Human Body, Encyclopaedia Britannica Films, Inc.

To Smoke or Not to Smoke, American Cancer Society.

To Your Health, Ideal Pictures.

Traffic with the Devil, Teaching Film Custodians.

What about Drinking? McGraw-Hill Book Company.

c. Filmstrips

Alcohol and You, McGraw-Hill Book Company.

Alcohol and You, Young America Films.

Alcohol and Your Health, Society for Visual Education.

Danger of Narcotics, Popular Science.

I'll Choose the High Road, American Cancer Society.

Narcotics and You, Young America Films.
Nature's Filter, National Tuberculosis Association.
To Smoke or Not to Smoke, American Cancer Society.

d. Posters

Best Tip Yet—Don't Start, American Cancer Society.
I Don't Smoke Cigarettes. American Cancer Society.
100,000 Doctors Have Stopped Smoking, U.S. Public Health Service.
This Chimp is No Chump . . . Don't Smoke, American Heart Association.

e. Records

The Drugs You Use, American Medical Association.

f. Comics

It's Best to Know, Connecticut State Department of Mental Health.
Where There Is Smoke, American Cancer Society.

g. Selected Stories for Children
(P) Primary Level, (I) Intermediate Level

Alcohol Talks from the Laboratory (I), H. Hamlin (The author, Columbus 12, Ohio).
Facts about Alcohol (I), Raymond McCarthy (Yale Center of Alcohol Studies).
Facts about Narcotics (I), V. A. Vogel (Science Research Associates).
Modern Medical Discoveries (I), I. Eberle (Crowell).

12. Consumer Health

a. Pamphlets or Leaflets

Consumer Protection—Drugs and Cosmetics, U.S. Food and Drug Administration.
Consumer Protection—Foods, U.S. Food and Drug Administration.
Facts on Quacks, American Medical Association.
Folklore and Fallacies in Dentistry, American Dental Association.
Food Values in Common Portions, U.S. Department of Agriculture.
Health Quackery, American Medical Association.
Hot Tips on Food Protection, U.S. Food and Drug Administration.
How Safe Is Our Food? U.S. Food and Drug Administration.
The Cold Facts about Safe Food, Equitable Life Assurance Society.

TV and Your Eyes, National Society for the Prevention of Blindness.
Read the Label, U.S. Food and Drug Administration.
Safe New Drugs, U.S. Food and Drug Administration.
Your Clothing Dollar, Money Management Institute.
Your Food Dollar, Money Management Institute.
Your Health and Recreation Dollar, Money Management Institute.

b. Films

Choosing a Doctor, McGraw-Hill Book Company.
Dress for Health, Encyclopaedia Britannica Films, Inc.
Folks, Facts, and Pharmacy, Lederle Laboratory.
Horizons of Hope, American Cancer Society.
How to Select Florida Oranges, Florida Citrus Commission.
I Have a Secret Cure for Cancer, American Cancer Society.
Medicine Man, American Medical Association.
More Food for Your Money, National Dairy Council.
Pork Around the Clock, National Livestock and Meat Board.
Pressure Steam Sterilization, Ideal Pictures.
Quacks and Nostrums, McGraw-Hill Book Company.
Science and Superstition.
The Best Way to Eat, Florida Citrus Commission.
The Meanest Crime, U.S. Food and Drug Administration.
To Your Health, National Council on Alcoholism.
Your Friend the Doctor, Coronet Instructional Films.

c. Filmstrips

Be a Balanced Wheel, National Dairy Council.
Health Helpers, Encyclopaedia Britannica Films, Inc.
Merchandising Beef, National Livestock and Meat Board.
Tale of a Toothache, Society for Visual Education.
The Little Pink Bottle, National Foundation.

d. Posters

What You Eat Can Make a Difference, Florida Citrus Commission.

e. Selected Stories for Children

(P) Primary Level, (I) Intermediate Level
Doctor John (P), F. Thompson (Melmont).

Doctors and What They Do (I), H. Coy (Watts).

Habits, Healthful and Safe (I), W. Charters (Macmillan).

Health Can Be Fun (P), M. Leaf (Stokes).

How Hospitals Help Us (P), A. Meeker (Benefic Press).

Linda Goes to the Hospital (P), N. Dudley (Coward).

Magic Bullets (I), L. Sutherland (Little).

The Hospital (P). M. Pyne (Houghton Mifflin).

We Went to the Doctor (P), C. Memling (Abeland Schumann Ltd.).

ADDRESSES OF FILM SOURCES

Association Films, Inc., 25358 Cypress Avenue, Hayward, California.

Avis Films, 2408 W. Olive Avenue, Burbank, Calif., 91506.

Bailey Films, Inc., 6509 De Longpre Avenue, Hollywood, Calif., 90028.

Canadian National Film Board, 680 5th Avenue, New York, N.Y., 10019.

Carousel Films, 1501 Broadway, New York, N.Y., 10036.

Charles Cahill and Associates, P.O. Box 3220, Hollywood Calif., 90028.

Churchill Films, 6671 Sunset Boulevard, Los Angeles, Calif., 90028.

Classroom Film Distributors Inc., 5620 Hollywood Boulevard, Los Angeles, Calif.

Coronet Instructional Films, 65 E. South Water Street, Chicago, Ill., 60601.

Encyclopaedia Britannica Films, Inc., 1150 Wilmette Avenue, Wilmette, Ill., 60091.

Eye Gate House Inc., 146 Archer Avenue, Jamaica, N.Y., 11435.

Ideal Pictures Corporation, 321 W. 44th Street, New York, N.Y., 10036.

International Film Bureau, Inc., 322 S. Michigan Avenue, Chicago, Ill., 60604.

Knowledge Builders, 625 Madison Avenue, New York, N.Y.

McGraw-Hill Book Company, Inc., 330 West 42nd Street, New York, N.Y., 10036.

Modern Talking Picture Service, 45 Rockefeller Plaza, New York, N.Y.

Moody Institute of Science, 12000 E. Washington Boulevard, Whittier, Calif., 90606.

Popular Science, 330 West 42nd Street, New York, N.Y.

Society for Visual Education, Inc., 1345 Diversey Park, Chicago, Ill., 60514.

Teaching Film Custodians, 25 West 43rd Street, New York, N.Y.

United World Films, 221 Park Avenue, South, New York, N.Y.

Walt Disney Productions, 800 Senora Avenue, Glendale, Calif., 91201.

Wexler Film Productions, 801 N. Seward Street, Los Angeles, Calif.

Young America Films, 330 W. 24th Street, New York, N.Y.

Selected References

Beyrer, Mary K. "Popular Literature: A Rich Resource for Health Education." *Journal of Health, Physical Education, and Recreation,* 32:31–32, March 1961.

Beyrer, Mary K., Nolte, Ann E., and Sollender, Marian K. *A Directory of Selected References and Resources for Health Instruction.* Minneapolis, Minn.: Burgess Publishing Co., 1966.

Harris, William H. "Suggested Criteria For Evaluating Health and Safety Teaching Materials." *Journal of Health, Physical Education, and Recreation,* 35:26–27, February 1964.

Osborn, Barbara M. and Sutton, Wilfred. "Evaluation of Health Education Materials." *Journal of School Health,* 34:72–73, 1964.

Evaluation in Health Education

CHAPTER 12

All measurement in health is concerned with orderly progress toward the goals of health education. Classroom teachers of health, therefore, want to know if their pupils are improving in health behavior—practices and attitudes. They want to see progress brought about as a result of having been exposed to their teaching. An uncertain knowledge as to whether a health program is successful or not actually frustrates the conscientious teacher. Only through a continuous appraisal of the results of teaching can information be obtained which will relieve frustration and doubt.

Purposes of Evaluation in Health

Health evaluation does several things:

It determines the health status of pupils. Learning in any area is limited by the presence of organic strains and drains, defects, and poor mental health.

It may be used to classify pupils for school activities. Pupils with chronic fatigue, faulty posture, or malnutrition often need a modified program.

It measures the efficiency of the total health program. The effective health services department, the healthful school environment, and the health teaching program all share in influencing the health status as well as the health practices of each pupil.

It measures teacher efficiency. Even the most elaborate health curriculum depends for its success on techniques and aids employed by the individual teacher.

It provides a basis for grading pupils in the instructional program; it is a means of reporting individual pupil achievement.

It contributes useful information relative to student knowledges, attitudes, and practices which may be of value when the curriculum or course of study is being updated.

Evaluating the Total School Health Program

It is a major undertaking to appraise the effect of the total elementary

386

school health education effort. The combined activity of many people is involved. The contributions of the classroom teacher are supplemented by those of the guidance and physical education personnel. In larger schools it involves not only the physician and nurse but also often involves a school dentist, school nutritionist, and psychiatrist actively engaged in promoting child health. There may also be an active health council. These persons work in the three areas of health education: health services, healthful school environment, and health instruction. Any measure of pupil improvement in health knowledge and behavior must, therefore, relate to the cooperative efforts of several forces within the school.

As previously indicated in Chapter 3, there are many ways a pupil's health status can be appraised. Much of this appraisal, when understood by the student, has a beneficial effect on health attitudes and practices. By the same token, the example of a healthful school environment does much in a quiet, even subtle, way to influence the formation of desirable health behavior (Chap. 4). Usually, any formal health effort beyond this becomes one of specific instruction in the classroom.

It is sound educational practice to periodically evaluate the total elementary school program in health education. This may be accomplished every two or three years by employing a specially prepared evaluation instrument. Several such instruments are available for the use of elementary school administrators. A few of the more complete ones are as follows:

Criteria for Evaluating the Elementary Health Program (California State Department of Education, Sacramento, Calif., 1962). This form is used to evaluate: Administration, Health instruction, Health services, and Healthful school environment. Each of the criteria are set forth as desirable practices. The quality of each practice is

judged for a particular school on a four-point scale: excellent, good, fair, and poor.

Evaluative Criteria, *Health Education*, NSSSD, American Council on Education, Washington, D.C., 20036.

LaPorte, William A. *Health and Physical Education Scorecard No. 1 for Elementary Schools* (Parker & Co., 241 E. 4th Street, Los Angeles, Calif.). An easy-to-use appraisal card which has been widely employed for many years and revised from time to time.

Los Angeles City Schools. *A2, A4 and A6 Health Tests* (Los Angeles City Schools, Division of Educational Services, School Publication 673, 1962). An especially useful test for grades two, four, and six. The pupils themselves respond to questions relative to their behavior and attitude.

Michigan School Health Association. *Appraisal Form for Studying School Health Programs* (Michigan School Health Association, 1962). A complete form covering all aspects of the health program.

Oregon State College. *A School Health Program Evaluation Scale* (Oregon State College, Corvalis, Ore., 1955). This scale, appraising the various aspects of the total program, permits numerical scoring of 1000 possible points. The points are distributed in three areas as follows:

Part 1. School health services	350 points___
Part 2. Health instruction	400 points___
Part 3. Healthful school living	250 points___
	Composite score___

Smith, Sara Louise. *Evaluation of School Health Program by Classroom Teachers*, rev. from (Florida State University, Tallahassee, Fla., 1959). The six-page forms are obtainable from the author at the University. This survey throws more light on a given topic than the ordinary "yes" or "no" answer. The author asks such meaningful questions as "What is the attitude of children toward staying at home when there is danger of spreading disease by coming to school?" Although answers to such questions are frequently difficult to tally for statistical purposes, they are individually informative in surveying classroom attitudes.

Texas Education Agency. *A Checklist Appraising the School Health Program* (State Education Department, Austin, Tex., Bull. 519, 1955). This is an example of an instrument that can serve as a guide to a good program. It may be reproduced and it is not difficult to complete. It covers eight areas of the school health program.

Problems in Evaluating the Health Instruction Program

> While health is not in itself the flower of life, it is the soil from which the finest flowers grow.
> — DUNCAN SPAETH

The very meaning of the above quotation suggests that the effect of good health teaching on human activity may be difficult to measure. This is true for several reasons:

The power of the human organism to adapt to the physical and psychological stresses placed upon it is most remarkable. All too often the apparently healthy person is harboring one or more potential killers. Heart disease, cancer, respiratory congestion, and kidney malfunction are all about us. The diseases of stress and the shades of malnutrition do not always manifest themselves so that they are easily observed. The line between adjustment and maladjustment is not always defined. Even "normality" is relative.

There is a "sleeper effect" in health teaching. What is learned today in terms of factual knowledge may not be applied until months or years later. Improved attitudes and habits make themselves known at a time when they do not seem to be directly related to

anything—least of all to a health course.

This chapter is chiefly concerned with appraising the *health instruction* aspects of health education. There is, here, a manifest interest in healthful behavior that is the result of health teaching in the classroom. The one big question raised is "Just how effective is health teaching?" Once the teacher secures the answer to this question she is in a better position to fulfill one of the major purposes of evaluation—that of program improvement. Deciding on health instruction objectives and selecting measuring instruments is not enough. One must appraise and interpret the results of measurement. The findings are then applied toward the improvement of the health instruction program.

Even under the most favorable conditions it will be difficult to fully appraise the health instruction program. Not all of the ramifications of a health lesson are statistically measurable. Very often health instruction goes far beyond the pupil and affects the behavior of his parents and other members of the community. Frequently the support which the public gives to a health project is at least partially the result of effective school health teaching. Even such community items as improved disease reporting, increased circulation of health literature in public libraries, reduced water pollution, the further installation of sanitary facilities, the increase in physical fitness tests and physical examinations, and the increase in newspaper editors who refuse to accept advertising for quacks and nostrums—all of these may be related to the efforts of the classroom teacher.

An accurate measurement of health attitudes and practices is difficult under the best of circumstances. It has always been rather simple to test for health facts, and considerably more difficult to sample attitudes or beliefs, or ascertain whether a pupil has shown the ability to apply health information in an effective manner.

Too many teachers through the years have simply handed out facts to their pupils and have received the facts back at examination time. Thousands of schoolchildren can spell, write, and recite the names of the vitamins and minerals found in specific foods; they can name the teeth, and diagram how the blood circulates in the body. Yet many of them do not choose foods wisely; they do not own a toothbrush, or appreciate the relationship of a sound heart to personal well-being in work and play. In short, they are rated as good students of health because they have given the teacher what she wanted to hear—health facts and figures.

These statements are not meant to imply that facts are unimportant in health teaching. Quite the opposite is true, for facts are always of value when it comes to specific knowledge and intelligent behavior. The quarrel comes when mere facts by themselves are the meat of the teaching and testing program. Personal involvement must be added. Students who *act* on facts during the teaching program are more apt to *behave* differently when habits and attitudes are appraised at a later date, Appraisal, therefore, involves pupil behavior and attitudes as well as a number of noteworthy facts. One of the specific findings in the Los Angeles study was that "how people *feel* toward health education" determines to a great extent what they do about their health behavior.[1] It takes time and a concentration of effort in school to develop *feelings* toward health. Research supports this view by showing that direct teaching is superior to integrated and correlated instruction.

The classroom teacher will evaluate

her health instruction by noting such concrete items as the increase in children having dental work completed, the number of improved habits relative to milk drinking, cleanliness, posture, and appearance, the increase in the sale of nutritious foods at the cafeteria, the reports on changed habits made by parents, the increase in the number of parents attending school health examinations of their children, the increase in the percentage of physical defects remedied, and many more such specific items.

There is a shortage of valid and useful elementary health education tests, scales, and other appraisal devices. While local knowledge tests are not difficult to construct, homemade tests of attitudes and practices are harder to come by. Even when there are fairly good tests, their usefulness is reduced by the fact that many teachers fail to determine what a pupil or class knows about a health topic at the beginning of the study. In other words, some *pretesting* or early appraisal is necessary before a particular unit of work is started. Shaw points out that this pretesting need not be elaborate; and it does not necessarily have to be in the form of a written examination—"even impromptu discussions at the beginning of a unit of study may partially serve this function."[2] The teacher's objective is simply to find out what the class knows and how it feels about the topic *before* instruction begins. Dearborn has shown that there is tremendous variation in initial health knowledge, not only between individuals, but also between classes and between schools.[3] Pre-testing provides the teacher with information relative to pupil inadequacies and strengths, and

[1] Johns, Edward B. "The School Health Education Evaluation Study, Los Angeles Area," *Journal of School Health*, 32:5-11, January 1962.

[2] Shaw, John H. "Evaluation in the School Health Instruction Program," *American Journal of Public Health*, 47(5):582, May 1957.

[3] Dearborn, Terry H. "A Plan for Pre-testing in Health Education," *Journal of Health, Physical Education, and Recreation*, 35:28-29, February 1964.

thus makes possible the selection of the most appropriate subject matter and the placement of emphasis to meet individual pupil shortcomings.

APPRAISAL METHODS IN THE CLASSROOM

Health appraisal is not something that is done after the instruction has been completed; it occurs simultaneously with teaching and learning. Evaluation is much broader than organized testing which takes place at specific intervals prior to sending report cards home. It is something that occurs whenever pupils are within the observation of the teacher. This permits the teacher to evaluate both the pupils and herself. In this way teaching techniques may be modified or better ones employed without too much delay.

A common finding in several studies, including the School Health Education Study, is that teachers tend to limit their evaluation practices to two or three kinds, when more ways of evaluating pupil behavior are called for. The popular use of paper and pencil test can be criticized if they are not supplemented by other evaluation devices. Veenker makes it clear that skillful oral questioning, particularly when accompanied by a satisfactory recording of results, yields valuable information relative to a student's real understanding of what he has been taught.[4]

Observation

To the teacher who knows what to look for, observation can be a most fruitful evaluation technique. It is sometimes held in low repute only because it tends to be subjective. It

[4] Veenker, C. Harold. "Evaluating Health Practice and Understanding," *Journal of Health, Physical Education, and Recreation,* 37:30-32, May 1966.

need not be, for observations can be made quite objective, especially if they are guided by the use of rating scales and check lists.

Classroom appraisal involves much more than tests as such. It involves the creation of situations which may be used to observe children. Observing how children go about a task, how they work together, how they discuss and share information and ideas, how they report, and how well they manage the transition from one health activity to another—these are examples of situations which may be created to appraise their behavior. Some of the individual pupil items which shed a good deal of light on the application of health knowledge, and may readily be observed by the teacher, are as follows:

Evidence of a cleaner and more attractive school building.

Increased cooperation in helping to maintain a healthful classroom.

Improved personal cleanliness—related to the use of the handkerchief, handwashing and toilet practices, condition of clothing, and eating.

Improved general appearance and posture, mental alertness, enthusiasm.

Better habits of oral cleanliness, e.g., rinsing mouth after meals.

Improved eating practices as observed at lunchtime: Increased consumption of milk during snack and lunch periods. Better lunches brought from home. Less food thrown away at lunchtime.

Evidence of attitude changes with respect to appreciation of the human body and its functions.

Evidence of practices to limit the use of sweets and carbonated drinks for class trips and parties.

Improved practices with regard to working and playing in good light and in properly heated rooms.

Evidence of greater awareness of others, of social adjustment, personal friendliness, more willingness to share materials and to help when help is asked for.

	Always	Usually	Seldom	Never
Are the hands, face, neck, and ears clean?				
Are the fingernails clean?				
Are the clothes neat and clean?				
Is the hair combed?				
Is a handkerchief or tissue carried?				
Are the hands washed before eating?				
Is the shower enjoyed following the physical education period?				
Is the mouth covered during coughing and sneezing?				
Is there good sitting and standing posture?				

Improved attitudes toward safety patrols, traffic officers, the handling of pets and animals, the handling of scissors, leaving materials and equipment where they may cause falls, and so on.

Improved behavior during safety and fire drills.

Evidence of increasing responsibility for planning a balanced school day by participating in rest, play, lunch, and work periods with decreasing assistance from the teacher.

Check Lists and Rating Scales. An observation of an individual or group will be much more revealing if the teacher has something to use as a guide. A simple list of things to look for when engaged in appraising pupils makes the difference between a thorough and objective evaluation and one that is weak and of limited value.

The check list or rating scale brings order and completeness to the observation. It is not difficult to make a list of the more important "behavior" outcomes expected for each unit or health topic. Once such a list has been formulated, however, it is then reworked into a list of expected day-to-day practices and attitudes. *The teacher's job is to fashion a simple check list of practical things that boys and girls actually do when they have a fairly good grasp of the subject taught.* Moreover, these "behavior signs" may be rated numerically or by words to indicate the degree to which the pupil complies with the item. A desirable outcome of a unit of personal appearance and cleanliness would be that the children assume responsibility for protecting their personal health and the health of others. On the teacher's check list under personal appearance and cleanliness would appear such questions as those mentioned in the accompanying list.

An example of a standardized check list which furnishes the user with a complete appraisal in a major health area is the *School Safety Education Checklist* which was designed to measure the effectiveness of the safety education effort.[5]

Most check lists and rating scales for elementary school health instruction are developed at the local level. This is necessary until such time as the curriculum topics and content becomes more widely standardized. Moreover, it provides a rough measure of the rate of improvement in health behavior, especially with reference to local health problems.

Health Records

In practically every elementary school, health records are available

_____

[5] National Commission on Safety Education. *School Safety Education Checklist.* Washington, D.C.: National Education Association, 1967.

for teachers to look over. Very often the school nurse will be able to interpret the physical examination in such a way that a good deal of meaningful information may be obtained. A review of individual pupil health records will reveal improvement in attendance, the extent to which remediable physical defects have been corrected, and the degree of personal illness. It will also show improvements in growth factors such as height and weight and the results of special screening examinations for vision, hearing, and mental health. Very often these is evidence of improvement of dental health status. Moreover, properly kept health records tell how much "follow-up" has been accomplished as a result of the discovery of organic drains, defects, or poor health habits and attitudes.

The cumulative record or anecdotal record has considerable value when it comes to pupil health evaluation. By making notations from time to time on the progress of a particular pupil, a record of lasting value is accomplished for others to use at a later date. Excellent examples of cumulative health record cards are found in the states of California and New York.[6]

Some classroom teachers prefer to keep a class chart which they call a Pupil Observation Chart. This lists the names of all class members in alphabetical order with space to the right for notations. Each day when the attendance is checked the teacher may make a comment if she feels that it is necessary. Such a chart tends to keep evaluation current with everyday teaching.

Another useful health record is one that may be kept by the pupils themselves and appraised periodically by the teacher. This includes diaries and other autobiographical records of pupils.

Performance Tests

One of the increasingly rewarding ways of appraising health status and health improvement in the elementary grades is to formally measure the *physical performance* of boys and girls. Those pupils who generally demonstrate a high degree of vigor, strength, muscular endurance, and enthusiasm usually possess a high degree of physical fitness. When they appear to "slow down" and become less vigorous and enthusiastic, it is time to check more closely for hidden organic strains and drains, physical defects, poor sleep and food habits, maladjustment, or something else.

In a number of elementary schools, tests of physical fitness are given by physical education teachers in cooperation with school health services personel. The findings of such tests almost always reveal information of value to the classroom teacher of health. The pupil whose physical performance is sub-strength and below par is in need of special help, part of which may involve the health instruction program.

A relatively simple screening device for physical fitness should be employed in schools where there is no physical education department, or where the appraisal of physical capacity is a responsibility of the classroom teacher. Such a test can be most revealing in pointing out those pupils who lack the "work capacity" to put in a full day of study and play. Such pupils are frequently underachievers who are existing at a point far below their potential level of intelligence and effort.[7] The classroom teacher

---

[6] Copies may be obtained from the Department of Education, Sacramento, Calif., and the New York City Board of Education, Department of Health, New York, N.Y.

[7] Among the better screening tests for elementary school-age physical fitness are the Kraus-Weber, Physical Fitness Index, AAHPER Youth Fitness Test, Indiana Motor Fitness Test, Oregon Motor Fitness Test, and the Washington Elementary School Physical Fitness Test.

should be able to check her boys and girls against the standards of the A.A.U. Junior Physical Fitness Tests. These are adaptable to any school situation and can be used with little motivation as self-testing activities.[8] The test standards are on page 393. Ideally, every elementary school pupil should have his level of physical fitness routinely appraised three times during the school year by a regular teacher of physical education who is able to employ more sophisticated measures and work with health service personnel to interpret the findings.

Another item that the classroom teacher is in an excellent position to rate on a day-to-day basis is *posture and general body mechanics*. She observes how pupils sit, stand, and walk. A child's postural attitude may be quite informative. It is related to many

[8] Free copies with full directions may be obtained from the Amateur Athletic Union, 233 Broadway, New York, N.Y.

things including disease, malnutrition, chronic fatigue, hearing defects, asthma, and mental disturbances. The teacher may appraise posture from a mechanical point of view by noting the position of the head, shoulders, lumbar spine, hips, knees, and feet. Essentially, a "straight line" type of posture is desired. This may be checked in the classroom as follows: The teacher holds a window pole or straight stick in a vertical position. The pupil to be checked stands with his side adjacent to the pole. Satisfactory posture is demonstrated when the vertical line of the pole falls approximately through the tip of the ear, the shoulder, the hip joint, the knee, and the external ankle bone above the foot. In the absence of a window pole or stick, a string plumb line may be dropped from the classroom ceiling. Even a vertical door frame may be used. This becomes both an object lesson in teaching and an evaluation technique.

A.A.U. Junior Physical Fitness Tests Standards — By Years

Event	Boys			Girls		
	6–7	8–9	10–11	6–7	8–9	10–11
Required events:						
1. Sprints	40 yd. 9 sec.	40 yd. 8 sec.	50 yd. 8 sec.	40 yd. 9 sec.	40 yd. 8 sec.	50 yd. 9 sec.
2. Walk and Run	¼ mile 5 min.	½ mile 8 min.	¾ mile 10 in.	¼ mile 5 min.	½ mile 8 min.	¾ mile 11 min.
3. Sit-ups	8	12	16	8	12	14
4. Pull-ups	(modified) 3	(modified) 7	(regular) 3	(modified) 3	(modified) 7	(modified) 8
5. Standing Broad Jump	3'	4'	5'	3'	4'	4'6"
Choose any one of these events:						
6. Push-ups	(modified) 5	(modified) 8	(modified) 13	(modified) 4	(modified) 7	(modified) 9
7. Playground Ball Throw for Distance	35'	65'	85'	20'	30'	40'
8. Continuous Hike for Distance	1 mile	2 mile	3 mile	1 mile	2 mile	3 mile
9. Running High Jump	1'6"	2'3"	2'9"	1'6"	2'3"	2'6"

There is one other performance test that is being used more and more in elementary schools. This is a motor skill *test for bicycle safety*. The children bring their bicycles to school and demonstrate how to turn, using appropriate hand signals. In the primary grades they demonstrate the method of getting on a bicycle, the means of guiding it, applying the brake, and the methods of stopping and parking. The National Safety Council has simple test suggestions to teach and appraise bicycle skills. An excellent bicycle skill test which may be set up on any elementary school playground is distributed free, complete with diagrams, by Aetna Life Insurance Company of Hartford, Connecticut. A guide entitled *How to Cycle in Safety* is also distributed for use with this test. These particular tests offer quite a challenge to youth and are a first-rate appraisal device for the teacher. (See bicycle safety section of Chapter 8, page 233, for a diagram of one of these tests. See also the diagrams for four bicycle performance tests widely used in Oklahoma City in *Safety*, February 1967, p. 20.)

Reports

The results of good health teaching may sometimes be demonstrated by the reports of local physicians, ophthalmologists, nurses, and dentists regarding the increase in medical and dental treatment of school-age groups. Through interviews with these professional people it is possible to become aware of the physical defects and other adverse health conditions that have been corrected or improved. Each year in the city of Cincinnati, Ohio, the school health director compiles an extensive breakdown of facts and figures relative to the health of the school-age children. This is used in a number of ways to improve health teaching at several grade levels.

Surveys

The survey is a formal approach to the topic of health appraisal. It may be community-wide and involve information secured from parents and others in the community, or it may be limited to the confines of the school. In either case it is an attempt to discover certain useful health information which may be related to health teaching. There may be a survey of the school cafeteria to check on the sale of milk, salads, fruits, wholegrain cereals, and enriched bread, or of a local restaurant, dairy, meat market, or grocery store. There are surveys of the school environment to determine such things as the cleanliness of shower and toilet rooms, and whether there are appropriate rest and relaxation periods for young children. But more important from a health instruction viewpoint is the survey that seeks to determine *pupil behavior* in shower and toilet rooms, and during rest and relaxation periods. Environmentally, there may be an opportunity to wash the hands before eating, but what does the survey show? How many children using a lavatory actually wash their hands before eating? The survey, therefore, may make known a real need which calls for a different health teaching emphasis.

There are so many excellent items that lend themselves to being surveyed that care should be taken to select the ones most representative of changes in health behavior in a major health area. In surveying the class as a whole, the teacher will ask herself such questions as the following:

Are the children eating or at least tasting foods they never ate before? Are they eating more leisurely? How many now have milk with every meal? Is there less eating between meals? How well balanced are the meals being consumed?

Does pupil absenteeism due to illness relate in any way to a lack of sleep? Is there any improvement in achievement and adjustment of pupils when sleep habits improve?

Do children willingly wear glasses after the physician recommends them? Is there any indication that children take more precautions regarding the prevention of physical injury to the eyes and ears?

Do children want to stay home from school at early signs of head colds or other illness?

Do health records indicate any improvement in recommended immunizations and vaccinations?

Are there evidences of good manners while playing and sharing with others? Has there been an improvement in the respect shown for the feelings and viewpoints of others?

Is there evidence that the pupils are learning to accept their own limitations?

Is there less daydreaming, crying, timidity, "tattling," and hostility?

Do the results of a bicycle inspection indicate that adequate equipment is being used and that there is proper maintenance such as good brakes, lubricated chains, and proper air pressure in the tires?

How many class members have seen the dentist during the last six months?

It is becoming more and more common to ask pupils what they think about a certain happening or item of learning. When such questions are organized, they frequently take the form of a *pupil opinion survey*. Fifth and sixth graders sometimes have a very definite opinion about the nature of specific health instruction — techniques, materials, content, and whether or not it is effective in changing their attitudes and habits. Such surveys may be carried out in special health areas with the help of record forms provided by interested companies manufacturing healthful products. Both General Mills and the Kellogg Company, for example, distribute health record forms for surveying food habits.

As in the case of check lists and records, the survey probably has its greatest value when the pupils help prepare the questionnaires and check list items, or engage in the observations and interviews themselves.

Parental Opinions

Very often when boys and girls apply their health knowledge, the alert parents are the first to notice it. Attitudes and practices relative to visits to doctor and dentist, foods, personal cleanliness, appearance, oral hygiene, and rest are concrete items that frequently cause parents a fair amount of concern. When children show increased cooperation along these lines at home, most parents will be aware of it and are happy to pass the information along to the teacher. One teacher in a small upstate New York town made it a point to talk to all 28 mothers of her second grade class. Using a simple check list she asked pertinent questions relative to home improvement in specific areas where health instruction had been given. After reviewing all the evaluation techniques that she had previously used, it was her judgment that the interview with the parents was by far the most fruitful and enlightening. As a specific example, it was found that following several lessons on activity, rest, and relaxation, a rather large number of children willingly gave up television and radio programs that might interfere with their sleep, and went to bed.

In the elementary schools of Los Angeles, California a definite plan is in operation whereby parents are asked to cooperate with the schools by keeping a check on the health habits of their children. A sample letter which was designed to accompany a kindergarten health check is

LOS ANGELES CITY SCHOOLS

Office of the Principal

....School

...............................Date

Dear Parents:

We want to help you teach good *health habits* to your child at home and at school. Together we should know your child's *health habits*, what he knows, and how he feels about his health.

Here are two pages of *health habits* which kindergarten children use at home. Will you make a check in the right place to show us how your child is growing in his health habits?

Sincerely yours,

....

Principal

illustrated on this page. The form attached to this letter consists of 40 clear and straightforward questions which may be answered with "Yes" or "No." Here are a few examples selected at random:

		Yes	No
1.	Does your child wash his hands before eating?	☐	☐
2.	Does your child wash his hands after toileting?	☐	☐
8.	Does your child use his own toothbrush?	☐	☐
14.	Does your child go to bed at 7 o'clock?	☐	☐
18.	Is your child happy at mealtimes?	☐	☐
39.	Does your child stay away from strange animals?	☐	☐

Tests of Health Knowledge

Since tests of knowledge are often limited by calling for straight health facts, it is reasonable to expect the better knowledge test to measure also some degree of understanding. A satisfactory test of health knowledge requires the student to think about the facts and apply them in a specific way.

The test question may be so worded as to set up a problem situation requiring an answer of the "What would you do?" type. The proper health knowledge test is constructed so as to determine both the information pupils have learned and their ability to apply this information. An example of a test question suitable for a sixth grade pupil studying foods and nutrition, is:

A variety of foods is available in the school cafeteria. Which of the following would provide the best balanced lunch?

    a. Roast beef, bread, pie.
    b. *Vegetable soup, cheese sandwich, and milk.*
    c. Ice cream, chocolate layer cake.
    d. Spaghetti, potatoes, pudding, a soft drink.
    e. Vegetable salad, crackers, iced tea.

Even a correct pencil and paper answer to such questions does not guarantee that the pupil will actually act as he indicates he will. But the teacher does have some assurance that the pupil knows something about the topic.

Teacher-Prepared Tests. In appraising the results of health instruction there is a need to stress concepts rather than facts. How do pupils *feel* about a topic? What does it mean to them? An appropriate examination would be one in which pupils are asked to support certain concepts with their background of factual information. In this respect, the well-worded essay exam has a new potential value in many classrooms. This free-response type of test can be quite objective — particularly if the instructor knows what specific information he wants to get from the examination.

Most elementary schoolteachers prepare their own test questions and ask them in a manner which benefits the local classroom situation. This is justified on the basis of varied pupil needs and individual differences at the local elementary level. However, test validity, reliability, and objectivity are sometimes sacrificed when local tests are employed. The homemade test will be the most valid when it is checked several times to see just how it is related to known behavior and attitudes.

Health tests, constructed at the local level—preferably by the teacher of the group to be tested—possess certain definite characteristics:

The test must measure, as far as possible, the attainment of all the objectives and not merely the subject-matter aim.

Tests must be simple, clear, and short, and contain a variety of types of questions which have previously been explained.

Tests must be constructed so that pupils have to recall health information and apply it to new situations, see relationships between facts, analyze data and draw appropriate conclusions from them, and make decisions on the basis of material read.

Tests appraise the success of the teacher as well as the learner.

Teacher-made paper and pencil tests fall into two categories: *free-response* and *choice*. The essay question, in which the pupil explains what he knows about something, has already been mentioned. Another example of the free-response question is the short-answer type:

Short-answer question: In a sentence or two, express your understanding of each of the following terms:

alcohol	dentine
wheat germ	bacteria
vitamin A	obesity
sodium fluoride	mental health
calcium	overweight

Choice or guided-response questions are valuable because they do not depend upon skill in expression and handwriting. They provide a relatively wide sampling of knowledge in a short time. Once a key has been prepared,

they encourage highly objective scoring.

Multiple choice questions are extremely adaptable and lend themselves to an unusually wide range of use. They have been used in many health knowledge and attitude tests. A carefully formulated multiple-choice question with several alternatives can provide the teacher with a basis for appraising errors in thinking. The following points apply to the construction of multiple-choice test items:[9]

1. Preface the question with a short, clear set of directions.

2. State a single, definite problem in the lead statement.

3. Include as much of the item as possible in the lead statement.

4. Make the alternatives consistent with the lead.

5. Make the alternatives reasonably similar. The choices open to the student must be very much alike in order for the discriminatory power of the student to be measured. In a five-choice question, at least three choices should be close so that only the student with real knowledge can select the most appropriate or best answer.

Example
Section 1—Multiple choice: Read each question carefully. Select the one item which *best* answers the question. Put the number of the item selected in the space in front of the question.

18. At what time of year does the weight of schoolchildren increase more rapidly?
    (1) summer
    (2) winter
    (3) spring and late summer
    (4) fall and early winter
    (5) no set period

True-False questions have their limitations. They have been "worked to death" as a means of measuring

---

[9] Willgoose, Carl E. *Evaluation in Health Education and Physical Education.* New York: McGraw-Hill Book Company, 1961., p. 41.

factual knowledge. A proper true-false question should be written in the language of the pupil. It should be as nearly true or false as it can be made. Sweeping generalizations should be avoided. Directions should be clear.

Example
Section 2—True and False: The letters T and F have been placed before each statement given. Draw a circle around the letter T if the statement is *True* and around the letter F if the statement is *False* or *Partially False.*

> T   F   12. Accidents in the community are still the greatest threat to schoolchildren.

Matching questions are another variety of guided-response tests which, if properly prepared, will save the teacher time. The "stimulus" column should appear to the left and the "response" column to the right. There should be some five to 15 items listed with more response items than stimulus items. Directions regarding matching should be clear, preferably preceded by an oral discussion before the examination sheets are distributed. A matching test works quite well with health information.

Example
Section 3—Matching: Match the food elements listed in the left-hand column with the foods listed in the right-hand column. Put the number of the food element in the parenthesis after each item.

1. Vitamin B	a. Roast pork ( )
2. Iron	b. Calves' liver ( )
3. Calcium	c. Bread ( )
4. Carbohydrates	d. Milk products ( )
5. Fats	e. Ham gravy ( )
	f. Onions ( )
	g. Oysters ( )
	h. Cabbage ( )

Standardized Tests. A limited number of standardized health and safety knowledge tests are available for elementary school use. They are as follows:

Adams, Georgia S., and Sexton, John A. *California Tests in Social and Related Sciences:* Part 3, Related Sciences: Test 5, Health and Safety. Monterey, Calif.: California Test Bureau, 1953. This 75-item test for grades four to eight is composed of multiple-choice and true-false questions designed to appraise knowledge in the areas of health and safety. A manual of directions and norm tables are available.

Crow, Lester D., and Ryan, C. Loretta. *Health and Safety Education Test.* Rockville Center, N.Y.: Acorn Publishing Co., Revised 1960. A 90-item multiple-choice test for grades three to six built to evaluate a pupil's knowledge, application of rules, understanding of cause and effect, and ability to select the best habits in health and safety. Directions and norms are available.

Dzenowagis, Joseph G. *Self-Quiz of Safety Knowledge.* Chicago, Ill.: School and College Division, National Safety Council. A test for fifth and sixth graders consisting of 40 safety misconceptions in safety preparedness. See *Safety Education,* 36:6–7, November 1956.

Elementary Health: Every Pupil Scholarship Test. Emporia, Kans.: Bureau of Educational Measurements, Kansas State Teachers College, 1960. This is a multiple-choice test of 60 items for grades six to eight designed to measure knowledge and attitudes relative to the rules and principles of healthful living.

Elementary Science and Health, Grades 4, 5, and 6. Columbus, Ohio: State Department of Education, 751 Northwest Boulevard. An Ohio Scholarship Test with amended norms available every year. Objective-type test items designed to measure health knowledge.

Klein, Walter C. *A Health Knowledge and Understanding Test for Fifth Grade Pupils.* Doctoral Dissertation, Indiana University, Bloomington, Ind., 1958. There are 60 best-answer type questions. Two forms. Norms and T scores are available. See *Research Quarterly,* 32:530–537, December 1961.

Los Angeles Health Education Evaluation Instruments. Los Angeles City School District, Calif. Excellent instruments for kindergarten and grades two, four, and six are available for the measurement of knowledge and attitudes. Contact Division of Educational Services, Los Angeles City Schools, P.O. Box 3307, Terminal Annex, Los Angeles, Calif.

National Safety Council Tests. Chicago, Ill.: National Safety Council, 425 N. Michigan Avenue. These tests are included in a series of school safety lessons issued monthly, September through May, for the lower and upper elementary grades.

Speer, Robert K., and Smith, Samuel. *Health Test.* Rockville Center, New York: Acorn Publishing Co., Form A, revised 1960; Form B, revised 1957. This test of multiple-choice and problem-type questions for grades three to eight is designed to measure pupil judgment, understanding and knowledge of health facts.

Yellen, Sylvia. *Health Behavior Inventory,* Monterey, California: California Test Bureau, 1963. A 40-item picture-question inventory for pupils in Grades 3, 4, 5, and 6 which relates to the major health areas of personal health, personal cleanliness, nutrition, safety, community health, infection and disease, mental health, and dental health.

There are also several useful tests of knowledge and understanding available for seventh grade pupils which may be of interest to sixth grade teachers and others employed in the middle school or the eight year elementary school:

Mayshark, Cyrus. "A Health and Safety Attitude Scale for the Seventh Grade." *Research Quarterly,* 27:52–59, March 1956. Two forms consisting of 60 situation-response, multiple-choice items.

Myers, Frank H. "Safety Attitude Scale for the Seventh Grade." *Research Quarterly,* 29:320–332, October 1958.

The attitude of the pupil is appraised by answers to behavioristic-type questions (situation-response). Forms A and B available.

Veenker, Harold C. "A Health Knowledge Test for the Seventh Grade." *Research Quarterly, 30:*338–348, October 1959. The two test forms of multiple-choice items are available from the author at Purdue University, Lafayette, Ind.

Colebank, Albert D. *Health Behavior Inventory,* Monterey, California: California Test Bureau, 1963. A 100-item test for grades seven, eight, and nine covering all major health topics.

The most complete set of health and safety tests are those developed by the Los Angeles City Schools for their evaluative survey. These were constructed for kindergarten, grades two, four, and six. In grade two, for example, health appraisal is made by means of a picture test—27 multiple-choice picture items. The teacher reads the item and asks the pupil to put an *x* on the picture which is the best answer. (A copy of the test pictures may be found in the appendix of the Instructional Guide, *Health in the Elementary Schools,* Los Angeles City School Publication No. EC-201, 1959.) As a result of using this test the schoolchildren were found to be in need of more health instruction relative to sleep and rest, grooming, growth, and disease control. Here is an example of what the teacher says and what the pupils see:

Teacher says:
 3. Now let's look at the pictures in row 3. On a hot day, we play quietly in the shade, run around in a

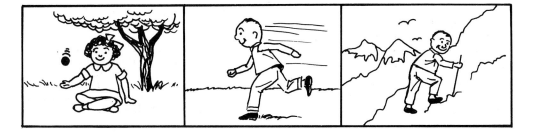

sweater, or climb a mountain.
Mark the best answer and put your
pencils up.

In the area of safety education there
are at least three excellent sources
of test materials for elementary school
use. One test for bicycle riders by the
National Safety Council is set up as
shown on page 235.

Another test, the *Bicycle Safety
Quiz,* is a 20-question true-false test
to be used in the classroom in connection with the moving picture, *Safe on
Two Wheels,* distributed by the Public Education Department of Aetna
Life Affiliated Companies. See 20
questions on page 401.

As a public service the National
Fire Protection Association distributes
free to school personnel their 20-item
test for boys and girls relative to home
fire inspection appraisal. This is part
of the SPARKY program; the questions
may be answered "Yes" or "No" and
are particularly well written. Here
are two examples from the battery:

3. Frayed electric cords often start
   fires. Are you sure all of the electric
   cords in your home are in safe condition?   Yes___No___
20. If there is a gas stove or gas heater
    in your home, do you know that you
    should call the gas company right
    away if you ever smell gas?
                     Yes___No___

The same organization makes available the *Home Fire Safety Quiz* and
the *Be-Prepared-For-Fire Quiz,* each
of which consists of ten excellent multiple-choice questions for teachers to
use in connection with safety education.

Knowledge testing may be made
more revealing when the results are
combined with teacher observations.
The kind of classwork that pupils
do — their drawings, projects, photographs, oral reports, and personal
questions — provide evidence which,

combined with formal test results,
frequently gives a good appraisal of
the health instruction efforts. It should
be pointed out that the manner in
which the various evaluation tools
and techniques are used is more important than the devices themselves.
Rugen and Nyswander warn that
"the best tools are ineffective instruments in the hands of the unskilled
worker. The 'measurement of understanding' demands thoughtful and
careful use of the tools just as does
effective teaching. Indeed, some of
the methods suggested could be employed as teaching aids as well as
for evaluation purposes."[10]

Tests of Health Attitudes and Practices

The formal measurement of attitudes and habits is difficult at best.
Whereas it is relatively easy to test
for factual knowledge, and only
slightly more difficult to search for
pupil understandings, it is considerably harder to obtain an accurate measure of health attitudes and health
practices. Classroom teachers deal
daily with attitudes of schoolchildren.
Attitudes are demonstrated by one's
bearing, feeling, or mood. They
change from time to time. And they
are influenced by a number of things
which may or may not be related to
health teaching.

What has been said in respect to
attitude applies equally well to the
appraisal of health practices. Practices
are a kind of behavior generally resulting from a balance of knowledge, understanding, interest, and attitudes.
Frequently the teacher is limited in
ability to attain firsthand knowledge

---

[10] Rugen, Mabel E., and Nyswander, Dorothy.
"The Measurement of Understanding," in the
National Society for the Study of Education,
Forty-fifth Yearbook: *The Measurement of
Understanding.* Chicago: University of Chicago
Press, 1946, Chapter XI, p. 219.

Is your bicycle 100 per cent safe? Take this test and see how you stand:

If your bike has: *Give yourself:*

1. Good brakes .... 20 points
2. A horn or bell that works .... 20 points
3. A light that works .... 20 points
4. A reflector 1-1½ inches in diameter .... 20 points
5. Tight seat and handlebars .... 10 points
6. Solid front and rear fenders .... 5 points
7. No loose spokes on wheels .... 5 points

                                      Total ....100 points

Bonus Points for:

8. Carrier on back or basket for heavy loads .... 10 points
9. Reflector tape on sides for added protection .... 10 points

---

Check (∨) if statement is True, or False

1. It is safe to learn to ride a bicycle on a busy street. ( ) True ( ) False

2. Bicycles, like autos, should keep to the right side of the road. ( ) True ( ) False

3. Bicycle riders should know and obey all traffic signs and lights. ( ) True ( ) False

4. People who are walking do not have the right-of-way on sidewalks and cross-walks. ( ) True ( ) False

5. Bicycles should be walked across heavily traveled streets. ( ) True ( ) False

6. A bicycle in poor condition is safe if the rider is careful. ( ) True ( ) False

7. It is safe and proper for a bicycle rider to carry a passenger on an ordinary bicycle. ( ) True ( ) False

8. Bicycle riders may hitch to a moving truck if it is traveling less than 20 miles per hour. ( ) True ( ) False

9. Riding in a single line is the sensible thing to do. ( ) True ( ) False

10. Night riding with dark clothing and without a front white light and a rear reflector is dangerous. ( ) True ( ) False

11. When tired, the rider should rest by taking his feet off the pedals. ( ) True ( ) False

12. Bicycle riders should be very careful and give the proper hand signals before making turns or stopping. ( ) True ( ) False

13. It is only necessary to look straight ahead when crossing streets. ( ) True ( ) False

14. The size of the bicycle makes no difference if the rider is skilled. ( ) True ( ) False

15. All bikes should have a horn or bell, rear reflector and front light. ( ) True ( ) False

16. As soon as you can balance your bike you are ready to ride in heavy traffic. ( ) True ( ) False

17. When passing a parked car, you should ride three feet away from it and give a warning with your horn or bell. ( ) True ( ) False

18. When entering a street from a driveway or sidewalk the bicycle rider has the right-of-way. ( ) True ( ) False

19. Bicycle riders should carry books or bundles in one hand if they must be carried on a bicycle. ( ) True ( ) False

20. Bicycles should be kept in good condition at all times and repaired by a mechanic when necessary. ( ) True ( ) False.

NOTE TO TEACHER: { Allow five points for each question. Have each pupil correct any questions he may have answered wrong.

of health behavior. If little Tom says that he regularly sleeps well, or has milk with his meals, or brushes his teeth after eating, the teacher must decide whether or not to assume he is telling the truth.

It is more difficult to construct local tests of health attitudes and practices than to construct tests of knowledge and application. This is even more difficult at the elementary school level. There are, therefore, very few standardized tests for use with elementary schoolchildren. The few that exist may be used to note tendencies toward optimum habits and attitude. In any field of endeavor no one test is accurate enough to be trusted completely. Tests and measures, at best, are only a limited means of appraisal. Test results coupled with teacher observations – as in the use of check lists and rating scales – tend to improve the evaluation.

Self-Testing Activities

When pupils attempt to evaluate their own health improvement, and actually enjoy doing so, there is an opportunity for a more accurate kind of appraisal and a more effective kind of teaching. The student's own immediate problems and how *he* evaluates them is of great interest.

Self-testing activities provide the pupil with a chance to measure progress in terms of his own potential, as well as to compare himself with his classmates. The child as well as the adult wants a certain amount of recognition, status, even prestige – all of which are dependent upon the acquisition of good grooming skills, social poise, proper health habits, and mental well-being. He wants these things because his feeling of adequacy, security, and acceptance are contingent upon them.

Adjustment or self-realization cannot be taught, except by providing materials, opportunities, conditions, and experiences whereby, *through self-activity,* the individual reaches the desired goals of achievement. It is not uncommon, therefore, to find that personal health inventories and self-rating charts have been used for some time with varying degrees of success. If the chart is one developed by the student himself to measure his own advance toward an accepted goal, or if the chart represents group decisions concerning items to be evaluated, it is likely to be more meaningful to the students involved than a printed or standardized chart.

As younger children learn to read, they help the teacher plan simple rating scales for evaluating group or individual health behavior. Primary grade children evaluate in simple ways, as when they select a food to eat, choose a story to hear, an activity, a color to use in painting. They make such judgments as "We cleaned the room very well today" or "We liked playing with the other children." From such beginnings come standards and expectancies.

Older pupils may discuss the kinds of health tests they need, or develop a set of guides for personal behavior on a bus, field trip, or in the school cafeteria. Later on the same pupils help construct check lists and questionnaires on objective health matters, keep health diaries, and take a critical interest in judging their performance about the school and community.

A pupil may rate himself on posture skills, food habits, attitude toward others, personal appearance, and several other such items. The accompanying check list, simple as it is, was worked out by second graders.

There are a number of sources of free and inexpensive self-rating charts which may be obtained in quantity for classroom use. The National Safety Council, for example, distributes a self-appraisal device entitled *Are You*

How Do I Look?

Do I stand tall?	Yes	No
Do I smile?	Yes	No
Are my hands and face clean?	Yes	No
Are my clothes clean?	Yes	No
Am I happy?	Yes	No
Is there dirt under my fingernails?	Yes	No
Is my hair combed?	Yes	No
Are my teeth clean?	Yes	No

Doing Your Part? It also supplies another form, *Keeping Accident Records,* with which pupils may make notations of accidents.

Evaluating a Health Lesson

There is another kind of evaluation that one should not lose sight of. This applies more to the teacher than it does to the pupils as such. It is concerned with appraising the actual instruction at any one time. The teacher should ask herself some rather definite questions as to whether the health lesson was properly conceived and carried out. Was there pupil interest, and did it grow? Was there satisfactory student participation? Was attention given to the individual needs of certain pupils? Was there time to think? Did the pupils help in the planning of the lesson? Was the lesson content adapted to the ability of the group? And finally, did the pupils enjoy the lesson?

EVALUATION – A CONTINUOUS PROCESS

Every conscientious teacher of health looks for ways and means of making the instruction more effective. She continually appraises the results of her teaching; and the more scienti-

fic she is the better. A little research may go a long way toward improving the program.

There is a tendency for some teachers to think of research as a kind of magic done in mythical ivory towers — something strictly divorced from the classroom. This is a species of romantic nonsense. There is no magic in research; nobody waves a wand, and there are no tricks. Research is just plain hard work by competent and dedicated teachers in the fields of their choice. Few elementary schoolteachers are asked to make a significant and scholarly contribution in health, but it is a rare teacher who does not have to ferret out health information, think about it, put it together in a new form, and use it. It is through this kind of activity that health curricula and methods are modified, and programs move in the direction of the preconceived aims and objectives of health education.

Evaluation is an ongoing process. So is education itself. Man and his leaders continually strive to balance his total well-being through a critical appraisal of his physical, mental, social, and emotional health. This is not easy, and it never will be. Yet, as Trow said almost four decades ago:

> If enough good food, rest, sunshine, and so forth, are obtainable, so that the physiological organism is strong and healthy, if there is sufficient opportunity for free activity, for strivings for ends which he considers desirable, and for the appreciation of things which are to him beautiful; and if in the eyes of his comrades, there is something of respect for him; and if there are those in whom he can confide and those whom he can in some way serve, man may experience that feeling of happiness which has been the goal of life for untold generations.[11]

---

[11] Trow, W. C. *Educational Psychology.* Boston: Houghton-Mifflin Co., 1931.

Finally, it is encouraging to note that real progress continues to be made in child health. The mortality among children one to 14 years of age has had a decided downward trend since 1950. Although much of this is due to a decrease in infectious diseases and accidents, a good share of this steady progress may be attributed to health and safety education as it influences man's hierarchy of values and general standard of living.

Questions for Discussion

1. If you were teaching a class in health, where might you begin to evaluate the effects of your instruction?

2. What is the relationship between curriculum improvement and the outcomes of evaluation? Give examples.

3. What seem to be the chief values obtained when grade school pupils appraise their own health instruction program? How does this differ from a typical self-testing activity?

4. What is the value of an individual pupil conference in appraising the health instruction program? Would you say that it represents an economical use of time?

5. Why is learning in health education difficult to measure accurately? Support your answer with specific illustrations.

Suggested Activities

1. Practically every source on the Selected References list has to do with appraising student health behavior, rather than with knowledge by itself. Most authors also point out the *difficulty* involved in evaluating health behavior. Look over some of what has been written and formulate a list of reasons why health practices are so difficult to measure. Later, compare your findings with those of your classmates.

2. Select a major health area in which to appraise pupil health practices. Construct a check list of significant items which should help you identify pupil strengths and weaknesses. The items included on the check list should be "behavior items"—action evidences of health understandings.

3. Prepare six multiple-choice questions on a health topic of your choice. Prepare the same number of true-false questions on the same topic.

4. Get together with three or four of your classmates and discuss the difficulties involved in appraising health practices in a given school-community setting. Are the problems any different in an urban setting than a rural or suburban location?

5. Ask several elementary school teachers to indicate how effective they believe the school health education program to be. Do they feel that the health service function is worth the money it costs? Are they happy with the results of their own health instruction efforts?

6. Prepare a short survey form which can be used to appraise the health teaching program of a school. If possible, arrange to try it out in a school.

Selected References

Anderson, C. L. *School Health Practice*, 4th ed. St. Louis: C. V. Mosby Co., 1968, Chapter 17.

Clarke, H. Harrison. *Application of Measurement to Health, Physical Education, and Recreation*, 4th ed. Englewood Cliffs: Prentice-Hall, Inc., 1967.

Cornely, P. B., and Bigman, S. K. "Some Considerations in Changing Health Attitudes." *Children,* 10:62, January 1963.

Fodor, John T., and Dalis, Gus T. *Health Instruction Theory and Application*. Philadelphia: Lea and Febiger, 1966.

Gavras, Emma B. "Searching for the Truth: Evaluation of Evidence in Health Education." *Journal of School Health,* 32:108–112, March 1962.

Irwin, Leslie W., Cornacchia, Harold J., and Staton, Wesley M. *Health in Elementary Schools*, 2nd ed. St. Louis: C. V. Mosby Co., 1966, Chapter 13.

Mayshark, Cyrus, and Foster, Ralph H. *Methods in Health Education*. St. Louis: C. V. Mosby Co., 1966.

National Commission on Safety Education. *School Safety Education Checklist*. Washington, D. C.: National Education Association, 1967.

Osborn, Barbara M., and Sutton, Wilfred. "Evaluation of Health Education Materials." *Journal of School Health,* 34:72–75, February 1964.

Sliepcevich, Elena M. *School Health Education Study: A Summary Report*. Washington, D.C.: School Health Education Study, 1964.

Smolensky, Jack, and Bonvechio, L. Richard. *Principles of School Health*. Boston: D. C. Heath and Co., 1966.

Sollender, Marion K. *Evaluation Instruments in Health Education*. Washington, D.C.: American Association for Health, Physical Education, and Recreation, 1965.

Willgoose, Carl E. *Evaluation in Health Education and Physical Education*. New York: McGraw-Hill Book Co., 1961, Chapter 5.

Willgoose, Carl E. "Needed Research in Health Education." *Journal of School Health,* 32:421–423, December 1962.

APPENDIX A

A Graduated List of Knowledges and Understandings for the Major Health Topics, Grades 1–6

PERSONAL CLEANLINESS AND APPEARANCE

Grade 1

Knowledge and understanding about:

Appearance, cleanliness and grooming for school: hands, nails, face, hair, teeth

When and how to wash hands

Hanging up clothing

Dressing appropriately for the climate and weather for school and play

Grade 2

Knowledge and understanding about:

Use and care of personal articles

Carrying a handkerchief and blowing the nose

Proper toilet habits

Posture and appearance

Grade 3

Knowledge and understanding about:

Cleanliness and disease control

The necessity for regular bathing

The care of the skin and nails

The care and appearance of clothing and shoes

Grade 4

Knowledge and understanding about:

Keeping the school environment clean

A well-balanced schedule of personal health habits

Good grooming for personal appearance

Sitting, standing and walking posture and how it reflects feelings of the moment

Preventing skin and scalp infections

Grade 5

Knowledge and understanding about:

The reasons for frequent baths and shampoos

Hair styles for girls and haircuts for boys

The relationship of appearance to success in everyday living

The wearing of eyeglasses

The selection of clothes for durability and style

Grade 6

Knowledge and understanding about:

Illness prevention through individual and group cleanliness

The role of personal responsibility in maintaining good health

The elimination of body wastes and body odors

Ancient civilizations and cleanliness

PHYSICAL ACTIVITY, SLEEP, REST AND RELAXATION

Grade 1

Knowledge and understanding about:

How to play, rest, and sleep for proper growth

How to enjoy activities such as fundamental

rhythms, singing games, dances, stunts, and games of low organization

Grade 2

Knowledge and understanding about:

Hours of sleep needed a night
Sleep and rest as factors in avoiding disease and fatigue
Appropriate evening recreation, especially before retiring
How to exercise for fun and health: stunts for fun, animals to copy, etc.

Grade 3
Knowledge and understanding about:
The reasons for physical strength and endurance
The different ways of building, and maintaining physical fitness: rhythms, dances, games, rope jumping, swimming, hiking

Grade 4
Knowledge and understanding about:
How to measure individual physical fitness
Alternating vigorous physical exercise with rest

Why it feels good to be "physically fit"
Physical fitness and total health: exercise, diet, rest, medical check-ups

Strengthening exercises to improve posture in sitting, standing, walking, and working

Grade 5
Knowledge and understanding about:
The effects of exercise, sleep and rest on digestion
How to plan recreation for personal physical fitness
The causes and correction of poor posture
The meaning and wise use of leisure time
Learning how to gain a wide variety of skills

Grade 6
Knowledge and understanding about:
The place of sports in the American culture
The reasons for participating in sports and team activities
The means of preventing injuries from physical activities
What physiology is involved in physical conditioning
Factors contributing to an adequate night's sleep

NUTRITION AND GROWTH

Grade 1
Knowledge and understanding about:
Why people eat (energy, growth, pleasure)
The importance of a good breakfast and lunch
Fruit juices and milk
Candy and in-between meal snacks
Pleasant, happy mealtime
Clean foods and utensils
The need for pure water to drink

Grade 2
Knowledge and understanding about:
Recognition of a wide variety of foods
Individual differences in the rate of growth
Foods that help you grow
Foods that help you "go"
Sweets in the diet
Beverages for children

Grade 3
Knowledge and understanding about:
Good habits of eating: chewing, tasting, eating leisurely
Improving the appetite
The importance of well-balanced meals
Using foods in many ways: milk, fruit, etc.
Eating at regular hours
The make-up of a good school lunch

Grade 4
Knowledge and understanding about:
The four basic food groups

The essential function of carbohydrates, proteins, fats
Vitamins and mineral sources
The relationship of food to proper body weight
The effect of cultural differences, customs and environment on eating habits
Growth through a balanced diet

Grade 5
Knowledge and understanding about:
The mechanics and elemental chemistry of digestion
The variety of daily eating practices
Family mealtime practices around the world
How to promote good digestion
The value of good nutrition to growth and physical fitness
Food excesses and deprivations and the relationship to growth, repair, energy, etc.

Grade 6
Knowledge and understanding about:
How basic foods contribute to growth
The similarity of animal and human requirements
The nature of malnutrition
Food charts and the use of calorie measurements
Balanced menus at home or in a restaurant
Fallacies, fads, and superstitions that distort food facts
Proper elimination of the end-products of digestion

DENTAL HEALTH

Grade 1
Knowledge and understanding about:
When and how to brush the teeth
Loss of baby teeth and appearance of first 6-year molar
Why people visit the dentist

Grade 2
Knowledge and understanding about:
How to use powder or toothpaste
The function of teeth in diet and appearance
Care of toothbrush
How raw foods help keep the teeth clean
How sweets affect teeth
The need for regular dental inspections and care

Grade 3
Knowledge and understanding about:
How teeth may be cleaned without brushing
Foods that build strong teeth and bones
The appearance of clean teeth
The causes and prevention of toothache

Grade 4
Knowledge and understanding about:

The basic structure of the tooth
The value of sound teeth for both talking and digestion
The harmful effects of tooth decay
Practices that may injure the teeth
The function of the school dental hygienist

Grade 5
Knowledge and understanding about:
The importance of orthodontics
The significance of malocclusion
Personal tooth care and regular visits to the dentist
The application of fluoride to the teeth to help prevent tooth decay

Grade 6
Knowledge and understanding about:
Progress of sixth graders toward the development of a full set of teeth
Water fluoridation and the reduction in tooth decay
Bone nutrition and tooth decay
Evaluating dentifrice advertisements

BODY STRUCTURE AND OPERATION

Grade 1
Knowledge and understanding about:
How children grow tall and strong
The reasons for health examinations and tests of seeing and hearing

Grade 2
Knowledge and understanding about:
How people look in a posture of sitting, standing, walking and running
How the body moves using bones and muscles
Exercises and games that show a wide range of human movements

Grade 3
Knowledge and understanding about:
How the eyes see and how the ears hear
The cooperative action between the five senses
How eyeglasses help correct visual defects
How to protect the eyes and ears from injury
The use of water by the body
How skeletal make-up functions to support the body and protect the organs
The function of muscles in good posture

Grade 4
Knowledge and understanding about:
The body's need for fuel
The work of the digestive system

The function of the skin, hair and nails
The structure and operation of the respiratory system
The nose, tonsils, adenoids, and teeth and how their function relates to speech
The function of the larynx and epiglottis

Grade 5
Knowledge and understanding about:
Structure of cells, tissues, organs, systems
The mechanics of growth through cell division
Enzymes at work
Health habits and digestion
The circulatory system and composition of blood
The interrelationship of circulation, respiration, digestion and elimination

Grade 6
Knowledge and understanding about:
The function of the central nervous system, brain and sense organs
How muscles, bones, nerves and glands work together
The elimination system
Diet, constipation and bowel movements
The reproductive structure of the body (referred to also under Sex and Family Life Education)

PREVENTION AND CONTROL OF DISEASE

Grade 1
Knowledge and understanding about:
Keeping hands clean and away from mouth
The need for regular health examinations
The importance of vaccination and immunization
Why it is wrong to share "bites," whistles, straws, glasses, etc.
How to drink from a water fountain

Grade 2
Knowledge and understanding about:
How to protect self and others from colds, sneezes, and sore throats
How to stay healthy through adequate amounts of food, water, sleep, and exercise
How some plants can make a person ill
What the hospital does for people

Grade 3
Knowledge and understanding about:
How people get sick—the germ theory
How germs are spread
Why some diseases are contagious
How to avoid illness through cleanliness, regular medical check-ups and immunization
How to prevent ear and eye infections
How the doctor helps to keep a person healthy

Grade 4
Knowledge and understanding about:
Harmful, harmless and helpful germs
What can be done in the school to prevent the spread of disease
What can be done in the home to prevent the spread of disease
Men in science, and what they have done to conquer disease

Grade 5
Knowledge and understanding about:
Sources of infection: bacteria, viruses, fungi; people, animals, climate, insects, water, food
The importance of keeping immunizations up to date
Preventing the spread of infections
How illnesses from food may be caused by faulty storage

Grade 6
Knowledge and understanding about:
Symptoms of common respiratory and childhood diseases
The care of the sick in the home
How the body builds its own immunity
How to recognize superstition and quackery in relation to disease control

SAFETY AND FIRST AID

Grade 1
Knowledge and understanding about:
How to proceed to and from school safely
General safety practices in the classroom
Safety during and after school hours
Particulars concerning personal identity when lost
Where to seek help for injuries or illness

Grade 2
Knowledge and understanding about:
How policemen and firemen protect children
How to use playground equipment
Treatment of strange animals and strange people
How to report accidents and illnesses
Safety on the water

Grade 3
Knowledge and understanding about:
Safe play in all seasons of the year
Bicycle safety: rules, skills, maintenance
Eyes, ears, and face protection
Fire prevention and fire safety
Personal responsibilities

Grade 4
Knowledge and understanding about:
Purification of drinking water
Elementary first aid practices
Safety out-of-doors (insect bites, sunburn, poison ivy, etc.)
Accidents in the community
How to assist younger children in accident prevention

Grade 5
Knowledge and understanding about:
Fire prevention at home and in the community
Water safety methods including artificial respiration
Leadership in safety patrols and school safety councils
How to prevent eye and ear accidents

Grade 6
Knowledge and understanding about:
First aid practices for minor injuries (cuts, burns, etc.)
Details of personal safety at home (medicines, automobiles, rugs, stairways, electrical outlets, etc.)
Safety in recreational pursuits
Food products safe to eat
Survival in the nuclear age

MENTAL-EMOTIONAL HEALTH

Grade 1

Knowledge and understanding about:

Getting to know and getting along with others

Developing new interests and new friends

Consideration for others

Enjoying and caring for pets

Working by oneself

Seeking help when needed

Controlling emotions of fear and anger

Grade 2

Knowledge and understanding about:

The need for a sense of humor

Sharing experiences and trying new things

Accepting new responsibilities

Winning and losing fairly, and having fun with others

Expressing feelings in an acceptable manner

Overcoming difficulties and adjusting to disappointments

Grade 3

Knowledge and understanding about:

Pleasure and satisfaction in helping others

Building self-control and self-reliance through work and play

Means of developing new interests: books, hobbies, skills, etc.

Wholesome characteristics that make for acceptance and friendship

Personal expression through speech, play and dance

Grade 4

Knowledge and understanding about:

Developing appropriate attitudes toward leadership and group participation

Evaluating personal capabilities and limitations

Human emotions as they have an effect on performance, health, and personality

Solution of personal problems and how to live with handicaps

Open-mindedness and personal receptiveness to suggestions of others

Grade 5

Knowledge and understanding about:

Personal contributions to the group; good leadership, good followership

Ways of making plans and carrying them out

Pleasure in solving pertinent problems

Pleasant and unhappy attitudes and how to overcome worry

Development of confidence and reduction of tension through definite accomplishment

Concern for the feelings of others

Satisfaction in acceptable social behavior

Grade 6

Knowledge and understanding about:

Relation of physical health to mental health

Relation of mental health to recreation, rest and nutrition

Values inherent in sharing ideas and experiences with others

Nature of mental illness

Emotional control and self-confidence

Relationship between the setting of personal goals and the attainment of good mental health

SEX AND FAMILY LIFE EDUCATION

Grade 1

Knowledge and understanding about:

How a happy home life depends upon the contributions of each member of the family

Cooperation in the home; sharing work as well as fun

Caring for pets in the family or at school

Animals as a part of family life

Grade 2

Knowledge and understanding about:

How animals protect and feed their babies

Recognizing that animals have babies like themselves

The many ways that happy families work and play together

The variety of good times found in home and family living

Grade 3

Knowledge and understanding about:

The way parents make a home a pleasant place

Elementary reproduction; all living things come from other living things—illustrated by baby animals, plant life, and mothers and babies.

Animals protect and feed their babies in different ways

Responsibilities in being a good member of the family through individual contributions; helping with family chores, caring for younger member of the family

Grade 4

Knowledge and understanding about:

Unique contributions of men and women to society

How children inherit the way they look from mother and father

The human body growing in the mother's abdomen—where life begins and develops

Different interests and choice of activities of boys and girls

The family as good neighbors

Grade 5
Knowledge and understanding about:
    Beginning of life and how the body starts from a single cell, which divides into two cells: terminology and structure
    Process of human growth and reproduction: egg cells, sperm cells, from egg to baby
    The elemental function of menstruation
    Growth differences from ten to fourteen years of age: boy and girl differences, more rapid maturation of girls

Recognizing the contributions of both sexes to family life and society

Grade 6
Knowledge and understanding about:
    The continuing process of physical growth toward manhood and womanhood
    Social, mental and emotional growth as an essential part of the process of maturation
    Meaning of adolescence

COMMUNITY HEALTH

Grade 1
Knowledge and understanding about:
    Means taken to keep the home, school and neighborhood clean
    How firemen and policemen protect children and adults
    The school physician and school nurse and the services they perform

Grade 2
Knowledge and understanding about:
    How milk is kept clean, fresh and safe to drink
    The community supply of water and how it is protected
    How pets should be cared for to provide health protection
    The duty that everyone has to help keep his community clean

Grade 3
Knowledge and understanding about:
    The control of insect pests
    The protection of the food we eat
    The many people and parts of the community that help protect the health of the citizens; physician, dentist, barber, etc.

Grade 4
Knowledge and understanding about:
    Health services in the community that work together to control the spread of disease; local government, professional personnel, and volunteer health agencies

How water is made safe for swimming and purified for drinking
Food inspections for handling, storage, and use
Playgrounds, parks and other recreational services which help build and maintain good health

Grade 5
Knowledge and understanding about:
    The role of voluntary health agencies
    The importance of public practices in chlorination, insect control, immunizations, x-ray screening, etc.
    How to purify water while on a camping trip
    The importance of fluoridation of the water supply

Grade 6
Knowledge and understanding about:
    School health services; their importance to the community and schoolchildren
    Rescue and ambulance services in the community
    The role of the community hospital; services, problems
    How individual concern and responsibility for the support of hospitals is vital to community welfare
    Individuals identified with the historic development of good community health practices

ALCOHOL, TOBACCO AND DRUGS

Grade 4
Knowledge and understanding about:
    Beverages that contribute to growth
    Why it is best to avoid coffee, tea and some cola drinks
    Precautions in taking medicine without the prescription of a physician
    The sound practice of never accepting anything to eat, drink or smoke from strangers

Grade 5
Knowledge and understanding about:
    The effects of tobacco smoking:
        Minor effects: throat, appetite, tooth stain, bad breath, taste, smell, etc.
        Major effects: heart, lungs, endurance, blood pressure, longevity, bronchitis, cancer, etc.
        Smoking and athletic performance: participation

The nature of nicotine

The wisdom of not starting to smoke; smoking is habit forming, serves no useful purpose and may contribute to serious disease of the heart or lungs

Tobacco smoking statistics and the prevalence of lung cancer

Grade 6

Knowledge and understanding about:

The nature of alcohol and its classification as a drug (narcotic)

Harmful effects of drinking alcohol; habit forming, effects the digestive system, circu-latory system, nervous system (thinking, acting, controlling), longevity, athletic per-formance, occupational performance

Alcoholism as a disease

Alcohol in industry and medicine

The nature and use of anesthetics

The difficulty of breaking smoking and drink-ing habits

Effects of narcotics in general

Laws governing the sale of drugs

The discovery of new drugs for the treatment of disease

CONSUMER HEALTH

Grade 4

Knowledge and understanding about:

How foods are purchased to provide well-balanced meals

The need for careful selection and purchase of clothing; how to aid parents in this process

Recognizing that everyone is a consumer of health products

How a bed mattress is selected for the pur-pose of providing an adequate night's sleep

Grade 5

Knowledge and understanding about:

A scientific way to buy: guides for consumer, law of cause and effect, difficulties with truth and half-truth

How a careful consumer eventually helps to make a careful producer or manufacturer

How to determine the value of a good tooth-brush and toothpaste or powder

Company costs of nutritious foods and food combinations

Learning the measurement of "fortified," "en-riched," and "homogenized"

The special work of different kinds of doctors

Grade 6

Knowledge and understanding about:

How to evaluate advertised health products: dentifrices, sports equipment, cosmetics, pain killers, cold tablets, "health" foods, vitamin pills, cigarette ads on TV, beer ads on TV, dietary substitutes, etc.

Reducing superstitions and fallacies brought about by ignorance and indifference; about food, clothing and health products

Dangers of self-treatment when ill—need to seek top professional care; the unique role of the specialist today, what he can provide

APPENDIX B

Competencies and Concepts in Health Education, Grades K to 6* (State of Washington)

ALCOHOL

COMPETENCY 1. *Understand the interrelationships of alcohol and the body.*
    Concepts (Intermediate level)
        1. The body rids itself of alcohol without digesting it and using it for food.
        2. Like most things that are taken into the body, alcohol affects the body.

COMPETENCY 2. *Understand the use of alcohol in our society.*
    Concepts (Intermediate level)
        1. Alcohol has been used in many ways throughout the ages.
        2. There are various reasons why some people choose to drink alcohol.
        3. There are various reasons why some people choose not to drink alcohol.

COMPETENCY 3. *Understand societal problems resulting from the misuse of alcohol.*
    Concepts (Intermediate level)
        1. When people misuse alcohol, problems may occur.

ANATOMY AND PHYSIOLOGY

COMPETENCY 1. *Understand and appreciate the basic structure, function, and development patterns of all living tissues.*

Concepts (Primary level)
1. The cell is the basic structural unit of life.
2. All parts of the body are made up of cells.
3. The skin is a protective covering.
4. The heart is a pump.
5. Muscles enable the skeleton to move.

Concepts (Intermediate level)
1. The cell is the basic unit of structure in all living things.
2. Cells may differ in order to perform different functions.
3. Tissues combine into organs.
4. Various organs and tissues work together to form body systems.

COMPETENCY 2. *Understand and appreciate the functions of the systems of the body.*
1. All the different cells, tissues, organs, and systems work together to make us a human being.

1. The skeletal system serves several purposes.
2. Two basic types of muscles perform a variety of body activities.

---

* Adapted from *Health Education Guide to Better Health*, State Office of Public Instruction, Olympia, Washington, 1966. Material used here does not include the excellent supplementary units on cancer, respiratory diseases and heart disease, nor any of the many sample learning experiences and resources.

414

2. Form and movement help or hinder how we look, feel and perform.
3. The body has special abilities called senses.

3. The skin performs several important functions.
4. The digestive system changes the food into a usable form for the body.
5. The respiratory system brings oxygen to the body and removes CO_2 from the body.
6. The excretory system takes care of the elimination of waste, liquids, solids, and gases.
7. The circulatory system transports supplies (food and oxygen) and waste products throughout the body.
8. The nervous system is a control center which receives, interprets, and transmits messages.
9. The endocrine system is the chemical regulator of the body.
10. The reproductive system provides the cells for producing a new person and the place for the developing embryo to grow until it is complete enough to survive in the outside world.

COMPETENCY 3.   *Evaluate continually available data to help understand the potentials and limitations of the body and appreciate the range of individual differences.*

1. A wide range of individual differences in size and shape is normal in growth patterns.
2. Development of our potentials is within the limits of design and age.

1. The function of the various systems can be interfered with by injuries, infections, and malnutrition.
2. Scientific research seeks better ways of helping us stay healthy.

COMPETENCY 4.   *Select health behavior which reflects understanding and appreciation of the human body.*

1. Exercise is fun and develops skills.
2. Rest and relaxation help the body to recover from fatigue and to grow.
3. Good posture helps prevent fatigue, enables the body to work better, and makes us more attractive.
4. Cleanliness is a factor in how we feel and how other people feel about us.
5. Body injuries from some hazards can be prevented.
6. Care of the body adds to effective living.

1. Exercise for fitness involves activities to develop strength, endurance, flexibility.
2. Good posture is the efficient way of using the body.
3. Personal cleanliness is an individual responsibility.
4. Practicing good health and safety measures helps insure our continued good health.

COMMUNITY HEALTH

COMPETENCY 1.   *Understand environmental factors which affect health.*

Concepts (Primary)
1. Water and air are important.
2. Clean food is important.
3. Clean and comfortable home conditions affect health.
4. Noise and space affect how people feel and respond.
5. Hazards in the environment can cause discomfort and problems.

Concepts (Intermediate)
1. Water and air are essential for life.
2. Waste disposal is an increasing problem.
3. Disease is transmitted in many ways.
4. Our surroundings, group activities, and group organizations affect us.

COMPETENCY 2.   *Participate in actions which influence community health.*

1. Many people keep water and air safe.
2. Many people help protect our food.
3. Individuals can improve their surroundings.

1. The safety of water and air depends on many people.
2. Many organizations try to improve sanitary conditions.
3. Many organizations help prevent and control diseases.
4. There are many ways of changing our surroundings.

CONSUMER HEALTH

COMPETENCY 1.   *Discriminate critically between reliable and unreliable health information and advertising.*

Concepts (Primary)

1. Physicians, dentists, and paramedical personnel are the best sources for health information.

Concepts (Intermediate)

1. There are sources of reliable health information.
2. Some superstitions are harmful to our health.

COMPETENCY 2.   *Use discriminating judgment in the selection and use of drugs and other health products.*

1. Safety precautions must be taken with medicines and other substances that we do not know about.
2. Medicines are to help get well.

1. Some health products are better than others.
2. Only medications prescribed for you by a competent physician should be used.

COMPETENCY 3.   *Avoid the danger of medical neglect, self-diagnosis, and self-treatment.*

1. We tell our parents or teachers when we are sick or hurt.
2. There are ways to protect ourselves and others from disease.

1. Following certain health practices when we are sick helps us get better.
2. Certain symptoms indicate that we need special health care.

COMPETENCY 4.   *Intelligently select and utilize qualified and competent medical, dental, and allied health personnel and services.*

1. The doctor, dentist, nurse, and other people who help keep us well are our friends.

1. Physicians help protect our health.
2. Many individuals have contributed to the good health we can have today.

COMPETENCY 5.   *Appreciate the roles and functions of health agencies and the responsibilities of citizens in supporting and promoting health programs.*

1. Rules help protect our health.
2. We can help protect the health of others at home, school, and on the playground.

1. Many health agencies and organizations serve, protect, and inform us to help keep us well.
2. Laws and regulations protect our health and the health of others.

DENTAL HEALTH

COMPETENCY 1.   *Appreciate growth and function of dental structures.*

Concepts (Primary)

1. Teeth have many uses.
2. Kinds and numbers of teeth vary with ages.
3. Teeth have structure.

Concepts (Intermediate)

1. Teeth contribute to general well-being.
2. Kinds and numbers of teeth vary with age.
3. The parts of the teeth have specific purposes.

COMPETENCY 2.   *Know and use information concerning causes, prevention, and correction of dental disorders.*

1. Daily care promotes dental health.
2. Foods affect teeth.
3. Dentists help maintain healthy teeth.
4. Safety practices can prevent dental accidents.

1. Regular personal care promotes dental health.
2. Foods contribute to dental health.
3. Regular dental supervision helps control dental disorders.
4. Safety practices can prevent dental accidents.

COMPETENCY 3. *Accept responsibility for meeting community dental needs.*

1. Community resources provide help for dental care.

1. Community resources provide help for dental care.

COMPETENCY 4. *Discriminate as a consumer of dental information, products, and services.*

1. Advertising affects choices of dental products.

1. Dental neglect is expensive for the individual.
2. There are many factors which influence choices of products and services.

DISEASE CONTROL

COMPETENCY 1. *Appreciate the historical aspects of prevention and control.*
Concepts (Primary)

1. Inquisitive minds seek ways to help maintain health.

1. Health heroes' efforts help us stay healthy.
2. We are healthier now than ever before.

COMPETENCY 2. *Understand possible causes and effects of disease.*

1. Germs may cause disease.
2. Diseases may be spread from person to person.
3. Illness makes us feel different.
4. Communication is necessary when we are ill.

1. There are many kinds of organisms.
2. Some of these organisms cause disease.

COMPETENCY 3. *Assume responsibility for prevention and control of disease within themselves and others.*

1. Good health habits help us keep well.
2. When ill, certain practices help us get well.
3. When we care for ourselves, we lessen complications from disease.

1. Our bodies help us fight disease.
2. Our bodies have help in fighting disease.
3. We can help prevent the spread of disease.

COMPETENCY 4. *Support programs organized to control disease, locally, nationally, and internationally.*

1. Your environment can affect your health.
2. We depend on others for good health.
3. You can help others and yourself stay healthy.

1. Community and world health problems affect us.
2. Individuals in our community and world carry on health programs.

FAMILY HEALTH

COMPETENCY 1. *Understand and appreciate the significance of the family in Western society.*
Concepts (Primary)

1. I am a member of a family.
2. Families do many things together.
3. I am a member of a school family (classmates, teachers, principal, custodians).
4. Animals are members of animal families.

Concepts (Intermediate)

1. Membership in a family can give one pride.
2. Family patterns differ throughout the United States and throughout the world.
3. Families may have problems, but they can work together to achieve a happy family unit (broken home, death, physical or mental handicap).

COMPETENCY 2. *Develop roles and responsibilities as family members.*

1. Grown-ups help me stay safe, happy, healthy, clothed, fed, and secure.
2. Girls and boys are alike in some ways and different in some ways.
3. My school community helps me to stay safe, well, and happy (friends, nurse, school patrol).
4. Girls and boys help at home and at school.

1. Each member of the family has certain responsibilities.
2. Joint planning and mutual confidences unite families.
3. Understanding among family members can help with problems of growing up.

COMPETENCY 3. *Understand interrelationships of family, cultural influence, and personal development.*

1. I am partly the result of family customs.
2. I learn about other countries and cultures at school.
3. School helps me learn about the culture I live in.
4. Families help others in the community.

COMPETENCY 4. *Continuously contribute to the development of happy and effective family life.*

1. Living things come from living things.

1. How life begins is a wondrous miracle.
2. Heredity partly determines who you are.
3. An egg grows into a baby.
4. When the baby has been in his or her mother about nine months the baby is born.
5. A baby grows into a school child.
6. Growth and development changes occur but with individual differences.
7. Puberty brings body changes including secondary sex characteristics.
8. Physical, mental, and social growth and maturity are interrelated.
9. Families may be strengthened or weakened by various factors (i.e., love, adoption, spiritual values, security, illness, fighting).

HEREDITY AND ENVIRONMENT

COMPETENCY 1. *Utilize the understanding of heredity and environment and their interrelationship to improve self.*

Concepts (Primary)

1. There are likenesses and differences among living organisms.
2. Living things are alike in many significant ways.
3. Living things are affected by their environment.
4. Living things can influence their environment.
5. Curiosity about our environment leads to a better understanding of the environment.

Concepts (Intermediate)

1. A living thing reproduces itself and develops and interacts in a given environment.
2. Organisms inherit traits which modify the environment, and they may become modified themselves.

COMPETENCY 2. *Understand genetic substances, their transmission, the basic laws of heredity, and the impact of this information on living things.*

1. There are male and female humans just as there are male and female forms in plant and animal life.
2. Each parent contributes something to its offspring.
3. Each species reproduces its own kind.
4. Related living things reproduce in similar ways.
5. Related living things develop in similar ways.

1. Each parent organism contributes its own peculiar characteristics to its offspring.
2. All living things develop from a single cell which is the unit of structure and function.
3. The pattern of the organism is passed along to new cells by duplication of chromosomes and their DNA content.

MENTAL HEALTH

COMPETENCY 1. *Understand and accept self.*

Concept (Primary)

1. "You" as an individual are important.
2. Every person has his own potential which increases with age; his success must be judged in terms of his own individual potential.

Concepts (Intermediate)

1. Increasing independence can be achieved (care for self and possessions, thinking for self).
2. Maintenance of self-control without loss of self-respect can be learned.

3. You can be proud of the things you do well.
4. Life has joy and pleasures and sometimes has sorrow and unpleasantness too.

3. Individuals can develop habits which help them.
4. Learning to evaluate is part of the growing-up process.
5. Skills can be developed to recognize, face, and solve problems.
6. A sense of imagination and creativity can bring self-satisfaction.

COMPETENCY 2.   *Understand and accept others as individuals.*

1. Rights and property of others need to be respected.
2. Sharing, taking turns, and giving in occasionally can give pleasure.
3. There is a difference between tattling and concern.
4. Ambivalent feelings are normal.

1. Respect for the differences in people is important.
2. Happiness is friendship.
3. Standards for acceptable behavior can be developed cooperatively.
4. Qualities of leadership and qualities of followership can be developed.
5. Older students' behavior and dress influence young children.
6. Growing up involves making constructive criticisms.

COMPETENCY 3.   *Attain a personal adjustment to a changing society.*

1. New experiences can give satisfaction.
2. The home, the school, the church, and the community can be nice, warm, and safe places to be.
3. There are reasons for most rules or laws.

1. Honesty and dishonesty influence you, others, and society in general.
2. Growing up necessitates adjustments to new situations and new ideas.
3. Self-respect comes from within you, not from material possessions.
4. Common courtesies help interpersonal relationships.
5. Decisions on rules and policies need to be carefully developed.

COMPETENCY 4.   *Understand factors which contribute to emotional and mental disability.*

1. Emotions are normal.
2. Such emotions as fear, love, hate, jealousy, and anger have a variety of expressions.
3. Anger, hate, frustration are caused by certain factors; ways to help one control or accept these emotions may be acquired.
4. There is a need for a balance of activities.
5. Certain traits may cause you to like or dislike someone (teasing, practical joke, sense of humor).
6. There are appropriate people to whom you can relate your problems.

NUTRITION

COMPETENCY 1.   *Know relationship of food, growth, and health.*

Concepts (Primary)
1. All living things need food.
2. Food helps us grow and do things.

Concepts (Intermediate)
1. We need a constant supply of food.
2. All nutrients are available through food.

COMPETENCY 2.   *Enjoy a variety of foods.*

1. Food is good.
2. There are many kinds of foods.

1. New and different foods can add interest to eating.
2. Many factors affect which foods we eat.

COMPETENCY 3.   *Critically evaluate food selection.*

1. Some foods may be better than others for you.

1. Some foods do more for us than others.

SAFETY EDUCATION

COMPETENCY 1.   *Prevent accidents through knowledge, attitudes, and skills.*

Concepts (Primary)

1. Safe practices get us to school and home safely.
2. Practices of safety and courtesy help prevent accidents at school.
3. Practices of safety and courtesy help prevent accidents away from school.

Concepts (Intermediate)

1. Extended mobility requires increased knowledge about safe practices.
2. School accident prevention needs understanding of rules of courtesy.
3. Most accidents occur in the home.

COMPETENCY 2.   *Assume individual and community responsibility for accident prevention.*

1. You can prevent accidents.

1. Freedom of mobility requires safety practices.
2. School accident prevention depends on you.
3. You can prevent many accidents in the home.
4. All emergencies are not mass made.
5. Knowledge and practice of safety rules in recreational activities prevent accidents.

INDEX

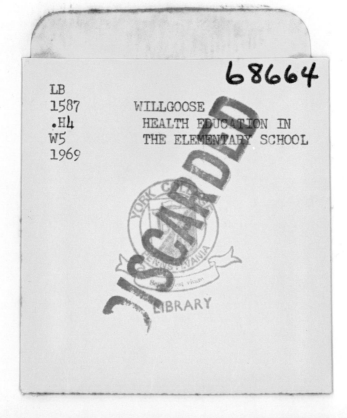